Key Ideas for a Contemporary Psychoanalysis

T0264819

André Green attempts the complex task of identifying and examining the key ideas for a contemporary psychoanalytic practice. This undertaking is motivated both by the need for an outline of the evolution of psychoanalysis since Freud's death, and by the hope of tackling the fragmentation which has led to the current 'crisis of psychoanalysis'.

In three sections covering the theoretical and practical aspects of psycho-analysis, and analysing the current state of the field, André Green provides a stimulating overview of the principal concepts that have guided his work. He draws on the work of Freud and his followers, along with his own experience of the practice of psychoanalysis to explore subjects including:

- Transference and countertransference
- Psychoanalysis and psychotherapy: modalities and results
- Language–speech–discourse in psychoanalysis
- The work of the negative
- Recognition of the unconscious

This unique contemporary perspective on the psychoanalytic enterprise will fascinate all those with an interest in the problems that face the field and the opportunities for its future development.

André Green is a member of the Paris Psychoanalytic Society and honorary member of the British Psychoanalytic Society.

THE NEW LIBRARY OF PSYCHOANALYSIS
General Editor   Dana Birksted-Breen

The New Library of Psychoanalysis was launched in 1987 in association with the Institute of Psychoanalysis, London. It took over from the International Psychoanalytical Library, which published many of the early translations of the works of Freud and the writings of most of the leading British and Continental psychoanalysts.

The purpose of the New Library of Psychoanalysis is to facilitate a greater and more widespread appreciation of psychoanalysis and to provide a forum for increasing mutual understanding between psychoanalysts and those working in other disciplines such as the social sciences, medicine, philosophy, history, linguistics, literature and the arts. It aims to represent different trends both in British psychoanalysis and in psychoanalysis generally. The New Library of Psychoanalysis is well placed to make available to the English-speaking world psychoanalytic writings from other European countries and to increase the interchange of ideas between British and American psychoanalysts.

The Institute, together with the British Psychoanalytical Society, runs a low-fee psychoanalytic clinic, organizes lectures and scientific events concerned with psychoanalysis and publishes the *International Journal of Psycho-Analysis*. It also runs the only UK training course in psychoanalysis that leads to membership of the International Psychoanalytical Association – the body which preserves internationally agreed standards of training, of professional entry, and of professional ethics and practice for psychoanalysis as initiated and developed by Sigmund Freud. Distinguished members of the Institute have included Michael Balint, Wilfred Bion, Ronald Fairbairn, Anna Freud, Ernest Jones, Melanie Klein, John Rickman and Donald Winnicott.

Previous General Editors include David Tuckett, Elizabeth Spillius and Susan Budd. Previous and current Members of the Advisory Board include Christopher Bollas, Ronald Britton, Donald Campbell, Stephen Grosz, John Keene, Eglé Laufer, Juliet Mitchell, Michael Parsons, Rosine Jozef Perelberg, David Taylor, Mary Target, Catalina Bronstein, Sara Flanders and Richard Rusbridger.

ALSO IN THIS SERIES

THE NEW LIBRARY OF PSYCHOANALYSIS

General Editor: Dana Birksted–Breen

Key Ideas for a Contemporary Psychoanalysis

Misrecognition and recognition
of the unconscious

André Green

Translated by Andrew Weller

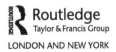
Routledge
Taylor & Francis Group

LONDON AND NEW YORK

First published 2005
by Routledge
27 Church Road, Hove, East Sussex, BN3 2FA

Simultaneously published in the USA and Canada
by Routledge
711 Third Avenue, New York, NY 10017

*Routledge is an imprint of the Taylor & Francis Group,
an informa business*

© 2005 André Green

Translation © Andrew Weller

Typeset in Bembo by
Keystroke, Jacaranda Lodge, Wolverhampton
Paperback cover design by Sandra Heath

All rights reserved. No part of this book may be reprinted or
reproduced or utilised in any form or by any electronic, mechanical, or other
means, now known or hereafter invented, including photocopying and
recording, or in any information storage or retrieval system, without
permission in writing from the publishers.

British Library Cataloguing in Publication Data
A catalogue record for this book is available from the British Library

Library of Congress Cataloging in Publication Data
Green, André.
[Idées directrices pour une psychanalyse contemporaine. English]
Key ideas for a contemporary psychoanalysis : misrecognition and recognition
of the unconscious / André Green ; translation, Andrew Weller.–1st ed.
p. cm. – (New library of psychoanalysis)
Includes bibliographical references and index.
ISBN 1-58391-838-8 (hbk) – ISBN 1-58391-839-6 (pbk)
1. Psychoanalysis. I. Title. II. Series: New library of psychoanalysis (Unnumbered)

RC504.G6913 2005
616.89′17–dc22   2004017857

ISBN13: 978-1-58391-838-8 (hbk)
ISBN13: 978-1-58391-839-5 (pbk)

To Jean-Claude Rolland
In fond friendship and with deep respect

It is time that I wrote my will;

I choose upstanding men
That climb the streams until
The fountain leap, and at dawn
Drop their cast at the side
Of dripping stone; I declare
They shall inherit my pride,

. . .

I leave both faith and pride
To young upstanding men
Climbing the mountain-side
That under bursting dawn
They may drop a fly;
Bring of that mortal mad
Till it was broken by
This sedentary trend

Now shall I make my soul
Compelling it to study
In a learned school
Till the wreck of body
Slow decay of blood
Tasty delirium
Or dull decrepitude.

W.B. Yeats, *The Tower*, 1926

Et l'on voit le vrai Citragupta
[le scribe]
surgir, répandre de l'encre sur
une feuille pour
y inscrire les faits et
gestes des
mortels, cependant que Yama
[le Dieu de la Mort], par un mouvement
symétrique, pose une feuille sur une
couche d'encre, pour faire savoir [. . .]
qu'il est bien Yama, c'est-à-dire Kala,
c'est-à-dire à la fois le Temps et le Noir.

. . .

L'écriture, la ligne d'écriture, devient la
métaphore des limites infranchissables
fixées par le destin, le temps ou la
mort: nul homme n'est assez habile pour
franchir la ligne écrite, ou tracée, par le
destin. Ce qui effraie dans l'écriture ce
n'est pas qu'elle soit lettre morte, c'est
qu'elle soit mortifère: comme si la ligne
d'écriture était par nature un dead line.

C. Malamoud, *Le Jumeau solaire*, coll.
Librairi e du XXe et du XXIe siècles,
© Éditions du Seuil, 2002

CONTENTS

Contents

Contents

FOREWORD

It is an honour for the New Library to publish the book that André Green says will be his last, and his 'will'. André Green is a leading figure of psychoanalysis in France and well-known in the world through his extensive writing. In *Idées Directrices Pour Une Psychanalyse Contemporaine*, Green presents a summary of the main ideas which he developed over nearly 50 years and the guiding concepts which underlie his work. This includes his notion of 'le negatif' (including his concept of 'hallucination négative' and 'la function désobjectalisante'), his views on temporality, on 'la tiercité' (thirdness, which need not be equivalent to the Oedipus complex in the strict sense) and on the centrality of sexuality.

Within French psychoanalysis, André Green had the merit and stature to free French psychoanalysis from the power of Lacan's writings. From a deep understanding of his work, having studied with Lacan until he broke with him in 1967, Green argues against certain basic tenets of Lacan's theory. He takes exception in particular to Lacan's claim that his theory is a 'return to Freud', to the role Lacan ascribes to language and to his assertion that the unconscious is structured as a language. He takes exception with Lacan for discounting the role of affect and he shows convincingly that in fact for Freud the unconscious includes the prediscursive phenomena. In particular he underlines the connection between the regressive mode of communication through free association and the mental state of reverie or even dreaming. A recognition of the specificity of this mode of communication in the psychoanalytic setting is absent from Lacan's writings.

Green also discusses his disagreements with the American schools and with the Kleinian school. From British psychoanalysis his appreciation goes to Winnicott in particular for his conceptualization of the role of illusion for the healthy development of the psyche, and to Bion for his theory of thinking.

In this book André Green gives his view on the state of psychoanalysis at the beginning of the twenty-first century, his thoughts about a 'contemporary psychoanalysis' and in particular its relationship to psychotherapy and to the neurosciences. Green himself always goes back to Freud, to the importance of Freud's discoveries, to retrieving his work from misunderstandings and to looking at what is left still to be understood. This brings him in particular to emphasize the role of object relations which Freud had underestimated and which British analysts starting with Fairbairn and Klein brought to the fore.

Green has made constant efforts to establish debates and exchanges between French and English psychoanalysis. In recognition of the many fruitful interchanges over decades, André Green was made an Honorary Member of the British Society in 2003.

Dana Birksted-Breen

PREFACE

Debts

This book would never have seen the light of day had a friend not once made me the suggestion – or challenge? – 'And why don't you write us an *Outline of Psychoanalysis?*' The idea took time to grow on me, for it was a bold undertaking, and it was quite clear that there could be no question of repeating what Freud had already done – and done well – in 1938. It could be interesting, though, at the beginning of this millennium, to take stock of the noteworthy acquisitions of psychoanalysis, theory and practice taken as a whole. The most difficult aspect of the task for me, used as I am to writing works of some length, is to be brief. I do not know if I will manage to do so. However long this work may turn out to be, it will nonetheless remain an outline.

Since then, our respective paths have diverged. My friend of the early years has responded increasingly to his long-standing inclination for literary psychoanalysis – not to be confused with psychoanalysis applied to literary works – of which he has become one of the dominant figures. His works – literary and psychoanalytic – have been consecrated by the success that they have met with in a public that only accepts psychoanalysis so conceived, presented and developed: in short, a 'soft' psychoanalysis. For my part, I had plunged ever deeper into psychoanalytic psychoanalysis. It is a difficult route, where language constantly comes up against its limits in its effort to explain the psyche, limits that are very different from those encountered in great literature. But I have not forgotten the time when we worked together, just as I have not forgotten all those who, over the course of the passing years, have given me the opportunity of conversing with them, in the psychoanalytic society to which I belong – the Société Psychanalytique de Paris (SPP) – and in others, both French and foreign societies.

I want to mention, in particular, Fernando Urribarri, to whom I owe the honour of having been named Honorary Professor of the University of Buenos

Aires. For several years now, he has been doing his utmost to make my works known in Argentina. He has contributed, indirectly, to the preparation of this volume by a series of meetings that we had together in 2001.

As I am about to write this book, I cannot help thinking of a remark made a long time ago by one of my former patients, who, having had the curiosity to read one of my books, said to me with a nuance in which one could sense a certain disappointment: 'You never let go of the handrail, do you?!' This observation was all the more justified in that, in her analysis, there was no handrail that I could make use of to help me analyse her. I am indebted to her, as well as to my other patients, especially those of whom Freud speaks in the *Outline* of 1938, for having oriented and guided me through the jungle of contemporary analysis, at my risk and peril. One cannot please everybody, and also one's father! For fathers I have had: some that I knew personally, others that I have only read. May their ashes rest in peace!

If I have stayed the course, it is also thanks to those who have shown attention and interest during the course of the seminars that I have given since 1965, with a few interruptions, in various places, but above all, in my society, at the Institut de Psychanalyse in Paris. Some of them have since acquired a certain acclaim, either within psychoanalysis or outside it in the world of culture. They have not forgotten me, just as I still remember them.

Finally, my gratitude goes to the publishers who have shown me their confidence by publishing me. I am thinking in particular of Jérôme Lindon, *primus inter pares*, who took the risk, in 1969, of opening the doors of the prestigious Editions de Minuit to me for my first book; and also of Odile Jacob, a long-standing friend. I trust I will be forgiven for passing over many intermediaries so as to avoid over-extending my acknowledgements and for coming directly to the last, Michel Prigent, who published my first work of 'pure' psychoanalysis, and who has never let me down.

I trust that the fact that I cannot name in person all the others to whom I owe something – friends, colleagues, collaborators – to whom I also offer my thanks, will not be taken as a mark of ingratitude.

I equally thank Chantal Nyssen for the untiring and generous help she has given me in finalizing the manuscript.

Last but not least, of course, my thanks go to Litza who, as usual, has given me the benefit of her invaluable advice. And also to Olivier, eagle-eyed and pitiless like all eldest sons towards their father.

Croagnes
July/August 2002

TRANSLATOR'S ACKNOWLEDGEMENTS

I would like to express warm thanks to Monique Zerbib for her support and assistance with this translation. I have also received assistance in different ways from Michael Zerbib and Paul Wolfenden. I also thank André Green for his help in clearing up the outstanding problems.

Andrew Weller
Paris, March 2004

PROLEGOMENA

PRESENTATION

The aim of this brief work is to bring together the tenets of psychoanalysis and to state them, as it were, dogmatically – in the most concise form and in the most unequivocal terms. Its intention is naturally not to compel belief or to arouse conviction.

> The teachings of psycho-analysis are based on an incalculable number of observations and experiences, and only someone who has repeated those observations on himself and on others is in a position to arrive at a judgement of his own upon it.[1]

This was how Freud expressed himself in July 1938, in the first lines of a preface introducing a work which death was to prevent him from finishing. It is a remarkable summary, gathering together in a few chapters the essence of his contributions.

Why an outline of psychoanalysis in 2002? Many arguments plead in favour of this formula. The first and the most evident is what is called, by general consensus, the crisis of psychoanalysis. It is a consensus that is none the less relative since there are some who say that this 'bad patch' cannot last as the intrinsic worth of psychoanalysis will enable it to come through it sooner or later. Not being a prophet, I shall not venture to predict the future, but will simply say that whatever fate the future holds in store for psychoanalysis, our present task is to fight for its survival today and for its victory tomorrow. One of the least contestable factors of the relative discredit into which it has fallen is the fragmentation of its knowledge, its dispersion, which has gone beyond tolerable limits because it calls into question its unity and exposes the absence of consensus among psychoanalysts. It is not the only one, but my aim here is not to denounce the causes of the problem exhaustively. Nevertheless, although I think the evolution of psychoanalytic thinking since Freud's death justifies an 'Outline', this work will not provide a summary of all the ideas that have been

3

defended since this date. Of course the role of other people's ideas in the elaboration of the concepts which I employ is by no means inconsiderable. I have already had occasion to acknowledge the ideas I have borrowed, often with reservations, from Winnicott, Bion, and Lacan. It would therefore be more exact to say that what the reader will find here, first and foremost, is an outline of the concepts guiding my own work. It will thus draw essentially on my own clinical experience and on what I have learnt from others. This is why I shall adopt a synthetic approach which will permit the reader to get an overview of the principal ideas which can be identified in my work.

This book does not claim to resolve all the problems which have contributed to the degradation of the situation of psychoanalysis and which have repercussions at every level of its institutional life, namely, training and teaching, so-called scientific exchanges, defining the codes of practice and the principles of professional ethics. My ambition here is more limited in scope: I hope that it will help the reader to see his way more clearly through the jungle of psychoanalytic literature.

The state of contemporary analysis is the result of a variety of forces. Leaving to one side an analysis of its relations with the various dissident movements which have separated from it in the course of its history (those of Adler, Jung, etc.), I will venture to define the contributions of certain leading authors within Freudian psychoanalysis, of whom the most famous in France is Lacan. The question will nonetheless be raised of the evolution of certain subgroups which have been formed like states within a state – if one can speak at all of a state to define the official psychoanalytic institution (International Psychoanalytic Association), whose authority is often questioned, not without reason. On the other hand, these diverse subgroups produce an output of literature – a body of knowledge – whose influence and radiance are neither limited nor limitable, since the publisher takes it upon himself to diffuse ideas which are not always welcomed as *personae gratae* within groups shut in on themselves. But this knowledge reaches us through our readings of authors considered as heretical; in any case, it provides food for thought.

Furthermore, a large diversification of practices has raised the question of the relations between psychoanalysis and derived techniques, whether they concern particular categories of patients (children, psychosomatic patients, psychotics, delinquents), or whether they are defined by procedures which deviate more or less from analytic treatment (individual and group psychotherapy, psychodrama, etc.). It would have been astonishing if this diversification of practices had left the unity of the theory intact. The final result accentuates an absence of homogeneity – a homogeneity that originally was due to the evolution of the classical treatment alone. All this has the effect of calling into question our relation to Freud and his work. Although, in certain institutes – fortunately quite rarely – reading Freud is proscribed (so as not to distort young minds which would be in danger of becoming resistant to a certain psychoanalytic modernity), elsewhere this same reading sometimes – though less and less – still has an air about it of the reverence that is due to a sacred text.

Psychoanalytic modernity has two sources. One is constituted by the contributions of post-Freudian authors, sometimes set up as dogmas whose exegeses have nothing to envy of those of the orthodox Freudians of an epoch which I think is now over. Particularly striking is the case of militant movements which are as far apart from each other as those claiming allegiance to Melanie Klein and Jacques Lacan can be. The other source of modernity is nourished by the epistemological horizon of our epoch. No one should underestimate the influence of the dominant ideas from 1900 to 1940 on Freud's work, even if the latter not infrequently made remarkable advances which transcended the bounds of what the spirit of the age made it possible to apprehend. Today, psychoanalysts are divided over the use that should be made of the prevailing concepts of contemporary knowledge, inasmuch as they can be brought together into a whole to which one can refer as if to norms of thinking. It is easier to agree on the critique that can be made of past ideas than on the adhesion to new ideas, which are far from enjoying unanimous agreement.

What we will encounter, then, is an a priori which we will try to transcend, using clinical experience as a major point of reference. Though the models arising from biology or anthropology cannot be overlooked, and though they always give the psychoanalyst the opportunity of reflecting on his knowledge, it is still the case that clinical thinking remains his prime requisite. It could exist comfortably alongside the hyper-complex thinking of our most avant-garde epistemologists who, it should be noted, do not treat the psychoanalyst with the same suspicion and mistrust as was customary for the scientists of the precedent generation – and with some of today's as well. In this respect, one cannot overlook, even if they have to be subjected to close examination, the relations of psychoanalysis with philosophy, past or present, making a necessary (and always debatable) selection amongst Freud's sources, certain of which have their origin in classical Greek philosophy and continue to play a part in contemporary thought.

The difficult task that lies before us, then, is one of identifying the key ideas for a contemporary psychoanalytic practice, submitting them to examination and actualizing them – necessarily in a schematic way – while trying to retain what is essential in them.

Note

1   Freud, S. (1938). *An Outline of Psycho-Analysis* [Preface]. *S.E.* XXIII, p. 144.

A BRIEF SUBJECTIVE HISTORY
OF PSYCHOANALYSIS SINCE
THE SECOND WORLD WAR[1]

The reader should not expect to find here a chapter by a historian, but rather a sort of recension which will bear the marks of the uncertainties of memory, written by a witness who cannot avoid the pitfalls of a subjective vision. More explicitly, the task I have set myself is one of painting a fresco of the recent history of psychoanalysis, arranging the acquired knowledge fragment by fragment, in the manner of secondary dream-elaboration, in order to attribute it with a certain coherence – even if it is seen as artificial or questionable retrospectively.

Where did psychoanalysis stand at the end of the Second World War? I will focus my remarks on four regions: North America, South America, England, and finally France. The North American continent was spared the upheavals of war. Just prior to its outbreak, the United States had gone through a period of uncertainty and instability. Reik's trial (he was not a doctor and legal proceedings had been brought against him for practising a discipline reserved for doctors in North America; he had also benefited from Freud's support, the latter being hostile to the monopoly of psychoanalysis by doctors) had made the headlines. The conflict between the American Psychoanalytical Association and the International Psychoanalytical Association resulted in a compromise granting the former a monopoly concerning the definition of its own rules in matters of training, whether they were in line or not with those of the International Psychoanalytical Association. Faced with the exclusive medicalization of psychoanalysis in the official institutions, the development of American culturalism gave birth to a dissident movement led by K. Horney, Fromm, Sullivan, etc., giving a boost to the revolt against Freud and his ideas in the name of a conception highly impregnated with socio-anthropology. The emigration (which had already begun before the war) of psychoanalysts from Germany and other central European countries fleeing from Nazism, modified the demographic equilibrium in America. Finally, the arrival of Heinz Hartmann on American soil in 1941 – hailed as a saviour of the Freudian tradition (he had the master's backing) – meant that so-called classical and orthodox psychoanalysis became centred around him. It was from this moment on that Hartmann began to deploy his ideas, assisted by E. Kris and R. Loewenstein (who played an important role in French psychoanalysis, before emigrating to the United States). One should also mention D. Rapaport, an important figure in psychology. The movement known as ego psychology gained ascendancy over American psychoanalysis, leaving far behind those, few and far between, who were not in agreement with its theoreticians. Martin Bergmann has carried out an in-depth and precise analysis of the scope of the movement, its advances and its errors of orientation.[2] In a word, it should be recalled that Hartmann had begun his work in Europe in 1938, well before he emigrated to the United States. Generally speaking, those who gave him their allegiance admitted that, as the id was unknowable, it was better to focus on the ego. Hartmann defended the existence of an autonomy of the ego, which did not depend on the id. In short, the autonomous ego was cognitive before the term had been coined; and it espoused the ideas of Piaget even though he was considered in Europe as an adversary of psychoanalysis. Nothing less was involved here than the promotion of a psychoanalytic *psychology* of the ego: an ego psychology.

Even if they did not die from it, many of them were sorely affected. Among those who adhered to this movement may be counted many authors whose ideas, in contradistinction to those of the leaders, continue to inspire the psychoanalytic world. The names of Edith Jacobson, Annie Reich, Greenson, Wälder, Rado, Loewald, H. Deutsch, Valenstein, Spitz, etc., may be mentioned. There is not enough space here to follow all the various movements within North American psychoanalysis which, notwithstanding the massive rallying to Hartmann, remains important. Let me simply say that the work of Hartmann and of his associates was extended by J. Arlow and C. Brenner, who were its popularizers for a long time thereafter. The latter has since distanced himself from ego psychology and has proposed a drastic reduction of psychoanalytic theory to the couple conflict/reaction formation. Non-medical psychoanalysts have succeeded in emerging from the batch who are more open to a psychoanalysis that is looking for its references on the side of phenomenology, among whom R. Schafer and Merton Grill, a merciless critic of Freudian metapsychology.

Then came the movement of the great revolution with Heinz Kohut which opposed self psychology to ego psychology. Kohut's thought cannot easily be summarized. In a word, he thought that Freud's theory of the drives was a lure. He attributed to it the failure of numerous analyses (the two analyses of M. Z . . ., in respect of which some say that these initials could hide a certain H. K . . .). He recommended giving the self a central role, dominated not by fixations to the drives, but by formations linked to narcissism (idealizations, mirror reactions, grandiosity), more connected with inhibitions of development. These ideas were welcomed favourably by some, while arousing resistances in many others. A long controversy was pursued between Kohut and Kernberg who was inspired by Edith Jacobson, the author of a theory of object relations. Kernberg's ideas eventually prevailed and spread throughout the United States. I think one can speak of a school of Topeka, which left its mark on all those who stayed for several years in the institution run by the Meninger brothers: Wallerstein, Kernberg, Hartocollis, and then G. Gabbard. On the west coast, the dominant ideas were those of R. Greenson who was considered as a master of the technique centred on the analysis of resistances and was engaged in a polemic with the Kleinians.

But the great event which gave a new direction to American psychoanalysis was the arrival in Los Angeles of W.R. Bion, who sowed confusion in the ranks of the Californian psychoanalysts (Greenson, Rangell, etc.). A local conflict, to which the administration of the International Association tried to put an end in vain, resulted in the creation of a local Kleinian antenna (Mason, Grotstein). This was the beginning of an evangelization of American psychoanalysis by a Kleinism adapted to local customs. Meanwhile, the monopoly of the American Psychoanalytical Association came to an end following difficult and expensive legal proceedings which led to the admission to the International Psycho-analytical Association of a few societies open to non-medical practitioners which had gained a serious reputation (IPTAR, New York Freudian Society, a Kleinian group in California led by Albert Mason, etc.). From that point on, American isolationism was destined to collapse under the pressure of those who wished to open their windows in order to breathe the air of European psychoanalysis.

Object-relations theory (according to Klein or Fairbairn) gained terrain over the drive theory. The other major writers of English psychoanalysis acquired an increasingly important status (J. and A. M. Sandler, H. Segal, B. Joseph, etc.). R. Schafer made himself the spokesman of Kleinian thinking in the United States. Broadly speaking, in spite of the fairly limited number of orthodox adepts of Melanie Klein, object-relations theory tended to impose itself, de-throning, for instance, in many places, Kohut's self psychology (T. Ogden, author of an original way of thinking) – even if it is true that, under his influence, the intersubjective movement was born of which Owen Renik is the leader, accompanied by other less charismatic figures (J. Chused, E. Schwaber, Greenberg and Mitchell, etc.).

As for French psychoanalysis (J. Chasseguet, J. McDougall, J. Laplanche, A. Green), it aroused interest mingled with curiosity with Americans who had a certain reticence in following the wild theoretical imaginings of colleagues too inclined, in their view, to complicate things and to express themselves in language lacking clarity. There is no philosophy class at the end of secondary education in the United States.

Let me say a word now on the interesting case of Canadian psychoanalysis. Placed at a meeting point of cultures, it succeeds as well as it can in enabling analysts from different countries to coexist. The Anglo-Saxon influence (English and American) was dominant outside Quebec, whereas the 'Belle Province' contained an important group trained in France in diverse rival societies. There were conflicts, notably on questions of training, in which Anglo-Saxon and French ideologies were opposed. A few names are noteworthy here: C. Scott, linked to the London Kleinians; Ch. Hanly, a non-Kleinian greatly influenced by English psychoanalysis; A. Lussier, who cast an eye towards France even though he was trained in England. Ultimately, this melting pot provided the only experience in the world of a cohabitation of ideas produced by authors of reference belonging to different traditions.

In Latin America, the story is less well known. I will be forgiven, I trust, for giving a succinct vision. The very general Kleinian orientation of Latin American, and especially Argentinian, psychoanalysis has often been noted. E. and A. Pichon-Rivière, Bleger, the Rascovsky brothers, Racker, have developed interesting theories which, in my opinion, bear the mark of a Hispanic Kleinism that is quite different from the London Mecca. The decisive influence of Willy and Madeleine Baranger should receive particular mention here. Willy Baranger, the author of a classical work on Melanie Klein,[3] has played a major role in the Argentinian Psychoanalytic Association, by stimulating an orientation focused on a 'return to Freud'. Furthermore, the Barangers have maintained contacts with their country of origin and have ties with Lacanian circles. Notwithstanding a strong Kleinian influence, the reference to Freud animated the central trend of the Argentinian Psychoanalytic Association (APA). Consequently, conflict (with numerous institutional resonances) with the pure, hard-core Kleinians became inevitable (Grinberg). The outcome was a split which resulted in the creation of the Buenos Aires Psychoanalytical Association (BAPA). Since then, subgroups have been formed within each of these two societies. At the heart of the APA there are those who have been inspired by the thinking of Winnicott, Lacan and post-Lacanians (Aulagnier, Laplanche, McDougall, Green, etc.), whereas the BAPA is divided into orthodox and moderate Kleinians. But generally speaking, a growing influence of French psychoanalysis is noticeable. Among those who take particular interest in it, one can mention M. Baranger, F. Urribarri, R. Serebryanni, Galvez, Lutenberg, Ahumada. Moreover, a significant Lacanian movement (L'Ecole de la Cause: J.-A. Miller) is seeking to integrate itself with the official institutions. Finally, let me mention, by way of conclusion, institutional psychoanalysis (Garcia Badarracco) which counts among the most original experiments in this domain.[4] The evolution of the political regime has led to the emigration of many analysts, particularly to Spain.

In Brazil, after a period of infatuation with Bion (via the intermediary of Frank Philips, in São Paulo), the movement diversified (Kleinians, Winnicottians,

Lacanians, Kohutians), creating a somewhat motley impression, fragmenting local psychoanalysis, in Rio notably, after an affair which had raised issues of psychoanalytic ethics. Lobo, an analyst in training, had been defended by Cabernite, his training analyst – and a big manipulator of the Rio Society I – accused of collaboration with the Brazilian authorities in the practice of torture. Long contoversies ensued, the adversaries of Cabernite accusing the IPA, at the very least, of negligence and bias. Whereas in São Paulo one was witnessing the end of the Bionian hegemony, which made way for multiple orientations (Kohut, Lacan, etc.).

The situation of psychoanalysis in Europe does not allow me to enter into details, owing to the multiplicity of societies and influences to which they have been subject. Germany took a long time to recover from the Nazi period when psychoanalysis there was under the thumb of National Socialism and was expurgated of its Jewish contributions. Today, Germanic psychoanalysis is emerging from its silence. At the end of the war, two main movements shared the European space. The first, and the strongest, the English movement, extended its field of influence into Northern Europe (from Holland to Scandinavia). The other, more modest, though not unimportant, originating in France, extended its influence in French-speaking countries and towards Southern Europe (Belgium, Spain, Italy, Portugal, Switzerland), even if in recent years, there has been a tendency to look more towards England.

Since Freud and his daughter decided to emigrate there (they were obliged to leave Vienna in 1938), England became the capital of psychoanalyis of the Old Europe. The history of English psychoanalysis has been through some tumultuous, but always rich periods. *The Freud–Klein Controversies 1941–1945*,[5] edited by Pearl King and Ricardo Steiner, constitute, in my opinion, the most important document of post-Freudian psychoanalysis. They give a precise and complete idea of the issues which divided the English psychoanalytic world. Melanie Klein, who had settled in London in 1926 thanks to Jones, did not look upon Freud's arrival favourably. It was almost as if she considered his landing on her territory as a betrayal by the very one who had facilitated her own emigration towards British soil, a few years earlier. Other emigrations followed gradually. A rift occurred in the British Society between those who were British by origin and the naturalized Europeans (above all Viennese). The *Controversies* enable us to get an idea of the different trends which animated this rift. I do not intend to carry out a detailed analysis of the political and institutional problems which tore the group apart. Among the non-Kleinian British analysts of great value were the Glover brothers, E. Sharpe, M. Brierley, S. Payne, then P. Heimann, who combined a deep knowledge of Freud's work with extensive clinical experience. As for the core of the discussion, let me simply recall that, after the enquiry, Edward Glover's accusations denouncing the investment and constitution of a Kleinian group at the heart of the Society were rejected. It remains the case today, however, that this accusation has been confirmed by the facts: the Kleinians dominate the British Society and the other groups. The Independents and contemporary Freudians cohabit with them, not always easily. In fact, each subgroup had its own evolution. Melanie Klein had a rich filiation: J. Rivière, Herbert Rosenfeld, Hanna Segal, Betty Joseph. E. Spillius[6] has traced the principal changes affecting the basic axioms, of which I will mention the one that seems the most significant to me: beyond the different conceptions concerning the chronological and structural relations of the schizo-paranoid and depressive phase, fresh attention was given to the Oedipal complex, revised and corrected by Kleinian theory.

Kleinism underwent an important mutation with the work of W. R. Bion, who completely reformed this theory. I even consider that Bion reversed the orientations of Kleinism, and it was in this way that Melanie Klein's work was re-evaluated from a Freudian perspective. Accordingly, many non-Kleinians adhere to Bion without necessarily accepting the basic Kleinian corpus. Let me sum up the situation by saying that, though the Kleinian movement as a whole has enabled the theory of psychosis and psychotic structures to make an important step forward, it was Bion who was most successful in throwing light on this new field thanks to a theory of thinking which was lacking in Melanie Klein's work, and it was by this means that the the link with Freud was re-established.

It is difficult to situate D. W. Winnicott, for if one wants to define him as a representative of the independent group – which he is undeniably – one can also see him as a Kleinian dissident, even though he was never admitted to their ranks. The large majority of the independents consider him as their point of reference, even if he never trained a pupil (how would an independent train pupils who would not themselves be independent?). The result is that the analysts of the independent group are not linked by a theory which they have in common. Those who have been seen to have affinities with Winnicott (P. King, Masud Khan, Marion Milner) cannot be looked upon as his disciples. C. Bollas denies this, claiming to be autonomous.

The group of contemporary Freudians was dominated, especially after Anna Freud's death, by the Sandlers (Anne-Marie and Joseph). Their ideas spread as far as the United States. After being appointed to a post at University College, J. Sandler inspired and furthered the psychological and objectivist tendency in which P. Fonagy gained renown before pursuing his own independent path. C. Yorke, A. Haymann and R. Edgecumbe should also be mentioned here. It is a great satisfaction to see the relations between British and French psychoanalysts becoming closer, denser and richer, not only in terms of a discussion of concepts but also in terms of a confrontation of clinical experience.

Finally, let us turn to France. It is clearly more difficult to describe the situation when it concerns one's own country. The overabundance of information, the necessity of reducing it to the essentials, and the danger of having a partisan view are all stumbling blocks. I would ask readers to make certain allowances for what follows, as it will be easy for each in turn to accuse me of being incomplete, partial, or misinformed.

The French psychoanalytic movement had two moments of birth. The Société Psychanalytique de Paris (SPP) saw the light of day for the first time in 1926, then in 1946, the war having thwarted its expansion. One point should be noted. A foreign psychoanalyst, Rudolph Loewenstein, who had settled in Paris, became the analyst of S. Nacht, J. Lacan, P. Mâle and D. Lagache. After fighting in the war from 1939–1940 in French uniform, he emigrated to the United States. In 1946, the second birth of French psychoanalysis took place. Notwithstanding the presence of Marie Bonaparte, who was analysed by Freud and was a family friend, it was S. Nacht who became influential in France, where he was recognized, almost unanimously, as having unquestionable analytic know-how. As it grew, the SPP thought about setting up a training institute. S. Nacht felt he was altogether suited for taking on its direction. Some suggest that he wanted to use it as a springboard for obtaining a university chair. D. Lagache, a former student at the École Normale Supérieure and a leading figure in the teaching of psychology at the Sorbonne, nourished the same ambitions. On another front, an original mind, J. Lacan, was trying to impose his ideas which he diffused with increasing success to numerous young people of philosophical, and often literary training, who were particularly receptive to his teaching at the SPP of which he became the president. It was he, moreover, who drew up the statutes of the future institute (in 1953). For reasons on which I shall not dwell, the relations between Nacht and his followers (Lebovici and others) and Lagache, who led the opposition with his own followers, became embittered. As for Lacan, the liberties he took with technique, which had repercussions for future analysts in training with him, brought him the disapprobation of his peers. After a series of warnings and promises of amendment on his part, and owing to his highly disrespectful attitudes towards regulations, he found himself obliged to resign from the presidency of the SPP.

A split now occurred which was triggered – for quite different reasons (the personal ambitions and authoritarian attitudes of Nacht) – by Lagache and his group which Lacan immediately joined. The Société Française de Psychanalyse (SFP) was thus established, with Lagache and Lacan as its leading lights. But those who had resigned were unaware of the maze of formalities necessary for admission to the International Psychoanalytic Association (IPA) as a dissident group. However, though Lagache benefited from considerable support from the administration of the IPA owing to the favour that Loewenstein continued to grant him, the same was not true of Lacan, who was little known in the circles of the International Association and not much appreciated when he was or became so. Thus began a long and scarcely glorious period for French psychoanalysis. After a good deal of tricky manoeuvring and backstabbing, the final outcome, in 1963, was the creation of a Study Group, led by Lagache, which was to become the Association Psychanalytique de France (APF). It was now that the Société Française de Psychanalyse (SFP) split up and ended. The Association only came into being after Lacan and those close to him had rejected a measure depriving him of the right to conduct training analyses, while allowing him to continue his Seminar. Those who were unable to accept this clause, rallying behind the master, did not therefore join the Association Psychanalytique de France (APF). They founded, under Lacan's high command ('Alone as I have always been, I found'), the Ecole Freudienne de Paris (EFP) which proliferated all the more quickly in that it admitted non-analysts into its ranks. At the APF, Lagache, surrounded by Lacan's disciples, Granoff, Anzieu, Laplanche, Pontalis, and joined later by Rosolato, was to constitute the young society which adopted the line of 'neither/nor': neither Lacan, nor the SPP. In fact, Lacan's influence continued to make itself felt for some time. Innovations, claimed to be revolutionary (this was the cultural revolution of Lacanism), were proposed concerning norms of training (the pass, where the analyst is judged by his analysand), which many found unacceptable.

Fresh dissidence followed: J.-P. Valabrega, F. Perrier and P. Aulagnier founded the fourth group, differentiating themselves from Lacanism and situating themselves outside the IPA. Lacan continued his Seminar. Driven out of Sainte-Anne (Lagache and Delay were colleagues at the Institute of Psychology there), he emigrated to the Ecole Normale in 1964, arousing the interest of those in the rue d'Ulm, disillusioned by Maoism, then, after being requested once again to leave, a few years later, he joined the Law Faculty. After 1968, the Department of Psychoanalysis was founded in Vincennes and entrusted to S. Leclaire. Lacan's influence grew exponentially. His students besieged the teaching posts in the Faculties of Letters and Human Sciences. He got a foot in the door of the publishers Le Seuil, publishing his *Ecrits* there in 1966[7] and his *Seminaires*, edited by his Normalian son-in-law, Jacques-Alain Miller, met with great success (but equally caused controversies). Nevertheless, after internal conflicts and the dissolution of the Ecole Freudienne de Paris, the Ecole de la Cause Freudienne was set up under the leadership of J.-A. Miller, who succeeded in eliminating his rivals. Neither Leclaire nor Melman were part of it. Dolto was practically excommunicated. Lacan died in 1980 without designating his successor, except for the publication of his works which were entrusted to the care of Jacques-Alain Miller who was accused by the other pupils of Lacan of misappropriating the heritage. Those among his disciples who did not join the Ecole de la Cause formed a group which, after multiple splits, fragmented into a vague collection of small groups directed by – just to mention the most important – Maud Mannoni and P. Guyomard, and C. Melman. Finding himself isolated, S. Leclaire suggested creating an Order of Psychoanalysts, in an attempt to kill two birds with one stone: to regroup the scattered Lacanians and to work towards a general reconciliation with the non-Lacanian groups. It was a failure. Currently, various attempts are being made to reintegrate the Lacanians within the psychoanalytic community and to have them recognized by this IPA (International Psychoanalytical Association) which they once vilified so much, to the point of seeking its destruction. *Delenda est Carthago*, Miller had proclaimed, aiming at both the SPP and the IPA. They are almost holding out their bowl to the authorities of the IPA in the hope of being allowed to sit down at the very same table as those they had formerly despised.

Throughout these years, the SPP survived the departure of its dissidents. Nacht's authority was reinforced at first, before it declined, the torch being passed on to Lebovici who was himself to be marginalized. With M. Fain, a rejuvenated team took up the reins of the Institute (De M'Uzan, David, Green). The SPP offered a diversity worthy of emulation, a principal source of its richness. One can identify schematically the clan of Nacht (Lebovici, Diatkine, Favreau, Benassy, etc.); that of Bouvet (Marty, Fain, Sauguet, Luquet, C. Parat); and the group of Pasche (with Renard and Mallet). Later, the group Lebovici, Diatkine, Favreau, E. Kestemberg took over from Nacht, abandoned and forgotten by his disciples. Grunberger, a maverick, benefited from a certain aura. A few older members enjoyed a reputation which earned them respect (Schlumberger, Mâle). After Bouvet's death in 1960, Marty founded the Ecole Psychosomatique de Paris (with Fain, de M'Uzan, David). Today, one can say that the SPP is still a society from which interesting personalities emerge and its merit lies chiefly in the clinical training it offers, preparing candidate analysts for their profession.

Such is the panorama. How can this evolution be summed up in terms of a debate of ideas? On Freud's death, psychoanalysis was divided between those who adhered to his ideas (with the exception perhaps of the death instinct and femininity) and those who wished to extend his work by going beyond it. As Martin Bergmann proposes, a distinction can thus be drawn between the *extenders* and the *modifiers*. The main characteristic of the post-Freudian evolution is that it has succeeded in keeping within the psychoanalytic community members who wish to rectify, more or less deeply, Freud's theories or to propose other principal or leading concepts. No split has occurred as a result of theoretical disagreements. Thus the Kleinian movement claims to be rooted in the Freudian heritage of which, it says, it is merely an extension. The theory of object relations has supplanted the drive theory which, however, constituted the pedestal of Freudian dogma. Today, those who still refer to it are almost a minority within the psychoanalytic movement; but, in spite of their orthodoxy, they cannot accuse the others of dissidence. All things considered, object-relations theory has become polysemic. There are very few 'Fairbairnians', even though he was at the origin of the concept. Its revision by Klein supplanted Fairbairn's ideas and became the implicit reference for this current of thought. Kernberg, after Edith Jacobson, adopted it, somewhat differently no doubt, as did Bouvet, who gave it a broader content than Klein. Even the Sandlers joined this movement. It seems that the idea of the analytic couple (two-body psychology) has imposed itself progressively, just as one speaks more often of transference/countertransference reactions than of transference alone.

It was inevitable that, ultimately, this accentuation of the object would produce, in return, a resurrection of the polarity linked to narcissism. But first, dissatisfaction with Freud's concept of the ego had to be given expression. As the latter was considered as insufficient, the Self, under the different colours of Hartmann, E. Jacobson, Winnicott and Kohut, was added to it. In fact, psychoanalysts were uneasy about the fact that they only had at their disposal one concept which, in Freud's eyes, had to sever its links with classical psychology *and only be considered as an agency whose meaning depended on its relation to the two others: the id and the superego.* Whoever says ego is alluding almost implicitly to a global concept identified with the person, the personality, the individuality, in the form of an ensemble containing the idea of a singular totality which can be opposed to that of a non-ego concerning, depending on the case, reality, objects, the Other. There is, therefore, in the employment of the concept of the Self, a surreptitious return to the ego of academic psychology as an autonomous entity.

In fact, as I suggested as early as 1975,[8] a new metapsychology was already in labour, centred on object–Self relations. Following this revision, there appeared, with different authors, adjacent concepts which were to have diverse fortunes: I, subject, person, identity, etc. The reference to the concept of narcissism, eclipsed by the object relation, was reinforced. It was not without good reason that Lacan refused to follow Bouvet – on the chapter of the object relation, among others – and that Grunberger, for very different reasons, wished to complete what, from his standpoint, Bouvet's ideas had overlooked.

In America, as I have already recalled, after the era of a Hartmannian ego (free of conflicts, that is to say, eluding the influence of the conflicts of the drives in the id and supposedly autonomous), one saw rising from its ashes an abandoned narcissism, revised and corrected by Kohut. I believe that it was this accentuation of the ego which served as a justification for all the developmental studies (Spitz, Mahler, Stern).

Within this general movement, I shall single out a few contributions. I have already mentioned the decisive role of W. R. Bion for his contribution to the metapsychology of thinking (alpha function, capacity for *reverie*). To this may be added Winnicott's theory of the transitional area and phenomena, which is very enlightening where symbolization is concerned. As for Lacan, he differentiated himself from the psychoanalytic movement as a whole by putting the accent on the subject's relation to the signifier, by proposing a theory of the unconscious structured like a language, by setting the symbolic in opposition to the imaginary and the real, by referring to the Name of the Father more than the real father, and finally, by rejecting as illusory all the theories of the ego. After him, Piera Aulagnier and Jean Laplanche extended the Lacanian theory, the former with reference to the pictogram as a psychic concept which is supposed to make up for the insufficiency of the concept of the signifier in psychosis; the latter by proposing a theory of generalized seduction on the basis of enigmatic messages coming from the mother's preconscious, which are supposed to transcend the same limitations of the reference to the signifier. Before that, S. Viderman had subjected Freud's work to the fine sieve of a critique without complaisance, drawing up a balance sheet of the certainties and uncertainties; but he left us unsatisfied with respect to the theory which should have replaced it advantageously.

From 1975 onwards, numerous studies highlighted the epistemologically requisite character of a theory of the analytic setting (J.-L. Donnet) and underlined its limits in face of the growing number of non-neurotic structures in analytic practice. Moreover, it was important to recognize the commonly acknowledged insufficiency of the Freudian theory to account for non-neurotic structures. The other existing theoretical corpuses scarcely commanded unanimity. The necessity of constructing a new theory on the basis of the experience of these new clinical pictures became evident. Finally, the question arose of the variations in analytic technique, or even of analytic psycho-therapeutic practice, in an attempt to find a way out of the impasses encountered in clinical work. These problems are the object of often lively controversies, diversely formulated, in psychoanalysis today, and they raise the question of its future.

Notes

1   I am indebted to Alain de Mijolla for much of the information contained in this historical overview. The aim of this chapter is not so much to retrace the history of psychoanalysis as to cast a retrospective glance on the one that we have internalized. Hence, the numerous approximations, or even inexactitudes.

2   Bergmann, M. (2000). *The Hartmann Era*. New York: Other Press.

3   Baranger, W. (1999). *Position et objet dans l'oeuvre de Melanie Klein*. Paris: Erès.

4   I am indebted to Fernando Urribarri for drafting this passage.

5   Tuckett, D., King, P., and Steiner, R., eds. (1991). *The Freud–Klein Controversies 1941–1945*. London: The New Library of Psychoanalysis.

6   Bott Spillius, E. (2001). Développements actuels de la psychanalyse kleinienne. *Revue française de psychanalyse*, special edition: 'Courants de la psychanalyse contemporaine' under the direction of André Green, pp. 253–264.

7   Lacan, J. (1966). *Ecrits*. Paris: Le Seuil.

8   Green, A. (1975). L'analyste, la symbolisation et l'absence. *La folie privée*. Paris: Gallimard, 1990. [English edition: The analyst, symbolization and absence in the analytic setting, tr. K. Lewison and Dr D. Pines. In: *On Private Madness*. London: Hogarth, 1986.]

PART ONE

Practice

1

THE WORK OF PSYCHOANALYSIS

No chapter of any general work on psychoanalysis has changed so much as that which concerns the psychoanalyst's praxis. And yet it remains surprising to read Freud's articles on technique (1904–1918, with the exception of the writings of 1937) which still have a certain contemporary relevance. Up until about the 1950s, psychoanalysis seemed to be quite a homogeneous discipline, with an indisputable identity, its purpose being psychoanalytic treatment *stricto senso*. The parameters of the latter could vary somewhat occasionally, but they rested on a set of propositions shared by all psychoanalysts. At the time, what was later called – depending on the country – orthodox classical psychoanalysis (United States) or the classical treatment (*la cure type*, France), constituted their activity almost exclusively. As time passed, the problems of the variations of technique were given consideration, but there was general agreement that psychoanalytic treatment remained the activity to which they devoted themselves. In recent years, the psychoanalytic field has been diversified by the progressive addition of derived techniques (group psychoanalysis, psychodrama, etc.) or again of applications of psychoanalysis (with ad hoc technical modifications) to different types of patients (children or adolescents, psychotics, psychosomatic patients, psychopaths), often practised in specialized settings (community clinics or hospitals, psychiatric hospitals, prisons, etc.). To avoid encumbering my exposition, and despite the interest presented by these technical innovations, I will confine myself to speaking of a more circumscribed field. I have proposed that a distinction be made between the following:[1]

1 *The work of psychoanalysis*: that which is carried out in the analyst's consulting room; it may be divided up into analysis properly speaking, analysis with temporary or permanent technical variations and, finally, a subject which deserves all our attention today, psychotherapies practised by psychoanalysts. I would add to this the centres of psychoanalysis or psychotherapy where an attempt is made to recreate, as far as possible, the conditions of private practice.

2 *The work of the psychoanalyst:* the work carried out by a psychoanalyst outside his consulting room, when he is part of an institution that is not exclusively devoted to psychoanalysis and psychotherapies, in which he collaborates with others by contributing his know-how and knowledge.

3 *The work of the person psychoanalysed (le psychanalysé):* this is the work of someone who, having undertaken an analysis, has not wished to become a psychoanalyst thereafter, but uses what has been acquired from this experience in his work which may be relatively far removed from psychoanalysis, or may even lie outside the therapeutic field.

I propose, then, to confine myself here to the work of psychoanalysis.

The classical treatment

While it is true that it no longer rules supreme in the activity of the psychoanalyst, it is no less true that the classical treatment remains for every psychoanalyst the indisputable reference for evaluating the kind of work to which he devotes himself. It is not because the necessities of practice oblige the psychoanalyst to take account of the limits of the application of his technique of reference that it is thereby relativised. It remains the yardstick with which other forms of therapy may be compared. How are we to understand the evolution which has led psychoanalysts to water down their wine and to give up a purism which ultimately lay in a stubbornness that was somewhat deadly? One can, of course, follow the literature chronologically with a view to detecting step by step the emerging facts which testified to a painful revision. It seems to me more interesting, as we look back, to ask ourselves what this transformation is due to.

Let us remember that Freud, from the beginning of his work, excluded the actual neuroses and the narcissistic neuroses from the field of application of psychoanalysis. The former suffered, in his opinion, from an insufficient elaboration of the libido which was discharged into the soma without involving any processes of symbolisation. The actual neuroses pleaded in favour of the absence of any real psychosexuality: in short, a libido discharging itself into the soma, which is quite different from a bodily libido undergoing conversion. As for the narcissistic neuroses, what they were lacking was the capacity of the libido to invest objects, apart from those of childhood, and its tendency to withdraw into the ego. One thinks of course of the process of turning away from reality that can so often be observed in psychotics. These formulations may appear old-fashioned today and too dependent on the 'hydraulic' model for which Freud has been reproached. In fact, if we think about it carefully, it is above all important to note Freud's concern to give a psychic treatment its maximum efficacy, as if he were trying to say that only what has undergone a process of 'psychization' can be treated psychically. This psychization manifests itself in two ways: on the one hand, by adopting a longer path than that which leads to somatization, the short path par excellence, and, on the other, by a capacity for mobilization enabling the subject to come out of himself and to leave behind his past fixations by investing new objects outside himself, a libidinal investment which brings sexuality into play and is capable of being displaced on to another person (this is transference: the primitive objects of childhood are replaced by projection on to the actual objects of the treatment). Freud was most probably interested in the neuroses because their structure was still the one, in the field of pathology, that was most reminiscent of the conditions of ordinary life. At the time, the main concern was to distinguish between neuroses and normality, even if Freud had already conceived of all the intermediaries existing between the normal state and the neurotic state. Certain privileged psychic structures formed a bridge between normal subjects and neurotics. Thus, acts of forgetting, slips of the tongue, bungled actions, in short, the entire psychopathology of everyday life, made it possible to understand normal subjects as neurotics without it being possible to make a clear separation between them. Furthermore, he did not hesitate to find in himself numerous traits belonging to neurosis. What is more, certain formations of the unconscious were common to the neuroses and normal people, for instance, dreams, phantasies, and even transference, which was scarcely confined to psychoanalysis. As psychoanalysis extended its interests, and as the patients who came to consult psychoanalysts began to fall somewhat outside the limits of the transference psychoneuroses, the discipline found itself faced with hitherto unknown difficulties. Not long after the 1920s, a great deal of activity was manifested by psychoanalysts who were concerned to improve results, which left something to be desired. This movement continued for a long time without anyone realizing that the difficulties encountered in the treatment stemmed from the fact that the categories of patients who were resorting to psychoanalysis fell outside the fairly strict framework defined by Freud. He had already paid a price for this himself in what was probably the most fascinating of the clinical cases he related, but also the greatest failure of psychoanalysis, namely, the Wolf Man. Freud was only interested in it from the standpoint of infantile neurosis, but it is considered by the majority of psychoanalysts today as a borderline case. One should mention here the inspirational work of Ferenczi, who mingled in a very surprising way technical aberrations, going beyond what is acceptable, with observations of great profundity which bear witness to his quality as a visionary and precursor of the entire field of contemporary analysis. However that may be, even if 'Analysis Terminable and Interminable' – Freud's testamentary text on the state of analysis on the eve of his death – gives a good idea of the problems encountered by analysis before the Second World War, it seems to me that it was above all around 1950 that a clear change occurred. The theories of Melanie Klein in England and those of Hartmann in the United States had doubtless already been developed, but it was certainly around this date that variations of technique began to be proposed.[2] Generally speaking, it was simply a question of improving the result of the psychoanalytic treatment by adopting more or less temporary appropriate methods, without modifying profoundly the guiding principles of transference, resistance and interpretation. It can be said that the authors were divided into two groups. In the first, they were content to commend such and such a variation without profoundly modifying the frame of reference. In the second, it was this very frame of reference that was modified – in Kleinian analysis, for instance, which proposed an altogether singular technique based on a theory which diverged considerably from Freud's. Thereafter, other major authors of psychoanalysis also proposed their conception of psychoanalysis, often calling into question the Freudian conception. It has to be said that there continued to be a marked change in the population of analysands. At a certain period, there was less and less talk of transference psychoneuroses and more and more of the new arrival in the field of psychoanalysis – character neurosis – even though it had been known about since Reich. A distinction was made between character neurosis and neurotic character, and the importance of pregenital fixations (Bouvet) was emphasized. The shift of emphasis on to the study of the ego was considered a good thing. The theoretical proliferation continued to manifest itself, each one hoping that his theory would be successful in resolving the practical problems in the face of which the theories of others had failed. I am skipping over many stages and avatars which, following psychoanalytic modes, place this or that concept in the limelight.

Psychotherapies practised by psychoanalysts

I will now turn to the present situation. One of the most important problems of contemporary clinical psychoanalysis concerns the psychotherapies. For a long time the psychotherapies were considered as a marginal activity, above all of practical interest (the famous brass in contrast with the pure gold) which could not lay claim to the same titles of nobility as psychoanalysis. The psychotherapies were above all designed for cases for which psychoanalysis seemed unable to give the desired results, on the basis of arguments which today appear highly debatable (weakness of the ego, strong pregenital fixation), and which called for an attitude that went beyond the usual neutrality. The psychoanalyst, for instance, would intervene actively by inviting the analysand to take such and such a decision, or even by injecting vigour into him in order to support his ego and to encourage him to get rid of his symptoms, or in a thousand other ways which did not have much to do with psychoanalysis. The psychotherapies took us back, whether we realized it or not, to the heyday of suggestion. I will not expand on the work of these courageous pioneers who accepted to take care of cases not considered 'worthy'[3] of analysis but which nonetheless required the help of analysts. Nevertheless, I am afraid that many illusions have been entertained about the empirical and pragmatic value of the technique in question, in the measure that the results obtained have been but transient, partial and without any deep modification. To be perfectly frank, I do not see how a result can be obtained short of an analysis as complete as possible of the unconscious conflict. I do recognize that such an analysis is very far from being easy, and that in many cases, it probably takes much more time than resolving a transference neurosis in a classical treatment. Still, this question of the psychotherapies did not arise from the resistance of certain patients to analysis, or from the scepticism of practitioners inadequately armed to deal with the difficulties of analytic treatment, but from the accumulation of disappointments which called for a thorough revision of received ideas. The problem of the psychotherapies rests on multiple findings which need to be distinguished. The indications for psychotherapy are:

1 People whose material situation or geographical location does not permit them to undertake a psychoanalysis. I shall not be considering these cases which involve material problems that are unrelated to considerations of the patient's analysability.

2 People for whom, manifestly, the depth, range and past history of the disorders is such that psychoanalysis cannot reasonably be envisaged. In certain cases where I have tried to carry out an analysis against my better judgement, I have observed a state of extreme disarray and deep distress which I have described under the name of *syndrome of psychic desertification*.[4] What we have to learn from these cases is that the psychoanalytic setting is not only a technical condition of the possibility of analysis or even a theoretical–clinical concept, but that it is in fact an incomparable clinical diagnostic instrument.

3 In another category we can put those cases where one or several psychoanalytic treatments carried out according to the rules of the art have only led to a very partial alleviation of the symptoms, and where the persistence of certain unresolved conflicts continue to trouble the patient a great deal, making the continuation of analytic work necessary. *In evaluating the number of psychotherapies practised by psychoanalysts, the portion which stem from the partial or unsatisfying results of one or several earlier analyses is greatly underestimated.*

4 Finally, there are cases which present good indications for psychotherapy and which can usefully take over from the indications for classical treatment insofar as they constitute the sector that is immediately adjacent to them.

It is clear that the polymorphism of the population of patients who are in psychotherapy with psychoanalysts, and *who do not wish to receive help from anyone but an analyst*, constitutes an original population with whom authentic psychoanalytic work can sometimes be achieved. *One can conclude that there is a new necessity in psychoanalytic training for psychoanalysts to learn how to practise psychotherapy*. If one fears amalgams with other psychotherapies and the loss of specificity which might ensue for the work carried out by psychoanalysts, other descriptive labels could be proposed which point up both the difference from classical treatment while, at the same time, linking these techniques to psychoanalysis. One suggestion has been 'psychoanalysis with a modification of the setting or with a modified setting'; I would readily propose: *psychoanalytic relation with an adjusted setting*. I am well aware of the difficulty of finding an adequate *appellation contrôlé*, but I do not think that the difficulty of finding the right term can be permitted to delay any longer the urgent need for training in the practice of a singular technique that is justified by the facts.

Notes

1   Green, A. (1994). *Un psychanalyste engagé*, p. 148. Paris: Calmann-Lévy.
2   Cf. A. Green, 'Mythes et réalités sur le processus psychanalytique. Le modèle de *L'interprétation des rêves*', *Revue française de psychosomatique*, 19/2001.
3   The expression, now obsolete, was in vigour in the 1950s. It was also said, concerning the failures of analysis, 'Many are called but few are chosen'.
4   Green, A. Preface to the book by François Richard et al., *Le travail du psychanalyste en psychothérapie*, Paris: Dunod: 2002; and, in the same work: 'A propos de certaines tentatives d'analyses entreprises suite aux échecs de la psychothérapie. Le Syndrome de désertification psychique'.

2

THERAPEUTIC INDICATIONS

When a patient meets an analyst, two cases can arise. In the first, it is an inaugural encounter; the individual requesting the consultation has never seen a practitioner of analysis before, nor has he had any prior experience of analysis. In the second, the patient wishes to have a new experience of analysis, feeling that there is still work to be done and so addresses himself, on the basis of various indications, to the person whom he hopes will be able to help him. Lacan has designated the analyst, in the patient's imaginary world, as the *subject who is supposed to know*. No doubt it is necessary, from the outset, for the patient to imagine that the person he is seeing knows something about the mind and that he can enlighten him about his own. But this definition seems to give more of a phenomenological than a genuinely psychoanalytical account of the situation, even if the question is one of who is supposed to know in the patient's unconscious. In any case, during the first encounters – indeed from the very first – the analyst is going to find himself, roughly speaking, faced with two different situations. In the first, he is going to be dealing with a person with whom the encounter will unfold on several levels at once which will all need to be linked up. Even if he does not speak about it, the patient will react to the analyst's presence, to the presence of this particular analyst. In this reaction there will be a mingling of elements which already constitute a pre-transference, combined with others which are related to the analyst's particular personality. As the consultation unfolds, the thread of the pre-transference which, in fact, is already a transference, will be apprehended more and more clearly, and will sometimes be perceived by the patient ('I don't know why, but you make me think of my uncle X . . .'). Within this transferential dimension, the patient, before or after talking about his symptoms and the reasons for his consultation, will tell a story, namely, that of his origins, his family or his parents, even though no specific question has been put to him by the analyst. He will himself react at certain moments of his story in what is sometimes an abrupt manner, which does not fail to surprise him. The evocation of an ordinary event of his infantile history will, for instance, provoke a sudden rush of tears. Another dimension is that the analyst will be attentive to the fluidity of the narration, to the patient's receptive attitude to what is happening extemporaneously in him and to the split which manifests itself between the one who is telling the story and the one – the same person or the analyst – who is listening and noting the effects that the narration have on the patient himself. All this allows the analyst to adopt an attitude which, from the outset, is close to that required by the analytic situation, namely, silent withdrawal, evenly suspended attention, and an attitude of benevolent neutrality towards what can already be glimpsed from the patient's free associations.

Another chapter has opened, that of the current situation and the conflictual knots which can be reactivated in the present: affective and sexual life, family and professional life, and social relations. All these diverse aspects become entangled in an indissociable whole; they are like a piece of music in which the analyst can already identify themes, counter-themes and variations, and can make out the contours of a childhood Oedipus complex, or even an infantile neurosis. But this ideal picture is rarely so harmonious and complete. On the contrary, one very often notices that the patient blocks out this or that aspect of his past or present life, or trivializes excessively such and such an event which, one senses, may have seriously shaken him. Very frequently, at the end of an hour's consultation, one notices that no mention has been made of this or that dominant figure of the Oedipal constellation. In other cases, one will be struck by the discordant note between the relative ease of the patient's discourse when he is speaking of this or that sector (professional, for instance) in contrast with others which affect him more closely and on which he hardly elaborates at all.

It is illusory to imagine one can put together a complete picture, which would necessarily be mythical. I have sketched this relatively eloquent picture of the first encounter simply in order to contrast it with a very different one, where the request for a consultation leaves the patient more or less mute in front of the analyst, prey to a major inhibition, incapable of expressing himself, living in a state that is not very far removed from one of terror. Needless to say, in this latter case, a transference as massive as it is indifferentiated inhabits the patient who is the first to be surprised by what is happening to him and sees no reason for this state of things. One often gets the impression that no sooner has he entered the consulting room than he is dreaming of leaving it and, in certain cases, there is no other choice but to resign oneself to this non-lieu. But before it comes to that, there are numerous cases where, if one proceeds deftly, in small dabs, one is able to orient the interview towards some level, whatever it may be, on which communication can be established. It is just a matter of grasping the most accessible thread in order to create a point of contact with the patient. The rest belongs to the future. Once communication has been established, it can be enriched progressively by punctuating the patient's discourse and dotting it with remarks based exclusively on what has been said. It is in these cases that it is often necessary to repeat interviews (three or four) before arriving at a conclusion and communicating it to the patient.

I want to stress two aspects which seem to me to be of great importance. The first concerns the evaluation of the subject's relationship to his own speech. That is to say, what relation does he maintain between what he says in his discourse and his subjective position? Likewise, I want to insist on what I call *indexation*, i.e. the connotation which the patient gives to the discourse; in other words, the way he marks it and indicates the price he attaches to what he says and to the revelatory value of what he says about himself. The second aspect concerns the analyst's evaluation of what the person who is consulting him seems to expect from analytic work. This appreciation may already reveal those areas of the patient's life in which he (or she) is hoping for change, in contrast to others to which his narcissism (or his masochism) is attached, and in respect of which he does not wish for change. Naturally, we cannot place too much value on these conscious aspirations, but although they need to be evaluated carefully, it is better to be mistaken than not to ask oneself questions.

A few decades ago, the question of the indications of psychoanalysis was posed, more often than not in nosographical terms (neurotic or non-neurotic structures, strength or weakness of the ego, and so on). Nowadays, it is rare for analysts to base their decision on such macroscopic criteria. Even taking into consideration the level of fixations (genital or pregenital) is not enough to establish a diagnosis of analysability. It is understandable, then, that when one has to decide whether analysis is indicated by asking oneself if the patient is going to be able to use the setting, it is not just a question of clinical reasoning, but truly of an examination by means of an *analyser of analysability* which must be submitted to a predictive hypothetical evaluation on the basis of the different elements of its applicability (the non-visibility of the object, the capacity to tolerate the analyst's attitude of withdrawal and waiting, the interpretation of the resistance and of the transference, the limited duration of sessions, their desirable frequency, the tolerance of separations, the attitude towards reality, etc.). It is not a purely empirical evaluation that is involved here. In fact the issue is to know whether the patient will be able to demonstrate a 'capacity for being alone in the analyst's presence' (Winnicott, Roussillon), and if, on the basis of this artificial solitude, he will be capable of a mental functioning akin to that which can be witnessed in dreams. After two interviews, one is generally in a position to tell whether analysis is indicated for the patient or not. I say two because, in general, it is always interesting to note the effects of the first interview in the course of the second, which is eventually supposed to complete it and has the purpose of setting up the conditions of the setting. When more than two interviews seem necessary, it means that there is a doubt in the analyst's mind, often motivated by the fact that he perceives a reticence on the analysand's part to undertake an analysis or himself harbours a reticence for other reasons.

I want to move on now to the question, much discussed in the circles of the International Psychoanalytical Association, of the number of weekly sessions. Though the French tradition is satisfied with three sessions per week, many analysts abroad consider that one can only speak of analysis if there are four or five sessions. Three sessions, they claim is a psychotherapy. It is a difficult question to settle; some say that, in fact, two different therapeutic processes are involved. I will put forward two arguments in an attempt to resolve the problem. In the first place, it seems to me quite unrealistic not to take into account the conditions of modern life and to require someone to see his analyst five times a week, considering the time outside the session (travelling time) which has to be added to its duration. The respect of this requirement would condemn psychoanalysis to only being able to survive by becoming a treatment for the well-off, which does not seem desirable to me. The second argument is that I believe much more in analyses of long duration, even if at a less frequent rhythm, than in analyses at a more sustained rhythm for a more limited duration. Experience shows that the process of change takes a long time to get underway, to establish itself, and to be maintained: the transference neurosis is a neurosis and, as such, it presents a resistant organization which requires time to be defeated.

When the analysis cannot be initiated immediately, it is postponed for a longer or shorter period of time; if this is then extended owing to the material circumstances either of the analyst or the patient, it is possible to suggest that the patient requests periodic sessions (if he is going through a difficult period) until the official beginning of his analysis.

As I have already pointed out, around 1950 a certain interest was being taken in technical variations.[1] As a rule, the issue concerned critical moments in an analysis which necessitated, on the analyst's part, the adoption, momentarily, of an appropriate attitude to facilitate the continuation of the analysis. I will not dwell on this question which has already been debated at length, and will adopt the conclusions of Bouvet in 1967 who only accepted as analytic those variations which contribute to 'an as complete as possible objectivation, and then reduction of the transference neurosis in the full sense of the term'.[2] The question has been posed with acuity in France owing to the technique adopted by Lacan, who, moreover, stepped well outside the framework of variations. His technique seemed unacceptable to the large majority of analysts of his time (short sessions, manipulation of the transference, no analysis of the negative transference, countertransference with violence exerted towards patients, an openly sadistic attitude alternating with charming seduction – without going as far as the sexual act – and so on). The problem of variations was not confined to the French situation and was also an issue in the United States, where the great question was to define rigorously the conditions of acceptability for the adoption of a parameter (K. Eissler). Likewise, in England, Winnicott was concerned with the same problem in an article dated 1954.[3] However, in this case, the question is less one of a selective variation of technique than of constant adjustments of the analytic setting by modifying the usual conditions (patient getting up and walking around the room in which milk is being warmed on a stove at his disposal, and so on). This whole period preceded what I shall not hesitate to call an explosion of the traditional analytic mould which led progressively, after 40 years or so, to the current situation.

Let us turn now to the indications for psychotherapy. I have just said that the reasons which plead in favour of a psychotherapy more than an analysis lie in the patient's more or less foreseeable intolerance for the analytic setting. Quite clearly, this intolerance is very often in keeping with a psychical structure far removed from the transference psychoneurosis (non-neurotic structure), the varieties of which are numerous (borderline, narcissistic patients, patients with a psychotic or perverse structure, psychosomatic patients, etc.). But here again, the nosographical criteria count less than others that are connected with the patient's *mental functioning* (frequency of the compulsion to repeat, tendency to act out, elaborative deficiencies marked by excessive frustrations, masochistic structure of the ego, importance of destructive positions, depth and tenacity of regressions, indifference towards his own psychic life, etc.). We have yet to speak of the frequency of sessions. Here, everything is a matter of nuance. Depending on the case, the analyst can propose periodic, isolated sessions or regular meetings the rhythm of which, it seems to me, cannot be established in a rigid fashion. In order to mark the differences between psychoanalysis and psychotherapy more clearly, the rhythm of analysis – several times a week – is frequently contrasted with the weekly session of psychotherapy. This attitude does not seem to me to be at all justified. In my experience, I have sometimes had patients in psychotherapy up to five times a week, whereas my analysands only disposed of three or four weekly sessions. What is essential is to determine, in the light of experience, the optimal number of times that these encounters can or should take place according to the needs and the tolerance of the patient. This will depend on his structure, his resistances, his demand, and his unconscious or manifest transference.

Another argument against training in psychotherapy in psychoanalytic institutes is to say that its technique is not codified. It is clear that the variability of attitudes and interpretations is greater in psychotherapy than in psychoanalysis. But I see this as a supplementary reason for being trained in practising psychotherapy owing to the fact that the choices to be made by the analyst are more aleatory and do not involve a pre-established recipe. Moreover, I would like to denounce the idea that was in circulation at a certain time that in psychotherapy, in contradistinction to psychoanalysis, 'anything goes'. Statements like this have been put about by analysts who are often scornful of what, for them, is nothing but a manipulative process of tinkering, and who do not hesitate to take liberties, examples of which I have already given, with what is expected of an analyst (by a sort of perversion of the method). They allow themselves to do more or less what they like depending on how the mood takes them. In fact, not only is anything whatsoever not permitted, but I would say, rather, that what is difficult to determine here is precisely what is at stake in the psycho-therapeutic situation where, *without doing analysis, one remains a psychoanalyst* (Winnicott). I will not insist on what is now an integral part of the experience of every analyst, namely, that it is possible to do excellent analytic work face to face which will sometimes take the patient further than if he was lying down. I think that the real problem is to determine what the optimal setting is for the patient, psychoanalytic or psychotherapeutic, while taking into account the importance of the face-to-face relationship where the analyst is visible and serves up his reactions to the patient.

A final argument consists in maintaining that, in psychotherapy, there is no psychoanalytic process. This is a particularly flimsy assertion for, in fact, I think there is always a process since, in all cases, there is a forward movement, but this assumes different tempos, modalities, rhythms and progressions depending on whether it is a classical analytical treatment or psychotherapy. Walking crabwise is still walking. What seems important to me is not to consider the relatively codified knowledge of the classical treatment as the only one that is certain in comparison with what still remains, to a large extent, a dark continent, namely, that discovered by psychotherapy. Instead of being disheartened by the absence of a map for venturing into these unknown regions, we should on the contrary set out to discover these little or poorly explored domains in order to assert the rights of analysis there. For I am persuaded that only analysts can understand these kinds of patients (moreover, the latter do not want any other help than that provided by an analyst) and help them to progress in the knowledge of themselves, without being satisfied with the role of distributing pills to which pharmaceutical psychiatry often confines them. I will not hide the fact that the work is often long, difficult, subject to many disappointments, reversals, repetitions, and so on. But provided that the analyst is determined to *hold firm*, at the end of efforts over several years, he arrives at a result which, though far from perfect, nonetheless allows one to think that the patient has gained an irreversible acquisition in respect of what has to be called his illness. Although the analyst does not always realize this, being a bit discouraged by the slow pace of progress, the patient, for his part, does. Notwithstanding his constant complaints and his denials, at certain moments the mask falls, and what he owes to psychotherapy, by his own admission, is impressive. What is more, I think that if psychotherapy did not bring him any benefit, he would have stopped coming a long time ago. It is not his fidelity, but his act of breaking off the treatment which should be attributed to his masochism.[4]

Notes

1 Cf. Green, A. Mythes et réalités sur le processus psychanalytique. Le modèle de *L'Interprétation des rêves*, *Revue française de psychosomatique*, 19/2001.
2 Bouvet, M. (1967). *Oeuvres psychanalytiques*, vol. 1, pp. 289–290. Paris: Payot.
3 Winnicott, D.W. (1954). Metapsychological and clinical aspects of regression within the psychoanalytical set-up. In *Collected Papers: Through Paediatrics to Psycho-Analysis*. London: Tavistock Publications, 1958.
4 I refer the interested reader to my work: Mythes et réalités sur le processus psychanalytique, *Revue française de psychosomatique*, 19/2001 and 20/2001.

3

SETTING – PROCESS – TRANSFERENCE

One can see how necessary it is to clarify our ideas concerning the conceptual tools of the psychoanalyst's work. The dispersion of the psychoanalytic field calls for a reunification. I have distinguished between classical treatment, treatment with selective variations, treatment with more or less constant variations and finally, the psychotherapies. Three notions need clarification.

The setting

It was introduced into psychoanalysis by two authors, independently, who proposed different definitions of it: Bleger, in Argentina, whose highly personal conception, linking it with symbiosis, only took hold in Latin America; and Winnicott, in England, whose conception has been widely adopted, in Europe at least. Let us note that the term used by Winnicott is 'setting' (*cadre*), which has much broader meaning than 'frame', for instance (also *cadre*). In French, it may be translated by *dispositif*. For my part, I have proposed a term that does not figure under this entry in the bilingual dictionary, that is, *montage*; but *cadre* is good enough. What is meant, in any case, by the term setting is the overall conditions of possibility required for practising psychoanalysis. This includes the material arrangements which govern the relations between analysand and analyst (payment of missed sessions, co-ordination of vacations between patient and analyst, length of sessions, mode of payment, etc.). These arrangements are fixed at the outset, constituting a convention between the two partners so as to avoid eventual discussions in the future. One has to distinguish, however, between this material setting, which serves as an analytic contract, and the *fundamental rule* on which analysts are divided. Some do not announce it, considering that they will have the opportunity of drawing attention to the patient's omissions and silences, whereas others, including myself, prefer to announce it as the only requirement laid down by the analyst concerning the analysand's work. It will be accepted by the patient, even if it proves impossible to respect in practice. But the rule plays yet another role, namely of inscribing itself as a third, as a law above the two parties, a law whose observance is necessary for the analysis to take place. It should be noted, in fact, that it is a complex injunction, for the patient is not only asked to say everything, including what seems to him to be the most absurd, the most contingent, etc., but *to do nothing*. Respecting the rule institutes *ipso facto* a modification of the psychical topography since it encourages a mode of waking reverie during the session. It is an exercise in soliloquy uttered out loud, even though the person being addressed is invisible, at once present and absent. In 1973, I described in detail the modalities of the analytic dialogue in *The Fabric of Affect in the Psychoanalytic Discourse*[1] (speech delivered in the lying position to a hidden addressee, with a loosening of the links of discourse).

More recently, I have proposed to distinguish within the setting between two parts:

1 The *active matrix*, composed of the patient's free association, floating attention and listening, stamped with the analyst's benevolent neutrality, forming a *dialogical* couple in which the analysis is rooted.
2 The *'casing'*,[2] constituted by the number and duration of the sessions, the periodicity of the encounters, the modalities of payment, and so on.

The active matrix is the jewel contained by the casing. One of the most remarkable phenomena of analytic speech is the patient's functioning via free association. In conjunction with the analyst's evenly suspended listening, this constitutes the dialogical couple which characterizes psychoanalysis. In my article 'The Central Phobic Position',[3] I put forward a model of free association which opens fresh horizons on mental functioning in the session. Free association does not suffice to define what the patient says in a linear manner, starting from the beginning and going to the end. On the contrary, underlying this conscious listening, a listening of another order (preconscious) allows the mechanisms specific to this mental functioning to be identified.

All reflection on the psychoanalytic process necessarily starts with the examination of its basic cell, namely, the analytic session. Reading the literature shows us that, even by going back to this psychoanalytic atom, the different ways of describing it, understanding it and interpreting it, face us immediately with an absence of consensus among the diverse groupings which currently make up the field of psychoanalysis. The same session seen from the viewpoint of an adherent to the ideas of ego psychology, a Kleinian, a Bionian, a Winnicottian, a Kohutian, a Lacanian, offers as many disparities as the examination of the various conceptions of psychic development based on the common reference to baby observation. I shall therefore have no scruples about adding my own, without attempting to conciliate everyone. The reference to the work of the session clearly shows that we are constantly concerned with following, as it progresses, the expression of an incessant process of transformation both from the angle of the relations of the *intrapsychic* and the *intersubjective*, and from the dual angle of *transference on to speech* and *transference on to the object*. This work of transformation is itself accomplished under the auspices of these contradictions. The analysand is divided, as I have said, between the desire to give expression to that which is most intimate in himself, and the least barred by censorship, and, at the same time, the fear that what is expressed in speech will become the object of a rejection or a sanction by the analyst, on the pattern of past internalized models, thereby giving the psychoanalytic discourse its self-contradictory dimension of being caught between the forward push of the already realized desire and the brake which restrains its progression, or even requires it to go backwards. No doubt the most interesting paradox of the analytic session is that this forward and backward movement is nonetheless marked by its temporal course oriented towards its end point. In other words, whatever contradictory tensions inhabit it, the session has a limited duration and moves, each time, towards its end in any case. And it is here that we need to be attentive. For, on the one hand, the more the session advances, the more one can assume that it is approaching its unconscious purposive ideal, and, as it moves ineluctably towards its own end, the more it refuses to accept that it must stop. In other words, the more one approaches the goal, the more this goal seems like the condensation of a sought after satisfaction and the end of all possibility of satisfaction. Winnicott used to say that the end of every session had to be considered, from the patient's standpoint, as the repetition of a rejection by the primary object. In short, each session is experienced as repeating a process of reunion–separation, the latter arriving after an attempt at reunion. But it is here that there is an alternative: either the separation constituted by the end of the session can lead to the hope of it beginning again and of the possibility of its continuation or, on the contrary, it is experienced as a traumatic abandonment which not only leaves no hope, due to the absence of any anticipation of a future session, but also has the effect of erasing everything that has been acquired during the work of the session.

Here mention can be made of the capacity to tolerate frustration and the Bionian dilemma which leads the subject to 'choose' between the recognition of frustration and its elaboration on the one hand, and its evacuation by means of excessive projective identification on the other. If the analyst wishes, from time to time, to know where he is at or, to be more exact, where his patient is at with him, he has no better means at his disposal than to ask himself what he thinks of the quality of the work of the sessions. Much more than any progress originating from outside or some sort of behavioural evaluation or an evaluation relative to the analysand's life, it is the potential fecundity of the session which remains the best criterion – in other words, what I call the *generativity of the process* during the session. It is in this way that new fields are annexed with many to-and-fros, but it is also a precious selective evaluation for, in analysis, there is something which resembles an interplay between hot and cold. The hotter it gets, the more the patient is confronted with the double contradictory desire, either to take the heat out of the conflict, to shut down, restrain or turn his back on his own creations, or to accept to tolerate the reactivation of the conflictual suffering in order to move forwards, to analyse it, and get beyond it.

It is plain that in the picture that I have just described one cannot make the analysand carry the whole weight of responsibility for the situation alone. It is here that the situation of the couple, which governs the process, acquires all its meaning. The analyst's attitude is also important for the development of the process, which it can just as easily facilitate or impede, stimulate or bridle to the point of extinguishing it. It is not easy to say on what condition one obtains the facilitation; it is not a simple matter, and under no circumstances can it consist of solicitations, encouragement or support in any form in order to help the patient have the courage to confront the obstacle, as Freud found in the early stages of his practice.

Nor is it recommended, it seems to me, to adopt a cold and indifferent attitude in the face of the patient's often distressing efforts. What one has to try and achieve is the classically recommended attitude of *benevolent neutrality*. Benevolence is not in contradiction with neutrality; nor the latter with benevolence. Benevolence consists, essentially, in an attitude of understanding receptivity (without this turning towards complicity) without giving way to discouragement or irritation, which, as a rule, only accentuate the patient's inhibitions. Receptivity, availability, evenness of temper, no doubt form the mental configuration of an ideal analyst who only exists in books and in the analyst's mind. And even if it is difficult for him to achieve this, at least he knows what he is striving at. However, when one speaks of receptivity and availability, it is not only a question of the analyst being open to what the patient is saying and to receiving his projections favourably, by virtue of an introjection which will give rise to identification. It is just as much a matter of receptivity and availability to the productions arising from the analyst's own unconscious which he will not only have to tolerate but to understand as well. Sometimes, para-doxically, it will be less damaging to the process to allow a lively transference reaction to be expressed, even if negative, in order to gain access to the internal movements animating the analyst. These are all evidence of the spontaneity of the manifestations which contribute, on his side, to the psychoanalytic communication, having more value for the patient than a conventional pseudo-tolerant discourse which will be experienced by the patient as artificial and governed by technical manuals. This is something that has been known since Ferenczi who denounced the often artificial character of the analyst's attitude. Nevertheless, following the logic of the pendulum, Ferenczi could not stop himself from pushing things to the opposite extreme in a manner which has as many drawbacks as the one that he was denouncing. There is no reason here to set up as a model the recommendations made by one analyst or the other, for all analysts have a tendency to sin depending on their individual complexion, their ideology, their personal morale, and their perversions. Accordingly, each one has to find his own way.

I will now make a more detailed description of the model of free association as I developed it in my work on the central phobic position.[4] I have described the phenomena of retroactive reverberation when certain words or certain ideas in the session evoke other parts of the material upstream with which they seem to be associated by various types of connections: similarities, symmetries, contradictions, antagonisms, and so on. In other cases, what the analyst hears are effects of anticipatory annunciation, as if the patient's discourse were playing the role of an announcement drawing the analyst's attention to what was going to follow. They give him no more than an intuitive and vague idea of it, yet make him feel that something is going to emerge in the discourse that is related to this announcement. *Retroactive reverberation and anticipatory annunciation* clearly indicate that behind the linear progression of the discourse, in its innermost reaches, a two-way causality is operating retrogressively and progressively in alternation. These two processes make it possible to speak of an *associative irradiation*, the words pronounced having an effect of resonance upstream and downstream within the statements of the discourse: such are the radiant effects of analytic speech, which, moreover, as I have said, *takes the mourning out of language*.[5] It is in this set of particularities that one recognizes the originality of the meaningful production in the session and the capacity of the discourse to mobilize the levels of the preconscious. Can these particularities go as far as influencing the unconscious directly? Though certain selective effects have to be acknowledged, we are also obliged to recognize the differences of structure between the preconscious and the unconscious, since we know that the preconscious can still contain linguistic phenomena whereas, at least in the Freudian conception, this is not true of the unconscious. This is one of the limitations of the Lacanian theory which has long sought to make us believe the contrary. Given the cardinal role played by free association and evenly suspended listening – which is simply the response adapted to speech uttered in a mode of free association – I propose to characterize the analytic situation by the denomination *analytic association*. This condenses in a single expression what we are accustomed to calling the therapeutic alliance, a very widely accepted concept but one which I have never really found convincing on account of its exaggerated optimism. Analytic association brings together two partners for the best and for the worst. For 'association' evokes 'dissociation', just as dissociation evokes, in turn, association. Once again we are in the presence of dialogical functioning.

Now, my thesis is that psychoanalysis (classical treatment) and psychoanalytic psychotherapy share many traits of the active matrix and differ, above all, concerning the 'casing' surrounding it. In effect, the aims of classical treatment and psychotherapy are the same. In both cases it is a matter of bringing the patient to the point of recognizing what his unconscious is saying to him – something he is unaware of as such, and hopes to remain unaware of by means of resistance. This process is based on transference and interpretation. Of course, the resistance, transference and interpretation differ greatly in the two situations. But though their appearances and even their nature are not the same, they pursue the same goal and have the same function. It is no longer a matter, then, of opposing pure gold and copper, but of recognizing their composite metallic nature, whatever the varieties of their alloy.

A question can be raised here. Though we attribute great importance to the concept of the analytic setting, what about situations in psychotherapy where it is modified to such an extent that it could be argued that it has disappeared in this technique? It is not easy to give an answer to this, but one does exist. Though psychoanalytic treatment allows for the setting to be established and 'embodied', the latter is not, however, absent in the psychotherapeutic relationship. Here an overly realistic interpretation needs to be avoided for, as we know, the setting only has value inasmuch as it is the metaphor of another concept (the dream-model, the prohibition of incest and parricide, maternal care, and so on). In psychotherapy, the absence of a setting analogous to that which exists in psychoanalysis obliges the analyst to refer to an *internal setting*, that is to say, to the setting which he has internalized during his own analysis. Even if it is absent from the analytic work in psychotherapy, it is no less present in the analyst's mind, governing the limits of the variations that he allows, making him protect the necessary conditions for the continuation of exchanges, and so on. This notion of an internal setting is an essential acquisition of the training analysis which must, therefore, be extremely rigorous so that the process of internalization can be accomplished.[6]

The process

It is remarkable to note that the expression *psychoanalytic process*, so much in vogue at the moment, does not figure in Freud's work. As is often the case, when an idea imposes itself in the post-Freudian literature, an attempt is made to look for its genealogy and ancestors, which are often more imaginary than real. Citations will thus be looked for in Freud which present analysis by comparing it to the development of a pregnancy, in order to sustain the idea that the psychoanalytic process follows a natural course. What is meant by that is that analysis progresses according to its own rhythm and that it is to be differentiated from the evolution of the transference, rather as one would distinguish between the background and the form. In reality, the idea of a 'natural history of the psychoanalytic process' appears in Meltzer's writings. The question that I feel justified in asking is whether the psychoanalytic process is the same irrespective of whether it is a Freudian, Kleinian, Winnicottian, Kohutian, Lacanian, and now Renikian, analysis? What can be said, in any case, is that the idea of a natural evolution comparable to the flow of a river which follows its course from its source at its estuary before flowing, like all rivers, into the sea, can only be validly maintained in the case of thoroughly adequate indications of analysis which go together with the idea that the analyst 'accompanies' this evolution, the main concern still being that his countertransference does not disturb the process in an inopportune way. Needless to say, the analysis of the forms that can be associated with non-neurotic structures by no means follows this cruising rhythm. The question of the process is not a simple one, for its content varies depending on the author, for instance in Sauguet[7] and in Meltzer.[8] The motor of the treatment can indeed be conceived of as an underground process. And one can contrast the neurotic process which moves, without too many pitfalls, towards its conclusion – *rebus bene gestis*, as Freud says – with the stagnant and repetitive chaotic forms, resembling the work of Penelope, of non-neurotic structures. But does this opposition not reflect, precisely, the very history of Freudian psychoanalysis which led Freud to modify his theory of the drives in 1920 and to change his first topography in 1923? I will deal with these questions in more detail further on. It remains clear that the negative therapeutic reaction and the compulsion to repeat were the decisive factors in what has been called 'the turning-point of 1920'. This did not prevent Freud, in his *Outline*, from recommending that psychoanalysts interest themselves in a class of psychical patients 'who clearly resemble the psychotics very closely . . . to see how far and by what methods we are able to "cure" them'.[9] In conclusion, I shall single out the psychoanalytic process as the exemplary model of psychoanalysis, paradigmatic in every respect, setting it in contrast with the varieties observed in the psychotherapeutic processes whose characteristics remain to be defined and which are an object of interest for psychoanalysts.

If one is seeking an element of coherence in the concept of process, it should be recalled that, originally, for Freud, analysis rested on a tripod: transference psychoneurosis, transference neurosis, and infantile neurosis. This can be easily seen if one examines the beginnings of Freud's work. Today, I would propose another tripod: the coherence of the relations uniting the setting, the dream, and interpretability. In effect, as I have shown elsewhere, though the model of the setting was not theorized by Freud, it is possible to find the justification for it in Chapter VII of *The Interpretation of Dreams*. That is to say, the setting reproduces an *analogon* of the psychical processes which govern the dream. And just as the latter can be interpreted through the associations which reveal the work of which it is the locus, similarly the homogeneous relation between setting and dream leads to optimal interpretability. Anyone who bases his reflection on this tripod is at once led to consider the process as an effect of these relations. In recent years, the experience gained from difficult analyses and non-neurotic structures has thrown light on the necessity of referring to the *mental functioning* theorized by P. Marty. It is precisely the differences, and sometimes the deficiencies of mental functioning in psychosomatic patients (irregularities of the preconscious), which make it possible both to understand the links between the symptomatic organizations and the way in which the latter are sensitive to analytic intervention. Clearly, the question of treatment by psychotherapy is being introduced here. At the same time, the differences between analysis and psychotherapy are highlighted. Those who want to oppose, often in a schematic fashion, psychoanalysis and psychotherapy, are led to sustain the idea that there is no identifiable and theorizable psychoanalytic process in psychotherapy. This opinion seems debatable to me; not because I deny that there are differences separating the psychoanalytic process of classical psychoanalysis and the diverse processes of psychotherapy, but because while the former can be identified with a model, the others only represent more or less extensive variations of it which can only be understood in relation to the model. Actually, it is not clear how a therapeutic relation of whatever kind could be devoid of processual considerations. Moreover, if one considers the evolution which marked Freud's approach, once it had made the turning of 1920 and introduced into the treatment the compulsion to repeat and the negative therapeutic reaction, it can be seen that the tranquil course of the psychoanalytic process was *ipso facto* relativized. One only has to think, once again, of the sad case of the Wolf Man, to notice the intermittent and alternating effects of resistance, repeated regressions, and the compulsion to repeat. The fact remains that, in the account he gave of the case, Freud did not seem to be aware of the problems that the patient presented in relation to the process. Admittedly, this negligence on his part does not constitute a justification. Nevertheless, if one looks at it from a contemporary perspective, one realizes that, in the case of the Wolf Man, the psychoanalytic process by no means follows a natural course, and that, whether one likes it or not, there is a 'process', that is to say, course or procession. So we should conclude from this that the question which interests us, for contemporary psychoanalytic praxis, for the evaluation of any kind of therapeutic relationship, concerns the idea that the analyst can form of the processual course of the treatment. When the latter does not conform to the so-called natural course, it raises questions about the nature of the fixations, the possibility that the ego is affected, the patient's non-neurotic structure, and requires the analyst to pay particular attention to the patient's mental functioning.

What I call the psychoanalytic process is the creation of a 'second reality' arising from an observation of the exchanges in the course of the sessions, which questions the evaluation of the mode of development of the relations between conjecture, which is constantly changing, what remains to be known, and, on the other hand, what makes interpretation susceptible to triggering disturbing effects which have to be warded off.[10]

39

To be trivial, is this not what the expression 'walking on eggs' means? The psychoanalytic process is based on the way in which the patient respects, and applies to himself, the analytic pact whose principal axis is the fundamental rule. The ramblings of the process can be related to the analysis of the work of the negative and of resistance. It is clear that the weight of the process can under no circumstances be evaluated in a way that does not take account of the network in which it is inscribed. The practice of psychotherapies and the questions that it raises – often broached in a polemical fashion – has initiated a process of reflection on this subject which is as yet far from exhausted.

Transference

A vast debate opens up before us here on the nature and the function of the transference. Let me just say, for the moment, that what I have just said about the process applies equally to the transference. In other words its evolution, its readability, its role at one and the same time as resistance and as a motor of the treatment remain within the limits of the 'playground' (Freud) in the classical analytic treatment and assume much more chaotic forms in the psychotherapies indicated, for the most part, in non-neurotic structures. It is remarkable to note that, in these latter cases, the patient is much deafer and more reticent in recognizing and identifying the transferential nature of the manifestations that he presents in the course of the treatment. Very often there exists a major defence against recognizing the transference which can however be lifted at certain moments, during certain indirect communications (written or telephoned messages, etc.). The soundness of the Freudian position is confirmed by the observation that destructivity infiltrates the transferential manifestations of non-neurotic structurings (destructivity that is frequently masochistic) to the point of masking expressions of the libido. Here again, the duration of the treatment is often much longer than with analyses. I would add, and I promise to come back to this, that from the contemporary perspective, the problem of transference can no longer be tackled without coupling it with its counterpart in the analyst, namely, the countertransference.[11] A distinction should nonetheless be made between the countertransference in the version that Freud gives of it, that is, of being an obstacle to analysing the transference, and the more recent version which confers it with a much wider function and meaning, even to the point of invoking asserting that the countertransference precedes the transference (Neyraut 1974).

We have arrived now at a point when certain conclusions can be drawn, while recalling the principal findings of our investigation. We should bear in mind:

• the diagnostic value (analyser of analysability) of predictions concerning the setting and the patient's capacity to submit himself to the conditions

- the existence of a de facto process for which the model, provided by classical treatment, merely constitutes a paradigm to be compared with other modes of progression
- the chaotic forms of transference putting to the test the countertransference of the analyst who, frequently, cannot avoid falling for the patient's very aggressive provocations. However, once again, the essential thing is to *withstand* this.

Let me add a further remark. In enumerating the components of the active matrix, I have made no allusion to the transference. This is because I wanted to consider them solely from the angle of the psychical characteristics of mental functioning. But it is obvious that the transference is part of these basic components, in the measure that it is it that mobilizes the associative work.[12] The essential point to be borne in mind is that all analytic work tends towards the same aim. That is to say, the aim it not so much the process of becoming conscious, as it is customary to say, as the recognition of the unconscious: *recognition because it emerges against a background of misrecognition*. The gap which separates the two terms of this couple is largely a function of what I have called the *work of the negative*, which I will return to later. When all is said and done, everything that I have just said only takes on meaning within a conception of psychoanalysis which recognizes within itself the existence of *clinical thinking*.[13] This means that we have to cease to see clinical work as a set of empirical findings in which theory simply precipitates (in the chemical sense), but rather to see it as comprising many forms of the psyche with its own specific mode of causal thinking which the analyst must detect and never lose sight of. On the contrary, it is by constantly bearing in mind the originality and the primacy of this mode of thinking that the analyst is capable of contributing to knowledge, without sacrificing anything of the complexity of the phenomena that he sets out to study.

Notes

1   Green, A. (1973). *Le Discours vivant*. Paris: Presses Universitaires de France, coll. 'Le Fil rouge'. [English edition: *The Fabric of Affect in the Psychoanalytic Discourse*, trans. A. Sheridan. London: Routledge, 1999.]
2   Translator's note: The French word here is *écrin*: a case, box, casket for jewels.
3   Green, A. 'The central phobic position: a new formulation of the free association method'. *International Journal of Psychoanalysis* 81, 429. (First publication 1988, *Revue française de psychanalyse*, 3/2000.)
4   Green, A. The central phobic position, ibid.
5   Green, A. (1984). Le langage dans la psychanalyse. In A. Green *Langages*. Paris: Les Belles Lettres.

6 Green, A. Le cadre psychanalytique, son intériorisation chez l'analyste et son application dans la pratique. In: A. Green et al., *L'avenir d'une désillusion*. Paris: Presses Universitaires de France, 'Petite Bibliothèque de Psychanalyse', 2000.

7 Sauguet, H. Introduction à une discussion sur le processus psychanalytique. *Revue française de psychanalyse*, 33. Paris: Presses Universitaires de France, 1969.

8 Meltzer, D. (1967). *The Psycho-Analytical Process*. London: Heinemann.

9 Freud, S. (1940 [1938]). *An Outline of Psychoanalysis*, p. 174. S.E XXIII.

10 Green, A. Mythes et réalités sur le processus psychanalytique. *Revue française de psychosomatique*, 19/2001, p. 72. I refer the reader to this article for more details on the question.

11 Green, A. (1988). Démembrement du contre-transfert, postface to: *Inventer en psychanalyse. Construire et interpréter*, by J.-J. Baranes, F. Sacco et al. Paris: Dunod, 2002.

12 Evelyn Seychaud has drawn my attention to this point.

13 Green, A. (2002). *La pensée clinique*. Paris: Odile Jacob.

4

TRANSFERENCE AND COUNTERTRANSFERENCE

Analytic listening

At the beginning of an analytic session, what state of mind am I in for responding to what the situation requires of me? I think I am adopting an analytic position when, having endeavoured to keep my attention as free floating as possible – we will see that it is not straightforward, and sometimes runs into serious difficulties – I hear the analysand's communication from two perspectives simultaneously. On the one hand, I try to perceive the conflictuality within him and, on the other, I consider it from the angle of the message, implicit or explicit, that it constitutes for me. The conflictuality to which I am referring does not concern the particular dynamic conflicts that could be identified by interpretation, but the way in which the discourse alternately moves towards and away from a meaningful nucleus or a set of meaningful nuclei which are trying to enter consciousness. It is not necessary to have a precise idea of what is activating or, on the contrary, inhibiting or diverting the communication, in order to notice the movement which sometimes carries it towards a more explicit or precise expression, and sometimes distances it from the verbalization of what is trying to communicate itself. One can, then, notice these variations intuitively even if one does not know the exact nature of the focal point around which they gravitate. This will appear more or less suddenly, sometimes perfectly clearly, and sometimes in a more accidental manner, in the course of the discursive process. It is in this latter case that floating attention undergoes a change of state and becomes investigative acuity, during a phase of reorganizing what has slipped under the fluidity of the 'suspended' reception of the analysand's more or less free associative discourse. In this description it is not just a question of naming the resistance, as it is encountered when activated moments of transference are approaching. I am referring to the background state against which movements of the discourse appear while waiting to be heard, or to the basic oscillation inherent in the analysand's impulse to speak, uncertain of its acceptability, both for the consciousness of the speaker and for that of the addressee. A convergent movement – but one that is far from being synchronous – thus causes the analyst's thinking to evolve from the identification of the analysand's punctual transferential position in the present moment towards a more global picture of his conflictuality insofar as the flux of the discourse allows it to be apprehended; or alternatively towards that which, at a given moment, bears witness on the one hand to the activation of a particular conflict and, on the other, to the manner in which this conflict stands out momentarily within a general configuration. The general conditions of verbalization, divided between that which seeks satisfaction through expression and that which translates a fear of expressing itself freely, are thus placed in perspective. In other words, there are two factors involved here: on the one hand, there is a particular local conflict relating to a more general state of conflictuality in the analysand which can be understood in the light of the relations between the parts of the discourse and the way in which the object's presence excites and inhibits their figures; and, on the other, an examination by the analyst of the significance of the present moment evaluated in terms of the general conflictuality of psychic life as it is expressed in the analytic relationship. The latter is caught between the ideal of a communication free of any censorship and the vicissitudes of a desire to speak, thwarted by imaginary fear and its consequences, which suggest that here speaking has lost, in part, its distance from doing.

When, changing vertex, I hear what is being said as something addressed to me, I focus on what I have heard from a perspective in which the internal conflict, in its attempt to externalize itself through speech, encounters a reflexive return towards the subject who is speaking. This transformation is produced by this publication of thought, which, by being addressed to another, retroactively engenders the echo of its words in the speaker, according to an effect facilitated by the setting. The singular alterity of the analytic relationship also engenders symmetrically the idea that the causality governing the words of the speaker modifies the status of the one to whom the message is being addressed. The latter, who is required to be a witness or object of a demand, is changed in the internal world and becomes, without the analysand knowing it, the *cause* of the movement animating his speech. This, indeed, is what lies at the bottom of every transference. The addressee – invisible in the analytic situation – falls back, so to speak, on the movement of speech, merging into it, and is from then on interpreted according to a double register. Though, originally, he was consciously defined as the one to whom the discourse – the singular mode of which he has fixed, moreover – is addressed in an attempt to approach the patient's inner world, unconsciously this condition of being the receiver of the message changes into that of being the one who induces it. He becomes the agitator through the presence of internal movements arising as much from what is addressed to him as from what has animated the analysand to make such remarks. The separation between the affective, internal movements of the subject and their objectivation through the discourse addressed to a third party no longer exists for the unconscious. A point is reached when the two become but one: the object to whom this discourse is addressed – that is to say, what the patient's demand, quest, hope expect from someone else – and its unconscious, instinctual subjective source become more or less exchangeable without the speaker being aware of it. At this level, the one who is being addressed through the verbalization of these internal movements is no longer separated by more than a thread from the tendency to see him as their causal agent. From this cause, consequences are expected, as the discourse seeks to provoke a response in the one to whom the discourse is being addressed. It is no doubt tacitly hoped, not only that his response will satisfy the demand which is being addressed to him – a demand that is inherent to the very process of undertaking the analysis – but, more particularly, that it will reveal to the one to whom it is formulated a desire related to the quest of which he is the object.[1]

I wrote these lines at the beginning of the report that I presented to the Congress of the International Psychoanalytic Association in 1999. It seems to me that they give quite a good description of the general atmosphere of the session and of the thought processes which unfold during it. Hitherto, my concern has been above all to describe the spectrum of situations in which psychoanalytic work occurs. Having considered the range of possibilities (or at least the main possibilities) with which the analyst may have to deal, I must return now to the paradigm represented by analytic treatment, where one has the possibility of having access to the optimal legibility of the psychic processes characterizing the psychoanalytic field.

It is remarkable that, in the year 2001, more than a century after the birth of psychoanalysis and more than 60 years after Freud's death, the International Psychoanalytic Association has felt the need to give the Nice Congress, which followed that of Santiago, the general theme of 'Psychoanalysis: Method and Applications'. This is revealing, and bears witness to a certain disarray in the face of the dispersion of the concepts of reference defining what the essence of psychoanalysis is today, as if we were being invited to stand back and to cast an eye retrospectively upon what psychoanalysis has become and to try and identify the essence of what it is. This was the thread J.-L. Donnet[2] followed in his pre-published report to which I refer the reader. Donnet deconstructs the method, with his customary precision, underlining the knots and contradictions in it. The method postulates an ego subject who is capable of a certain division and can thus allow into his consciousness that which reaches the surface of his discourse from his unconscious, while another part of this same ego can devote itself, with all the difficulties inherent in this task, to the observation of what is going on in it. Donnet had already made penetrating reflections in the past on the function of the fundamental[3] rule at work here. He pursues them by referring to the *function of creating a third object* ('*la fonction tiercéisante*', A. Green) underlying the dynamic of the processes. One of the important points of his contribution was to show that the method cannot be distinguished clearly from the object of analysis itself. It can thus be said, in a certain way, that the aim of analysis is attained when the method can be applied to the analysand's psychic productions by the analysand himself and when the analyst can listen to the material produced with the receptivity and sensibility which echo it. This makes it possible for psychic events connected with the transference – which are as unforeseeable as they are surprising – to come to light. It can equally be said that the transference is the result of applying the method or, inversely, that a 'good enough' transference is the condition *ipso facto* of applying the method.

The transference

We will see further on that a whole set of arguments, certain of which concern the transference itself, converge to explain the 'turning-point of 1920'. In fact, they were at the centre of a long period of questioning which culminated in impasses, the transference being seen initially as a resistance, before becoming the motor of the treatment. Freud's definitive description sees it as the result of the compulsion to repeat. Transference, whatever the form – positive or negative – stems from a compulsive factor which tends to repeat a constellation going back to childhood and which, unless it is analysed, will always tend to reproduce itself spontaneously. But what is important in this mutation is the idea that the repetition no longer occurs only in the name of the pleasure principle but also, where certain matrix forms are concerned, to repeat an un-pleasure. Freud is now 'beyond the pleasure principle'. It is interesting to follow the path he takes which, starting with the elective indications of psychoanalytic treatment, i.e. the transference psychoneuroses, conceives of these as psycho-neuroses *producing transference*, capable of libidinal mobility (from the somatic to the psychic and from one object to the other), and leads to the compulsion to repeat. Which means that what, at the outset, was a movement giving preva-lence to a dynamic point of view (one of Freud's articles is called 'The Dynamics of Transference') almost becomes an automatism. For a long time, the term 'repetition automatism' was used for 'repetition compulsion'. Here the dynamics become a constraint; and movement, instead of opening up the possibility of extending the field of investments, is transformed into the contrary, i.e. a sterilizing restriction of a compulsive (*com-pulsive*) nature.

I once remarked that we had seen how a *transference of thought (une transfert de pensée) gave rise to a transference-thought (une pensée de transfert).* The major modi-

46

fication – we will have the opportunity of returning to it often – is that of
the transition from a movement of desire (first topography) to the discharge
of an impulse through action (*Agieren*). It is this change of referent that makes
what is observed in the treatment pass from one model, at the centre of which
one finds a form of thinking (desire, hope, wish), to another model based on
the act (impulse as internal action, automatism, acting). We can see how the
general profile of analytic treatment is thereby subverted, to the extent that
the analyst now not only has to deal with unconscious desire but with the drive
itself, whose force (constant pressure) is undoubtedly its principal characteristic,
capable of subverting both desire and thinking.

The conception of the transference in the last part of Freud's work was
thus affected. It is remarkable that the technical writings of Freud stopped
in 1918, before he formulated the final theory of the drives and the second
topography. A very long interval would be necessary, during which the avatars
of the analysis of the Wolf Man played a not inconsiderable role, before Freud
returned, with his two articles of 1937, 'Analysis Terminable and Interminable'
and 'Constructions in Analysis', to the problems of analytic technique as part
of a general re-evaluation. One now understands better the place that Freud
accorded to the death drive in the treatment. We are familiar with the emotions
aroused by the publication of his article, sowing discouragement in analytic
ranks and giving rise to unofficial reactions with the internal circulation of
texts responding to the master's pessimism (this is the meaning of Fenichel's
article on the question[4]). Today one cannot say that the facts have proved Freud
wrong, even if there is discussion about the value of his explanation in terms
of the death drive which embarrasses a lot of people and deserves to be thought
about more deeply, perhaps implying eventually a modification of the concept
Freud proposed.[5] It seems to me that the dispersion, or even fragmentation
of psychoanalytic thought into as many opposing theories (ego psychology,
Kleinism, Lacanism, Bionian, Winicottian and Kohutian, etc.) could all be
interpreted as attempts to propose a solution to the limitations of the results
of classical treatment. An idea of considerable importance has been advanced in
certain schools of thought (which adhere to the conception of object relations).
It endeavours to prove that analysis is only efficacious if the analyst restricts his
interventions to formulating transference interpretations. This conception, much
honoured in England, particularly in Kleinian circles, is not, it seems to me,
without danger. Two drawbacks follow from it:

- a limitation of 'psychoanalytic respiration' favouring an atmosphere of
  confinement that is prejudicial to discursive liberty and spontaneity
- a danger of returning surreptitiously to suggestion in disguised forms.

Unlike the English school, which believes only in the virtue of transference
interpretations, the French school follows another direction. It makes a

distinction between interpretations *in* the transference and interpretations *of* the transference. All interpretations, whatever they are, are interpretations that occur within the framework of transference, even when they do not allude to it directly. They only have meaning when they are put back in this context; which is why some analysts are heavily criticized for giving way to the tendency to make interpretations outside the setting, that is, outside the conditions which govern their practice. On the other hand, the interpretations of the transference correspond to what is alluded to by the English school. In my opinion, what is in question is the recognition of the transference inasmuch as it is linked to the unconscious. This means that the analysand's discourse can follow a broken path or follow numerous meanders before arriving at a fruitful moment when the transference manifests itself fully. When I say fully, I do not necessarily mean to imply that this manifestation is noisy or dazzling or obvious. On the contrary, it can be very discreet. But it then becomes identifiable as such, recognizable in its value of repetition, with a specific connotation which makes it possible to recognize it.

It may be said that, from this perspective, the emphasis is placed predominantly on the patient's transference, whereas the examination of the countertransference is limited to the minimum or, in other cases, is translated by dazzling manifestations which cannot be ignored. This way of seeing things has often been reproached for a weakness which everyone recognizes in Freud's analysis; namely, that it presents a somewhat solipsistic conception which underestimates the effects of a situation in which both partners are immersed. This has led to talk of a *two-body psychology* or, to use an expression I prefer, *a dialogical situation.* It is true that this dialogical situation, which puts an analyst and an analysand at grips with each other, and is present in all the modalities that we have envisaged, can be identified in diverse ways. Was this not Freud's idea when he refused to grant narcissistic neuroses the benefit of psychoanalytic treatment? Even if we know today that transference is far from being absent in psychotic patients, it will always remain necessary to distinguish between transference and transference. For it would not occur to anyone to confuse the transference of the classical treatment of a neurotic, which serves as a basis of description for its study, and the transference, concealed behind its most noisy manifestations, of a schizophrenic patient or even that – which is more difficult to interpret – of a depressive, perverse or psychosomatic patient. The idea that I will try to elucidate throughout this work is that of envisaging concepts in relation to a gradient within a spectrum whose basic structure has to be broken down into its constituents. To paraphrase the well-known aphorism: all patients present transferences, but some transferences are more transferential than others. Such nuances are, I believe, indispensable. What is essential, then, is to try each time to establish the relative spectrum of the different constituents in the final picture. Certain questions are traditionally posed here.

48

How far does what unfolds in the treatment involve a repetition of the past and how far does it concern not what has been repeated but, on the contrary, what has never been experienced (Viderman)?

How far does the analyst's offer constitute an implicit invitation to form a transference, the demands of the analysand being for him secondary?

How far does the analytic setting itself participate in the production of the transference. This last question is extremely important and can only be resolved on the condition that we know what the requirements of the setting are.

Finally, and this is perhaps the most important question of all, can the transference be considered as the spontaneous and unipolar expression of a situation characterized by the exchange between two poles? This question can constitute a trap in many respects. First, it is perfectly evident that the cure and its setting establish a relation between two poles, as in any situation of communication or, more precisely, any relationship involving language. The modern epistemological point of view lays much stress on the dimension of the relationship, which must have prevalence over the conception of the definition of an object considered in itself. However, and it is here that the trap needs to be avoided, the asymmetrical dimension of the relationship has to be stressed. The aim of the setting is indeed to facilitate a topographical regression, as César and Sára Botella have clearly pointed out. Such a topographical regression links the discourse of the analysand, who is endeavouring to obey the fundamental rule, with the regression which occurs spontaneously in dreams. For my part, I have established a detailed parallel concerning the relations between mental functioning in the session and the characteristics of the dream model as constructed[6] by Freud in Chapter VII of *The Interpretation of Dreams* (1900).[7] If we turn now to the corresponding polarity in the analyst, that is, evenly suspended attention, it is not difficult to realize that the regression is much more limited here. In short, in the channel of analytic communication, there is a series of knots organizing the discourse:

- at one extreme, the dream in the context of the regression of sleep
- topographical regression in the waking state during the session
- the analyst's evenly suspended attention in listening
- the analyst's reflexive thinking, mobilised by listening.

One can see how this chain, which could be called the chain of the *discursive relationship*, is constituted not only by a series of organized traits but also by as many couples whose differential gap can be identified as ranging from the most unconscious towards the most conscious (the analysand's unconsciousness of the topographical dream-regression in the session, the analyst's evenly suspended listening, reflexive thinking). It follows that the transference cannot be envisaged as a uniform bloc or simply be defined in a way which stresses the repetition of the past in the present; it must, in my opinion, be envisaged in terms of a spectral analysis.

In 1984, in the course of a reflection devoted to the place of language in psychoanalysis,[8] I proposed the idea of a double transference. According to this conception, it is necessary to articulate:

1 *A transference on to speech*: it is the result of the conversion of all the psychic elements into discourse. It is what induces me to say that, in analysis, it is as though the psychical apparatus were transformed into a language apparatus. Since this intrapsychic dimension makes it possible to elaborate the psychic elements which do not belong to language into elements of discourse, it is also intersubjective, since language presupposes an enunciator and a co-enunciator.

2 *A transference on to the object*: admittedly, the object is necessarily included in the act of speech, for almost all speech is addressed to someone who is supposed to hear it; nonetheless, the idea of a transference on to the object implies that the transference comprises dimensions which cannot be contained by the discourse.

To put it in another way, the chain of the discourse is a chain which is attached to the agencies of the conscious and preconscious in the first topography and belongs to the conscious and preconscious ego and superego in the second, whereas the chain of the transference on to the object must be attached to the unconscious of the first topography and to the unconscious id, ego and superego of the second. Value is thus placed both on the cardinal importance of language in the analysand's discourse and in the analyst's interpretation, and it is recognized that this dimension is overwhelmed from all sides by the elements of the psyche that cannot justifiably be connected with language. It is by relating the repercussions of the events which take place in one of these two chains on those of the other that one gets a more precise idea of the nature, function and meaning of the transference. It should be pointed out – here I refer the reader to my work of 1984 – that both chains are connected to a central cell, that of the ego-subject, while each chain forms with this cell a circuit (action, reaction), and that they are governed by different processes (secondary, for the transference on to speech, and primary, for the transference on to the object). The central cell, known as the ego-subject, possesses self-reference.[9] It seems to me that these are the requirements for an updating of the problem of the transference of which the character, always strangely surprising, is nonetheless vividly present in the mind of every analyst. As I have pointed out many times, much later on, Freud, who did not much like getting involved personally in the therapeutic relationship, and did not wish to lay himself open to his patients' discoveries about him, defended a conception which has since been judged to be too monopolistic, attaching little importance to all the effects of the dialogical relationship that analysis has established.

The problem is by no means a simple one. Freud was justified in constituting the pedestal of his conception on instinctual life, which is both what is most primitive and most solipsistic in the psyche, as in principle it only knows the id. But in fact even in adopting this point of view, as I maintained in 1984, the drive reveals the existence of the object apt to satisfy it, just as in return the object reveals the drive. An unfounded quarrel eventually developed between the partisans of the drive theory and those adhering to object-relations theory. I have already had occasion to discuss the issues at stake here,[10] and concluded that the articulation of the intrapsychic points of view (where the instinctual component of the psyche is in the foreground) and the intersubjectivist perspective (whose foundations go back to object-relations theory) is inescapable. The drive–object couple, which constitutes the basis of the psyche, is henceforth indissociable.

But that is not enough. We cannot allow ourselves to be enclosed, in the name of a simplistic and naïve genetic outlook, within a dual relationship that is more or less condemned to circularity. Thirdness, the theory of which C. S. Peirce was the first to delineate, plays the role of an essential dynamic function and makes us sensitive to the influence of the third party in psychoanalytic theory. It is not only Oedipal triangulation that is being evoked here, but a supersession of the famous *here and now* by the reference, always implicit, of the third dimension *(elsewhere and in former times)*, which plays the role of a third dimension, always marked by absence, whether of the present or of the past and, of course, *a fortiori*, of the future.

The countertransference

It is necessary to return to the *analysing situation* (Donnet)[11] to complete the picture. One can say that today, and in a quite general way, analysts are sensitive to the importance of the countertransference. However, this sensibility does not exclude a very wide variety of opinions as to how the phenomenon should be theorized. As we know, countertransference is a reaction to the transference, the analysand's discourse producing effects of resonance and rejection on what has been insufficiently or poorly analysed in the analyst, pushing him to understand in a prejudiced and partial, in short, biased way, what the analysand is trying to communicate.

With the countertransference, the chapter was opened – and still remains largely so today – of the analyst's pathology, of the effects of what has remained unanalysed in him and is likely to disturb him in his analytic work which requires distance and sangfroid. This conception of countertransference is still valid. It can be observed particularly in the work of supervision during training and it continues to affect the analyst in his practice long after he has been accepted into the analytic community. Here there are, roughly speaking, two cases. Either the punctual effects of the analysand's communication finish by attracting the attention of the analyst who, after resorting to self-analysis, finally senses what is going on, in a given analysis, at a given moment. The analyst's recognition of his own unconscious can help him to untangle the situation and permit the process to continue. There was a time in analysis when it was in good taste to attribute all the impasses of the analytic process to a loaded countertransference. In the second case, either the situation cannot be untangled or, worse still, it tends to deteriorate, to multiply itself with other analysands – many patients giving the analyst the opportunity of rushing into the impasses that are only too frequent in treatments. When it is an isolated case, there always remains the solution – the best, ultimately – of speaking to a colleague about it (the third party yet again!); and often, a few sessions are all that is needed to remove the barrier. But if this situation repeats itself too often, the analyst has scarcely any other solution but to submit himself to a new period of analysis, especially if the countertransference has induced the analyst to act out! Did not Freud recommend the practice of periodically undergoing a new analysis. It is true that he had in mind a very short duration, a few weeks, rather like the periods of military service in force in certain countries.

Ferenczi played a major role in calling the countertransference into question. A reading of his *Clinical Diary*[12] is doubly instructive. On the one hand, it shows well just how far this neglected aspect assumes considerable importance in the treatment of so-called difficult patients presenting non-neurotic or even seriously neurotic structures. In this respect, Ferenczi was undeniably the precursor of modern analysis. But, on the other hand, the *Clinical Diary* also shows how the analyst can become truly alienated in his relationship with the patient when desires for reparation take centre stage and lead the analyst to place himself under the sign of a sacrificial vocation which, I believe, is inappropriate and ineffective. A reading of well-known passages of the correspondence between Freud and Ferenczi and the famous controversy which arose between them concerning Ferenczi's technique (everyone is familiar with the famous letter of the kiss dated 13 December 1931) gives a very poor résumé of what was really at stake in this debate. The *Clinical Diary* allows us to get a much more complete picture of it when one sees Ferenczi begin by according an equivalent period of time to his own analysis and to the analysis of his patient. Needless to say, this classic practice, which is theoretically conceivable rapidly becomes exhausting and artificial when it is applied. We then learn that, far from always giving the expected results, that is to say, an increase of lucidity in the patient, instead it simply excites his sadism, giving him the opportunity to rid himself of guilt ('You see . . ., it's you who . . ., because, as you have admitted . . .') and makes him grasp the line thrown out to him by the analyst, inviting him to martyrize him. Nevertheless, one has to recognize the exactness of some of Ferenczi's criticisms: not so much the one that made him famous, i.e. his calling into question of the analyst's distant and cold attitude, as certain reproaches that were addressed to Freud and his theory for being more concerned with intellectual coherence than with grasping faithfully the complex picture presented by his patients, where rationality has to be equal to this complexity.

A remarkable watershed occurred in 1950 thanks to an article by Paula Heimann[13] which is still famous today. This was the first time that it had been contended that the countertransference was the consequence of an unconscious desire of the patient to communicate to the analyst affects which he experienced but could neither recognize nor verbalize, and which he could thus only induce in the other. By examining her own reactions, Paula Heimann became aware of this communication by procuration. It is as though the analyst's psychical apparatus had, as it were, been rented by the patient in order to send the analyst messages which the patient could not permit himself to recognize and decipher himself. Still later, the sphere of the countertransference was extended to all the psychic processes experienced by the analyst, including those of his readings or exchanges with other colleagues. And the countertransference was even claimed to have precession over the transference (M. Neyraut) – a logical position, since an analysand begins an analysis with an analyst at a given moment in the latter's relationship with his unconscious, which is never resolved once and for all and continues in him, undergoing constant modifications. Two opposing positions are present here: one is Freud's, which is precise, circumscribed and limited; and the other is contemporary, diffuse, encompassing, with somewhat hazy limits.

In fact, there is another way of conceiving the problem which is by looking at it from the angle of a position of principle. In conformity with modern epistemological observations, the relation between two terms is something more than the sum of the attributes of each of the objects included in the composition of the relationship. Something more and something else. This is what characterizes the analytic session when the process is underway. It is stamped with an indefinable quality which is rendered imperfectly by any attempt to describe it; this is not only because one is referring to an indescribable affective quality concerning the intimate nature of the exchange, but also because one finds oneself here – a bit like with Heisenberg's uncertainty principle – in the impossibility of defining the corpuscle and the wave at one and the same time. If attention is focused on the corpuscle, the movement of the wave is disturbed and so it can no longer be defined; and if one only thinks about the wave, one sacrifices the definition of the corpuscles. Such is the paradox of the analyst who may, during the session, regret the patient's presence, for if he was not there, he could jot down on paper rich and fruitful thoughts, something the situation prohibits him from doing. And when, finally, he finds himself alone again, trying to make sense of what happened in the session, even a recent one, he regrets that the patient is no longer there to rekindle his memories and to give them the living quality that his actual presence gave them.

At the present time, a new movement – the intersubjectivist movement – which I will only mention in passing, is spreading like an epidemic in the

United States. This movement has many branches which are all different from each other, have their origins in each other, and are sometimes even opposed to each other; which is why it is difficult to give a univocal vision of them. Let us say, to clarify our ideas, that the intersubjectivist movement is the result of a reaction against the current that was dominant in the United States, that is to say, ego psychology, which was reproached for its attitude marked by authoritarianism and an absence of self-criticism, resting on a tendency to objectivism, too closely linked to medicine and its criteria. Already, Hartmann, in wanting to add the self to Freud's ego, which he considered insufficient to fulfil its functions, had undermined the coherence of Freud's ideas. Multiple conceptions of the self flowered thereafter. It was already a surreptitious return of the pre-Freudian academic psychology of the ego. Following this, and wishing to accentuate his difference, Kohut pushed the theory of the self to the extremes which we are familiar with. But there is always someone more radical than oneself! It was in the wake of Kohut that the movement centred on intersubjectivity developed. Other influences can be recognized in this tendency that are less directly perceptible in the partisans of object relations. Moreover, this seems to be borne out: as soon as the dimension of the object is developed in an excessive way in psychoanalysis, in the shorter or longer term, the birth of a movement is provoked which sets itself up as the adversary of the precedent movement, advancing a complementary and, at the same time, antagonistic dimension. I am referring to conceptions that are centred on narcissism, the self, the subject, and so on. This is the sense of what I have called the *intersubjective contestation*.

It is not my intention here to enter into the detail of this movement of which Owen Renik has become the most renowned representative. If I wanted to enlarge further on the theoretical characteristics of the theses postulated, I would be confronted with a mixture of ideas, sometimes drawn from a phenomenological basis, sometimes elaborated on the basis of fashionable scientific models very far removed from psychoanalysis, and sometimes inspired by a pragmatism which has little concern for theoretical coherence, possessing obvious traits of schematization for use by the uninformed psychoanalyst. Let me emphasize, first of all, that the concern with taking the countertransference into account is in the foreground. It is nonetheless a particular type of countertransference highlighting *enactment* and affirming bluntly that *insight*, on the part of the analyst, is always preceded by a behavioural manifestation. In this conception, the symmetry between analyst and analysand is pushed to the extreme, for it is said 'that an analyst cannot, when all is said and done, know the patient's point of view; an analyst can only know his own point of view'.[14] The idea prevails that the analysand knows as much about himself as the analyst. The resultant technical attitudes overstep the customary reserve required in analysis: they do not shrink from a pragmatic analysis of the behaviour of patients, active recommendations, requests for interventions by other therapists, and so on. There is much insistence on the necessity for the analyst to seem 'real'.

In fact, what we are dealing with here is a neo-psychoanalysis. Seen with hindsight it is possible to detect a certain logic in this deviation. One starts out by refusing or rejecting the concept of the drive. Too biological, and what is more, mythical. Did not Freud confess to as much? So, let us lean, then, towards the theory of object relations. A new movement. The object is fine, but we are forgetting narcissism, the self, the subject, etc. Let us push the object towards the exit. A subject is better than an object; but it would be even better if it were given a companion so that it does not get bored; so two subjects, united by subjectivity. So there is the solution. It is as though it were necessary to bury the drive ever more deeply in order to prevent it from ever surfacing again. And long live psychology!

There are three possibilities in the future: either intersubjectivist analysis will go out of fashion after a while, like many other analytic vogues, or it will progressively conquer the terrain of American psychoanalysis (in Europe, it would seem that its impact remains weak), eliminating its rivals. This is not impossible inasmuch as American practitioners see in it an opportunity to win back lost ground and to attract once again the patients who are deserting their couches. Or, the third and final possibility – in my opinion the most probable – is that after a period of infatuation, it will take up its place in the psychoanalytic scene, adding one more movement to those that already exist. What will be will be!

In an earlier work,[15] I proposed a conception of countertransference derived from a general model based on the couple drive–object, according to the views of Winnicott. If one presupposes a situation which plays the role of a model, i.e. the process in the child of the investment of the object by the id, this investment, arising from the instinctual impulse, must be conceived as a movement towards the object, impelled by a pressure, that is to say, a force. However, there are two situations involved here. In the first, this investment leads to satisfaction; the experience of satisfaction creates a psychic constellation which will induce desire to seek out this experience again with the pleasure that is associated with it when the investment achieves its aim. But this simplified model partakes of the solipsistic spirit which has been denounced. Namely that the object plays an inert and passive role in it, letting itself be invested without the contribution it makes – or does not make – to the result, that is, to the experience of satisfaction, being taken into account. From a more Winnicottian perspective, the question of the investment of the breast by the infant and of the movement which carries it towards the object of satisfaction is maintained. But the object will respond to this subjective polarity, anticipating the infant's desire, anticipating its search, by its tolerant attitude towards its aggressive manifestations, its availability, etc.

Meaning is linked to the anticipation, within the object's proximity, and along the trajectory which carries it towards the object, of the object's reaction, owing to the preservation and transformation of the operative force creating what it is expecting. In short, this means that the phantasy of the object's response to its proximity precedes and takes precedence over what its objective reaction will be; or, more exactly, that the relationship between the expectation of the object's response and this response itself will become a model for the couple anticipation-realisation, producing agreement or disagreement.[16]

As we know, the instances in which the response does not conform to the expectation are more frequent than those that do; that is to say, the realization is far more frequently out of harmony with the anticipation than the contrary. This is the second situation to which I was alluding earlier. But everything depends, then, on knowing if such a gap (in the equilibrium) can be corrected by the subject who can compensate for it with phantasy, or if, on the contrary, for reasons which reside as much with the infant as with the mother, this gap is transformed into an abyss and cannot be put right. Indeed this is why Winnicott does not speak of the good mother, but only of the good enough mother. The infant or the subject, as the case may be, can himself make use of his internal psychic object to construct a subjective pole which meets its expectation and constitutes the nucleus of a purified pleasure-ego.

Julia Kristeva, endeavouring to make up for the omissions of Lacanian theory concerning the premises which govern the organization of the signifier, proposes the idea of a *chora*, the maternal receptacle necessary for receiving impressions, sensations, affects, all preforms contributing to the elaboration of the symbolic function: 'a matrix-like space that is, nourishing, unnameable, prior to the One, and to God, and that thus defies metaphysics.'[17]

From the example that I have given, it is quite clear that this model can easily be generalized for a theory based on the search for satisfaction, and that it can be extended to the different registers of libidinal satisfaction, from the most elementary to the most developed. It is also plain that solipsism is overcome by introducing, from the first, the couple drive–object. It is equally evident that we continue to think of this couple as being asymmetric, and that its functional value resides in the child's capacity to restore the equilibrium by making use of his psychic activity of phantasy in order to make up for the disappointments of experience. The creation of transitional objects depends on this. In other cases, on the other hand, the model enables us to understand the reactions of panic, helplessness, and the sense of being overwhelmed, which mobilize increasingly desperate defences in order to cope with the traumatic situation. These reactions can even include the disorganization and disintegration of the ego which is prey to distress (*Hilflosigkeit*) without having any way out of the situation.

It is in these cases that the analyst's countertransference must be put on alert and must detect, by virtue of a hypersensitive receptivity, the traces left behind by such experiences in childhood. These experiences have since been overcome;

all that remains perceptible is their scars which can reopen at the first opportunity. By inviting the subject to abandon the mechanisms of control, the analytic situation, assisted by regression, can revive the traumatic situation by reopening highly sensitive wounds which one thought to be closed. Such are the *limit situations* (R. Roussillon)[18] we are faced with which mean that the analyst can be induced to take decisions which oblige him to renounce the analytic setting in favour of others where the perception of the object is maintained. It is not only that the analyst, in the context of psychotherapy, embodies reality more directly; it is above all that perception entails a modification of the psychic economy; for, very often, these patients present a dysfunctioning in their functions of representation. In other words, it is the entire function of phantasy which is affected here, and, of course, projection. This is often massive, shows scarcely any capacities for distance and rectification, and remains insensitive to interpretation. The projection is lacking certain traits that would make its analysis possible. It is often perceived as being an indubitable reality, taking over from repression: what is most immediately striking is negative hallucination, which can even affect the patient's thought processes. I will come back to this in more detail later on.

Conclusion

We see, then, that examining the couple transference/countertransference has allowed us to adumbrate new ways of envisaging the analytic treatment and of thinking about the function of the setting. This chapter cannot be concluded without speaking of a form of transference and countertransference which is referred to increasingly frequently nowadays – namely, transference and countertransference *on to the setting*. In other words, one has to analyse how the setting is experienced and given meaning by the analysand and by the analyst, his unconscious function. Of course, the situation is asymmetrical because the analyst has already been analysed. One still needs to know whether his analysis has enabled him to examine the signification of the conditions of this experience. We know that Freud did not feel motivated to theorize the setting which he had brilliantly invented. As I have indicated, I have been able to establish a parallel between the conditions of the setting and those of the dream as described in Chapter VII of his major work of 1900. But since then, other interpretations have been advanced – which, moreover, had not been proposed at the time – in which the analytic situation has been compared to that of the prohibition of incest and parricide, or again to a metaphor of maternal care. I continue to think that it is still the model of the dream that seems to be the most pertinent; on the condition, however, that we bear in mind that today the dream is only considered as one of the aspects of the dreamer's psychic life. For if anxiety dreams can be attached to the dream function in general, this is no longer the case for the nightmare. Other modalities deserve to be taken into consideration insofar as they can constitute paradigms: nightmares, nocturnal terrors, the dreams of stage IV, blank dreams, somnambulism, etc. In all these cases, there is both a failure of the dream function and, very often, correlatively, an impossibility for the setting to serve as a facilitating experience for the mutual benefit of the analysand and the analyst.

Notes

1 Green, A. Sur la discrimination et l'indiscrimination affect-représentation. *Revue française de psychanalyse*, 1/1999; reprinted in *La pensée clinique*. Paris: Odile Jacob, 2002.

2 Donnet, J.-L. De la règle fondamentale à la situation analysante. Report published prior to the 2001 Congress. *Revue française de psychanalyse*, 1/2001, pp. 243–257.

3 Donnet, J.-L., ibid.

4 Fenichel, O. A review of Freud's 'Analysis Terminable and Interminable'. *International Review of Psycho-Analysis*, 1974, pp. 109–116.

5 Green, A. (2000). La mort dans la vie. *L'invention de la pulsion de mort*, ed. J. Guillaumin. Paris: Dunod.

6 Green, A. Le silence du psychanalyste. *Topique*, 1979; reprinted in *La folie privée*. Paris: Gallimard, 1990.

7 Freud, S. (1900). *The Interpretation of Dreams*. S.E. IV and V.

8 Green, A. Le langage dans le psychanalyse. In: *Langages*. Paris: Les Belles Lettres, 1984.

9 This general model was inspired by an analogous schema used for other purposes by Heinz von Foerster.

10 Green, A. L'intersubjectif en psychanalyse. Pulsions et/ou relations d'objet, Lanctôt, 1998; Reprinted in *La pensée clinique*, Paris: Odile Jacob, 2002; Trs. A. Weller: The intrapsychic and the intersubjective in psychoanalysis. *Psychoanalytic Quarterly*, LXIX, 2000.

11 Donnet, J.-L., ibid.

12 Ferenczi, S., (1932) *The Clinical Diary of Sandor Ferenczi*, ed. J. Dupont, trans. M. Balint and N.Z. Jackson. Cambridge, MA: Harvard University Press, 1988.

13 Heimann, P. On countertransference. *International Journal of Psychoanalysis*, vol. 31, 1950.

14 Renik, O. Analytic interaction – Conceptualizing technique in the light of the analyst's irreducible subjectivity. *Psychoanalytic Quarterly*, vol. 72–74, 1993.

15 Green, A. (1998). Démembrement du contre-transfert, ibid.

16 Green, A., ibid. p. 152.

17 Kristeva, J. (1993). *Les nouvelles maladies de l'âme*, p. 302. Paris: Fayard. [English edition: *New Maladies of the Soul*, p. 204. Tr. Ross Guberman. New York: Columbia University Press, 1995.]

18 Roussillon, R. (1991). *Paradoxes et situations limites en psychanalyse*. Paris: Presses Universitaires de France.

5

CLINICAL WORK

The organizing axes of pathology

As for technique, if one compares the current situation with that which existed at the time of Freud's death, psychoanalytic clinical work is a domain that has been modified and enriched considerably. There are multiple reasons for this, but the principal cause of this enrichment is the interest psychoanalysts have taken in pathological structures that had originally been excluded by Freud from the indications for analysis. When one compares the indications that he proposed for analysis at the beginning of his work and those that he announced in the article for the *Encyclopaedia Britannica* of 1926, it can be seen that the list has grown considerably longer. There is a paradox here; for, though Freud seems on the one hand to have been emboldened and to have considered that psycho-analysis could achieve interesting results in a certain number of non-neurotic states, on the other he had also just described the compulsion to repeat and the negative therapeutic reaction (1920). However that may be, it was mainly after Freud, with the contributions of Melanie Klein and her pupils, that the field of therapeutic indications was extended in the direction of the non-neuroses. Melanie Klein did not trouble herself much with nosographical considerations. Following in the wake of Freud, she revised his ideas, underlining the regressive aspects that he had overlooked. This was the case with the Wolf Man. Between 1960 and 1970, some remarkable works appeared, the majority of which came from the Kleinian school, which could not fail to arouse the admiration of the reader. Certain bold and even adventurous therapeutic undertakings were reported concerning patients that few analysts had the courage to take into treat-ment. Herbert Rosenfeld, Hanna Segal, Betty Joseph, W. R. Bion were the heroes of this epic period in the discovery of unknown territories.

I have the feeling that although the adventure made the journey worthwhile, for it has taught us many things about psychotic functioning, the results have perhaps not always lived up to expectations. But it is psychoanalysis as a whole that has benefited from these explorations which have made it possible to get a better understanding of the psychotic base in numerous patients who did not present manifest signs of psychosis. Alongside these innovatory endeavours, the evolution of pathology in the ordinary population of analysands led analysts to investigate forms that were for the most part unknown to the previous generation (with a few exceptions). It was in this way that there was a renewal of interest in character neurosis, described by Reich much earlier, with ephemeral success, while experiments were being made in the domains of psychiatry, so-called psychosomatic medicine, or with delinquents.

Today, there is a need for the different aspects of our knowledge to be brought together and articulated in a coherent manner. My purpose, then, in this chapter will not be so much to rehearse facts that everyone is familiar with as to define domains of pathological organization, while trying to draw out their meaning and the connections that exist between them. Let me say right away that this updating will lead me to register my agreement with Freud's final theory of the drives and with the foundations of his second topography. This does not mean that I will be respectful towards any kind of orthodoxy whatsoever but that I will try to achieve the highest degree of coherence that I can. I shall distinguish several sectors:

1 Sexuality.
2 The ego.
3 The superego.
4 The disorganizations produced by destruction oriented towards the outside.
5 Internal destruction in the principal forms of negative narcissism and primary masochism.

From sexuality to desire

When it was decided that the principal theme at the Barcelona Congress in 1997 would be 'Sexuality in Contemporary Psychoanalysis', a colleague from across the Atlantic commented on the news by expressing a certain surprise: 'I thought we had got beyond that!' Strange as an observation of this kind may seem to a French psychoanalyst, it is a common occurrence in certain international psychoanalytic circles. In the United States, a not inconsiderable movement considers that sexuality comes far behind troubles of a different order. The role of the ego (in neurosis) and that of the self are invoked, as well as many other factors which deflect the psychoanalyst's interest from his primary purpose, as Freud conceived it. In England, particularly under Melanie Klein's influence, the emphasis placed on destructivity eclipses the interest taken in sexuality. The latter is accordingly obliged to face up to the combined attacks of ego psychology, self psychology, intersubjectivity, and the object-relations perspective. French psychoanalysis can pride itself on the fact that beyond its divisions (Lacanian or non-Lacanian), all the currents agree in recognizing the major role played by sexuality, even if this role is interpreted in different ways. As for me, I had already drawn attention, before the Barcelona Congress, to this desexualization in the theory of psychoanalysis.[1] There are many reasons pushing French psychoanalysts to consider sexuality as a fundamental domain of the psyche – not just the pathological psyche, but the normal psyche as well. Must we remind ourselves of the oft-neglected Freudian distinction between genitality and sexuality? It is the link uniting sexuality and pleasure which forms the foundations of the sexual in psychoanalysis. In short, sexuality is the 'pleasure of all pleasures', just as the prohibition of incest is the 'rule of rules'. Since Fairbairn, some have wanted to replace the Freudian theorem of psychic activity conceived of as *pleasure seeking*, proposing in its stead another idea, more innocent and less disturbing, that of psychic activity as *object seeking*. Furthermore, the Freudian idea of the pleasure/unpleasure principle has been radicalized in the expression of its negative polarity. Unpleasure has given way to much more disorganizing forms (psychic pain, threat of annihilation, catastrophic anxiety, tortuous suffering, fear of breakdown, etc.). At the other extreme, the quest for pleasure has been surpassed by a much more radical concept too, observed in the domain of social transgressions and criminal sexuality, where carrying out the transgressive act is accompanied less by pleasure than by an effort to ward off a threat of disorganization to the ego, even to the point of depersonalization, and to struggle against internal terror (C. Balier). Lacan extended Freud's thought by proposing the concept of jouissance to characterize these extreme forms which can equally include clinical forms of masochism. It may be concluded that when Freud chose neurosis and placed the experience of satisfaction and the pleasure/unpleasure principle at the centre of his theorization, he was interested in average values that psychoanalysis could work with. He left on one side the experience of pain or other more extreme forms of pleasure; perhaps because he thought that they eluded the work of analysis. But later, during the modifications which accompanied the creation of the second topography, he was himself obliged to recognize much more raw unconscious forms in which the *drive in action* makes its pressure felt in the psyche, engendering clinical manifestations and symptoms.

To stay in the habitual domain of psychoanalysis, it is plain that sexuality is to be considered as a source of pleasure. Via the intermediary of the erotogenic zones, it provides the satisfactions that the subject is seeking. To avoid fastidious repetition, I will not recapitulate on the very familiar stages of libidinal development (oral, anal, phallic and genital). Nonetheless, it is important to understand the varied nature of their interest:

1 They attest to the presence and importance of the body as an erotogenic body.
2 In these regions, the envelope of the skin-ego is extended via the mucous orifices.
3 These orifices put the inside of the subject's body in contact with the outside.

These findings, though they may seem elementary, nonetheless presuppose a highly elaborated organization.

Just as I have insisted on the fundamental value of the drive–object couple, along with Paula Aulagnier, I would also underline the role of the complementary object zone. If we push this line of speculation further, it will not be difficult to understand that, among the bodily functions, sexuality – aiming at pleasure – is the one that is searching for an object in order to satisfy itself. The auto-erotism of the early stages is indeed obliged to make room for the object of satisfaction situated outside the subject's limits. But the fact that the subject is capable of choosing an object on his own body is already indicative of the highly substitutable role of the object in the domain of infantile sexuality. Sexuality evolves towards its crowning achievement, from the infantile period to the Oedipal organization, and, beyond that, to the definitive object choice at puberty, which often leads to genitality. This means, in short, that sexuality possesses a richness that is incomparable with the other bodily functions. It should never be forgotten that one speaks of *psychosexuality* – the complexification of the psychic organization that is destined to find the object capable of procuring satisfaction justifying the Freudian definition of the drive.

There are still other reasons why sexuality-pleasure plays this major role in the psyche; for lack, that is to say, the search for an object capable of procuring the satisfaction of the pleasure that is not immediately accessible, opens up the dimension of desire. Here tribute should be paid to Lacan who, at a time when the analytic world as a whole was turning away from this orientation, reminded us of the place of desire, already observed by many philosophers in the past and superbly forgotten, over the course of time, by psychoanalysts. With the dimension of desire, we are touching upon the essence of anthropology. Lacan developed this point, showing that it is not only desire that is sought after, but *desire for the desire of the other*. This affirmation is open to little doubt. Its only limitations can be seen in the face of certain pathological organizations which do not seem to be in a position to attain such reflexiveness, although it is the most general sign of the human condition. Freud postulated that neurosis is the negative of perversion. He was referring, with regard to normality, to the polymorphous perversion of the child who aspires to the satisfaction of the multiple erotogenic zones of his body born prematurely. In the course of the evolution of infantile sexuality, fixations create particular points of appeal which become as many occasions for 'elective affinities'. The child is thus induced to seek in an obstinate manner, more insistently and more repetitively, the pleasure linked with certain fixations. Later, faced with situations of conflict that are difficult to overcome, he will seek to return to earlier fixation points (regression). When one reflects on the Freudian theory of sexuality, one cannot help but be astonished by its coherence and depth. Even when Freud felt the need to present his last theory of the drives, he carried out revisions – a point that is not given enough attention – making modifications to the pole of Eros, in which sexuality was included. One sentence stands out as particularly rich:

> The greater part of what we know about Eros – that is to say, about its exponent, the libido – has been gained from a study of the sexual function, which, indeed, on the prevailing view, even if not according to our theory, coincides with Eros.[2]

Eros, a metaphorical concept, is unknown as such, and unknowable directly:

- recourse to the libido, which plays the role of an exponent, is necessary
- this exponent points to the sexual *function*.

Metaphor, exponent, function.

The *Outline* announces a notable change. The theory of the drives treats of the two fundamental drives: Eros and the destructive drive. As for sexuality, it is now a function that is no longer directly attached to the theory of the drives. It is quite clear that by concerning himself with the neuroses, Freud wanted, by analysing the unconscious, to elucidate the pathological forms closest to normality. This means that his field of investigation – neurosis – extended in two directions: one, towards pathology (the other neuroses, perversion, the psychoses, etc.); the other, towards normality. This situation resulted in a remarkable decompartmentalization, to the extent that pathology and normality were no longer separated by a watertight frontier.

Nevertheless, the description of all the constituents of the field of Eros enables us to understand, as I have already contended, that here the vision centred on a particular element, however important it may be, needs to be replaced by the concept of an *erotic chain*. This chain starts with the drive and its instinctual impulses, extends to that which manifests itself in the form of pleasure and unpleasure, deploys itself in the state of expectation and quest for desire, nourished by conscious and unconscious representations, organizes itself in the form of conscious and unconscious phantasies, and branches out into the erotic and amorous language of sublimations. Clearly, all this relates to the essential question of the relations between sexuality and love, relations that raise yet many further questions. A twofold movement is at work here whose purpose is sometimes to make them coincide, and sometimes to dissociate them. The richness of Freud's contribution to this problem constitutes the hard core of psychoanalysis. The necessity of taking into account states that are situated beyond neurosis does not do away with the cardinal role of sexuality considered from the anthropological standpoint. In the part of this book that deals with modern anthropological references, we will see the late, but essential recognition of the role of human sexuality in the defence of social organization and in its production. Progress in reflection has given rise to elaborations which show just how far social imagination is nourished by phantasies related to sexuality, whether they be of reproduction, filiation or the beliefs which are involved in the bodily conception of the sexual, or the values of amorous relationships.

As we know, Freud began with the theory of seduction, an idea that he was to abandon *partially* later on (1897). What was important in the theory of seduction, beyond the transgression that it implied, was the premature excitation of erotogenic zones aroused by the adult-seducer. Subsequently, he opted against trauma in favour of phantasy. In fact, throughout his entire work, he returned occasionally to seduction by the adult in childhood. But this was, as it were, a variable, whereas the theory of phantasy was a constant. At the end of his work, he adopted a nuanced and precise position. In *Moses and Monotheism* precious indications can be found concerning the traumatic role of seduction. However, in the *Outline*, when he was describing the most normal of relations between the mother and child, he detected without difficulty a relationship of seduction. He asserts that the mother is the child's first seducer via the maternal care she gives him and the general attitude that she has towards him. Several ideas are intertwined here:

1   As in the early theory of seduction, there is the arousal by the mother of the child's erotogenic zones when she is caring for his body. Nonetheless, it is the mother's aim-inhibited impulses that are involved here, in contradistinction to traumatic seduction.
2   This erotic relationship fits into a context clearly marked by the stamp of love. Mother and child are reciprocally in love with each other. This is true to such an extent that there can be rivalry between the impulses at play in the mother's love for the child and those which are part of her genital sexual relationship with the father.
3   It is plain that this situation attributes to the other an essential role in the awakening of the erotogenic zones (polymorphous perversion). This does not, however, prevent the constitution of an auto-eroticism in which the child, during an experience of lack, can find his object on his own body.
4   The inscription of the traces of this experience is preserved in the unconscious and never disappears. It will, however, change in nature and form after puberty. This opens up the vast question of *pre-sexual sexuality* which Freud broached in his first works but never took up again in detail.

This picture, described by Freud, has given rise to important revisions in the evolution of post-Freudian theory. Though mother–child relations have been the subject of a large number of studies, mobilizing the interest of psychoanalysts, one is surprised to note, even in the best, the disappearance of this erotic dimension connected with the exchanges between the mother and the child. This is quite remarkable in the Anglo-Saxon literature, for multiple reasons in which puritanism has its part to play. It is as if Anglo-Saxon mothers did not make love. On the one hand, under Melanie Klein's influence, attention was turned towards the vicissitudes of the destructive drives. On the other hand, at the opposite extreme, the ego attracts to itself the full interest of investigators who valorize the non-erotic aspects of the relationship (capacity to tolerate frustrations, need for security, etc.). Freud's drive theory has undergone a true repression in psychoanalysts, quick to seize all available opportunities to get rid of it.

For his part, Jean Laplanche has defended a theory of generalized seduction in which he stresses the sending of enigmatic messages by the mother towards the child – as much for herself as for the child – arising from her preconscious, which will constitute a source-object. Laplanche clearly seeks to circumvent the role of the drive or, at least, to restrict it considerably, objecting to the solipsistic character of the Freudian construction. However, if it is accepted, as I suggest, that the solution to the problem is not to be found either on the side of the drive alone, or on the side of the object alone, but rather that it is the drive–object couple that should constantly be kept in mind at all stages, then I think we will be in a much better position to account for clinical material. What is more, when Laplanche draws on Freud's letter to Fliess of 6 December 1896 to give support to his theory of seduction, one may point out that in this same letter Freud considers this idea as part of the superstructure, and feels the need to base it on organic foundations. Rightly or wrongly. Once again, we can see that Freud's constant concern to forge links between the psychic and somatic orders has been left on one side in modern psychoanalysis which is turning more and more towards a psychological or, if you like, exclusively psychical theory, accentuating the hiatus between the participation of the soma and that of the psyche. Likewise, when reference is made to the object (to the other), a complementary movement completes the minimization of the role of the drive, considered as a source of errors, tending to biologize the psychic and to overlook the relational dimension. Now, once again I do not think that there are grounds for opposing what pertains to the Self and what belongs to the Other. Self and Other are also in a relation of complementarity which means that they must both be distinguished and related to each other. The extension of these confusions can be seen in the so-called intersubjectivist theories where the relation between two subjects accentuates even further the tendency to give prevalence to the relational pole over all others. Let me point out in passing that the most glaring paradox of this theory is that it never sheds the slightest light on the conception of the subject to which it refers. It is evident that, whatever theme we touch upon, we come across all the contradictions that contemporary analysis lays before us without always being aware of them. This backs up my idea that Freudian theory, notwithstanding its insufficiencies and with the proviso that it is appropriately updated, is still the one that gives most acknowledgement to the said contradictions.[3]

The ego

The ego is a concept in psychoanalytic theory which has been the object of incessant metamorphoses. I do not intend to take up its detailed and complicated study here, and will simply emphasize certain particular aspects.[4] All the exegetes of Freud's work acknowledge that there are two theories of the ego in it. The first is anterior to the presentation of the second topography. It presents the ego as a global agency, not very different from the academic conception, except for the emphasis Freud places on its antagonistic role in relation to sexuality. Even before the theory of narcissism, the ego was presented as a concept related to self-affirmation. Freud even lets it be understood that a portion of the affects associated with hate could be attached to it. Let me cite again his very sharp observation according to which the ego's development is in advance of that of sexuality in obsessional neurosis. Nevertheless, it is above all with the second topography that the concept of the ego takes on new relief. The very title of his work of 1923, *The Ego and the Id* (with the curious omission of the Superego), clearly shows the central role that Freud gives it. But before that, the major mutation, at once decisive and yet only temporary, was the creation of the concept of narcissism in 1914. Here the change concerns the fact that the former distinction opposing the self-preservative instincts and the sexual instincts is no longer sufficient. Though it is not customary to qualify the period from 1913 to 1920 as that of a second theory of the drives, before the formulation of the last one, which was to oppose the life drives and the death drives, it seems to me that this denomination would be entirely justified. From thereon, then, Freud was to establish an antithesis between the ego-instincts and the object-instincts. Narcissism was born. In my opinion, it is one of Freud's richest concepts which had been present in an embryonic state from the beginning (in particular in the denomination of a category of neuroses: the narcissistic neuroses). The stage of 1914 seems to me to have been one of cardinal importance, with Freud proposing a categorial opposition, namely, ego-object, which can be seen today to traverse the fields of neurobiology and even those of philosophy, with different senses, but referring to an axiomatic source material which remains constant. Freud's text on narcissism is one that can be constantly read again with profit. Narcissism is a concept that covers the diverse domains of perversion, psychosis and love life – just to stay within the limits of psychoanalysis. Now, what is most remarkable is the way in which this concept would be subject both to eclipses and returns in post-Freudian psychoanalysis. Already in Freud's own work, as I have already pointed out, the formulation of the last theory of the drives relegates narcissism, i.e. the *libidinal investment of the self-preservative instincts*, to employ Freud's definition, to the background. For, on the one hand this restricted conception of narcissism drowns it within Eros of which it is no longer any more than a partial sector; and, on the other, it says nothing of the impact of the theory of the death drives on narcissism. One cannot fail to be struck by what seems to have been a case of surprising negligence on Freud's part, which is no doubt explainable by the fact that he was too busy revising the psychic phenomena that he had described earlier from the angle of the last theory of the drives.

After Freud, the theory of object relations, promoted by Fairbairn and Melanie Klein, meant that narcissism would practically disappear from the map of psychoanalytic theory. One had to wait until 1971 for a Kleinian, Herbert Rosenfeld, to re-establish its importance and to give a version of it centred on destructivity.[5] For its part, American psychoanalysis, with Hartmann, more or less played with narcissism. Finding that the conception of the ego proposed by Freud was much too narrow, Hartmann proposed to add to it the Self, which comprised a much vaster theoretical field in which the place of narcissism was recognized. This, however, was still not enough, and there followed a new psychoanalytic mutation due to Kohut. The Kohutian Self exploded Freud's and Hartmann's theories, relegating the drives once again to a secondary role. The intense controversies between Kohut and Kernberg are familiar ground, with the latter, inspired by Edith Jacobson, pleading for a theory of object relations which would acknowledge the role played by the erotic and aggressive drives, in antagonism with narcissism. This resurrection of narcissism came as no surprise for French psychoanalysts who had always maintained a very lively interest in this concept. Lacan's work would be incomprehensible if one did not refer to it; the mirror stage shows this very clearly and his conception of love confirms it. In his wake, Grunberger developed his personal view which made narcissism an agency. For my part, I have proposed a dual conception of narcissism, opposing a life narcissism, attached to Eros, aspiring to a unity of the ego to the detriment of the object, and a death narcissism, which I also call *negative narcissism*, as a manifestation of the destructive drive tending towards the zero level of excitation and aiming at the disappearance of the ego itself. This conception was received favourably, inasmuch as it was able to account for clinical phenomena that are difficult to explain.[6] At any rate, whatever the vicissitudes of narcissism in his theory, Freud never abandoned the category of the narcissistic neuroses. However, whilst these included the psychoses in the initial phase of his work, subsequently, in 1924, he was to reserve the denomination for melancholy (and for its inverted double: mania). From then on he considered the psychoses, apart from manic-depressive psychosis, as an expression of the predominant action of the destructive drives. I think that this last rectification is justified; for, even if we step outside the limits of psychosis, the consideration of depression, in general, invites us to recognize the predominant role of narcissism in it. In a still more general way, since it leads us to the domain of normality, the phenomenon of mourning itself gives rise to the same observation. We know, moreover, that in contemporary praxis, an interminable state of mourning shows through in many non-neurotic structures, the role of which is more marked than the anxieties that can otherwise be noted.

Clinical experience with borderline states has led analysts to be attentive to the role of the ego and to the concept of limit in eponymic conditions. I have described two forms of anxiety which are met with particularly frequently in the study of borderline cases: (a) separation anxiety, which has been given abundant treatment in the literature; (b) its symmetrical and complementary opposite, intrusion anxiety. Winnicott was the first to underline its importance. It is understandable that, caught between these two combined dangers, the ego of the borderline subject lives under the permanent threat of being abandoned by its objects, and/or of their encroachment on his subjective individuality. In these conditions, its dependence on the object and on the distance from the object, greatly reduces its freedom of movement. I have suggested that these two forms of anxiety be considered as the equivalent, at the level of the ego, of what castration anxiety (in men) and penetration anxiety (in women) are at the level of the libido.

The second topography has unfortunately been a great source of misunderstandings. We know that it has given rise to simplifications and schematizations that have been harmful for psychoanalytic thought, with the conceptions of ego psychology. One frequently hears it said in America that it was Freud who invented ego psychology with his second conception of the psychical apparatus which, under the influence of Hartmann, Kris and Loewenstein, became the structural conception of the psychical apparatus. Such assertions produce in the French reader a real sense of stupefaction inasmuch as, most of the time, he or she considers ego psychology as such a profound alteration of the Freudian corpus that it deserves to be qualified as an abusive interpretation of Freudian thought. It is true that a superficial reading of Freud can invite, if not such an interpretation, at least an inflection of his thought in this direction. And Freud is not totally innocent of what he is being made to say. But the parallel should not be pushed too far. The idea of an ego with an origin which is distinct from that of the id, with an energy free of all conflict, said to be autonomous, is very far removed from the Freudian vein of inspiration. One only finds an allusion to the idea of a neutral energy in respect of the transformation concerning love into hate in the chapter on the ego's states of dependence in *The Ego and the Id*; nothing in any case that justifies the introduction of a new concept, which was nonetheless received extremely favourably in the United States. Here again, it was just a question of minimizing the influence of the drives, and it was commonly asserted that, since the id is unknowable, and the ego is the necessary passage for approaching it, there is good reason to focus all one's attention on the ego. It seems to me that reflection on this topographical conception of the psychical apparatus – I will come back later to its theoretical analysis – fails to appreciate the importance of the Freudian affirmation according to which a very important part of the ego, whose significance Freud is far from limiting, was conceived of as being unconscious. This seems to be the major lesson of, and justification for, the second topography.

Before bringing this chapter to a close I want to indicate the extent to which the study of the ego suffered after Freud. For psychoanalysts have sometimes tried to return to its pre-psychoanalytic sense, giving up the originality of their conception in order to get a better hearing with the supporters of non-psychoanalytic, academic conceptions; while sometimes, on the contrary, studies of the ego have been affected by a sort of prohibition of thinking, promulgated by Lacan, on the pretext of avoiding falling into the errors of the past. Indeed, since the publication in 1936 of Anna Freud's work – most probably supervised by her father – on the ego and the mechanisms of defence, a large proportion of analysts have taken this path. Freud himself, in *Inhibitions, Symptoms and Anxiety* (1926) turned his attention to the mechanisms of defence, distinguishing those of hysteria and those of obsessional neurosis. However, it should be noted that what is sometimes described in 1915 in the *Papers on Metapsychology* under the denomination of 'Instincts and their Vicissitudes' was later reformulated in *The Ego and the Mechanisms of Defence* (1936). Analysts, particularly American analysts, found much material in it to be exploited and did not fail to develop it. In American psychoanalysis, R. Greenson made himself the herald of the analysis of resistances.[7] There was consequently a danger of shifting the accent from the analysis of the transference on to that of resistances, with the drawback that this risks turning the analytic situation into a power struggle which is somewhat reminiscent of the problems encountered with suggestion during the hypnotic period at the beginning of analysis. This was one of the reasons for the success of the intersubjectivist mode, which took the opposite view to this position. It is not because one gets the better of others that one can always avoid also being in the wrong oneself. It would seem that this whole evolution and the changes to which it gave rise, misunderstands Freud's innovation to the effect that *the ego is unconscious of its own defences*. The real question is this: Is the technique for making the ego conscious of its own defences and its resistances the same as that for interpreting the content? And, if the technique of the analysis of resistances can be criticized, what is the alternative for promoting this recognition? The problem, it seems to me, is still with us. Perhaps it has been given clearer relief by the recent contributions of Bion and Winnicott, who concerned themselves, respectively, with analysing thought processes and defining the function of transitionality. The anathema pronounced by Lacan against ego psychology, not altogether without justification, does not permit us in any way to shirk the necessity to examine the concept of the ego, whose disturbances are obvious in clinical work. And one cannot thank Lacan for having discouraged any study in this field. For Lacan, as we know, the ego is a captive of the subject's imaginary identifications. This theory can hardly be contested, but does it suffice to account for all the manifestations that are encountered in clinical work and which are connected with the ego? Let us not forget that Freud himself considered that clinical work with psychoses called the ego very directly into question. It is thus not surprising that borderline cases concern what may be called the pathology of the ego. It has only been possible, I think, to continue to block out this weak point in Lacanian theory by denying the relevance of the notion – albeit very generally accepted – of borderline state. The negation of clinical evidence can only last a certain period of time; and this period of time is largely exhausted today.

The superego

When considering these organizing axes, the pathology of the superego needs to be taken into account. Its effects are well known, ranging from the sense of guilt, in its most general forms, to guilty anxiety or anxiety in face of the superego. They open out on to the mysterious unconscious sense of guilt – one of the arguments often raised by Freud apropos of the existence of unconscious affect. Moreover, he admitted his preference for the formula 'a need for self-punishment'. The superego can manifest itself simply in the form of an internal tension, a sense of unease, without further precision. Freud devoted much reflection to its study at the end of his work. It was while he was studying primal masochism that its role was reconsidered. It was then that Freud discovered libidinal co-excitation, and he did not cease to study the relations of pleasure and pain. One particular fact struck him forcefully – namely, that masochism could not be reduced to a reversal of sadism. But other distinctions have to be made; in particular those that concern the relations between the super-ego and the ego ideal. They are defined by the following formula: the superego is heir to the Oedipus complex, and the ego ideal to primary narcissism. Guilt is the pathognomonic sign of the first, and shame of the second. Another distinction is that which separates the superego, a form bound by the destructive drive, finding an outlet in guilt, from the destructivity which spreads throughout the whole of the psychical apparatus ('Analysis Terminable and Interminable 1937c'). The first can be encountered in the form of repetition-compulsion. This remains decipherable and its meaning can be guessed, whereas the second seems to be devoid of intentionality. One of the most remarkable transformations in Freud's thought is the way in which guilt – which, originally, was attached to the prohibition in relation to sexuality – slips towards the prevalent role of aggressivity and the destructive drive. This is rarely given any emphasis. But the anthropological role of *guilt* cannot be minimized; it is the foundation of all religions and participates in the most ordinary constitution of the superego. For guilt is founded on identification. From Freud to Klein, guilt was transformed into reparation, a consequence of acceding to the depressive position when the infant expiates the 'bad' that he has inflicted on his objects in the paranoid-schizoid phase and tries to repair them. An important issue proceeds from this concerning the resolution of the Oedipus complex. For Freud it is marked by guilt, and analysis will enable the subject to get rid of his excessive sexualization though masochism. Masochism re-sexualizes morality. For Kleinians, on the contrary, the work of reparation, which is never achieved, condemns the subject to perpetual expiation. It seems to me that the goal of analysis lies more on the side of the Freudian position than on that of the Kleinian theory of reparation.

In fact, there are numerous discussions in Kleinian circles concerning the successive order of the paranoid-schizoid and depressive phases. Though for Melanie Klein they followed each other, her point of view was later contested. It is as if there was a preference for speaking of a permanent oscillation between the two. This modification corresponds in part to the observation, in certain patients, of a truly persecutory psychic activity of the functions linked to the superego. A superego which, beyond the caricatural and even derisory aspect that it can assume in obsessional neurosis, has become completely devoid of meaning, forbidding all thought activity (Bion), as well as any psychic development, susceptible of elaboration.

But there is a theoretical finding to which Freud attached great importance, but which is not so clearly set out by other authors. The genesis of the superego depends on a phenomenon of splitting (Freud does not employ the word) between one portion of the ego and another, highly idealized part, which will play the role of evaluator, censor, critic, examiner, and so forth. We know that, at the outset, Freud distinguished poorly between the ego ideal and the superego. Be that as it may, the embryonic superego is assumed to be formed in the image of the parents' superego (and not of their ego). Freudian theory took an important step forward here: identification does not occur with a 'concrete' part of the parental objects related to their person, but to a metaphorical, abstract entity, existing in absentia. It is thus in the light of this internal split and the way in which the two parts can coexist, or even live on good terms with each other, that the function of the superego can be appreciated. It will evolve towards anonymization. I have examined the complicated relations between masochism and narcissism in the negative therapeutic relationship.[8] One further point by way of conclusion: the superego is an absolute novelty of the second topography. It has no equivalent in the first topography.[9] The question is applicable today to the domain of the cultural superego.

Destructivity towards the object

Let us return now to the last theory of the drives with a view to considering the phenomena related to destructivity. There is no need to dwell at length on the variety of destructive forms of behaviour towards the object. My purpose is more to make what seems to me to be an important clarification. It is indispensable to distinguish between aggressivity and destructivity. Aggressivity, as we have known since the early days of psychoanalysis, is linked to sadism and attached to the stages of the evolution of the libido, i.e. the anal-sadistic and oral-sadistic stages. During the first of these, the tortures and torments inflicted on the object are one of the expressions of the wish to master it so as to ensure one's absolute control and domination of it involving a *jouissance* that is only equalled in its inverted aspects, that is, in masochism. When one is dealing with destructivity turned towards the object, it is commonly confused with sadism. And it is not easy to dissociate them. It seems to me that unlike sadism, destructivity does not imply the unconscious *jouissance* of the complementary polarity. In other words, the sadist takes unconscious pleasure in his object's masochism via identification. In destructivity, it is the narcissistic dimension that prevails: the destructive subject wishes to destroy his object's narcissism. In other words, it is omnipotence more than *jouissance* that is involved. For there can be omnipotence here that is not necessarily accompanied by *jouissance*. I have described under the name of *primary anality*[10] a singular clinical manifestation in which the subject's narcissism is in the foreground, engaged in an endless struggle with an internal object to which he is ultimately subjected owing to a solidly anchored masochistic organization, ensuring a dependence which is aimed at maintaining a state of non-separation with it.

Since Winnicott, we know that destructivity does not necessarily imply contact with the object. On the contrary, disinvesting the object can involve the satisfaction of destroying it by making it feel that it does not exist. Making the other experience this sensation of non-existence can become, in the strategic indifference of which these subjects are capable, a more murderous weapon than tearing it to pieces.

Destructivity oriented towards the inside

Here it is self-hate that dominates, and it is often difficult to distinguish narcissism from masochism.[11] Confinement within repetitive forms of behaviour that are masochistic in character can lead one to raise the question of unconscious *jouissance*. In my view, the narcissistic confinement specific to repetition-compulsion seems to predominate over the *jouissance* that is derived from it. I will come back to all these problems when I turn to the study of the dis-objectalizing function. It is clear that, in these last two chapters, we are once again faced with the question of the avatars of narcissism. It is difficult to know whether, as Freud thought, the orientation of destructivity is always, in the first place, internal, or whether it is primitively directed towards the outside.

The definition of these organizing axes is obviously related to Freud's conception of the psychical apparatus. The pathology of the superego, it seems to me, can be divided up according to the four fields individualized by sexuality and the ego. Since we know that the superego has its roots in the id (sexuality and destructivity) and, furthermore, that it results from a division of the ego which is divided into two parts, it is necessary, if we are to offer a global vision, to refer to the concept of the *work of the negative* in which splitting plays an important part. For the moment, I will just mention the neurosis of depersonalization described by Bouvet.[12] In a general way, depersonalization is a symptom affecting the ego, dividing it into two parts. One part experiences, with anxiety, the operation of transformations in its sense of unity, its coherence, and its familiarity with itself, frequently liberating an image marked by infiltrations of instinctual impulses experienced as being very dangerous. The fear of self-transformation, of his own behaviour involving a tendency to act out, evokes in the patient's mind a threat of madness, though there is nothing really to be feared in this respect, since the ego preserves its integrity in spite of these distressing but temporary transitory states, which only seem psychotic to the patient. Literature is decorated with famous descriptions of such states: Maupassant's *Horla* is the most extreme example, along with the works of fantastic literature which have the double as their theme. One part of the ego, then, experiences its transformation with anxiety – and who can escape a sense of anxiety when witnessing the changes affecting Grégoire Samsa? – whereas another part is simply a powerless spectator of the other part. Alienation is the explicit theme in this pathology. As far as alienation is concerned, its conceptual centrality can be invoked well short of, and well beyond, depersonalization. In effect, though transitory episodes of depersonalization can occur in an ephemeral manner in normality, and even more so in the course of every analysis, certain analysts, such as Michel de M'Uzan, attribute alienation with a central role in the psychoanalytic process. It should nonetheless be added that depersonalization can also be present in dramatic clinical manifestations found in schizophrenia.

I have now defined the principal domains of the organization of pathology. We have yet to grapple with certain general notions running through them. As far as sexuality is concerned, I have mentioned and justified the reasons for the existence of fixation and regression, as well as their relation to the polymorphous perversion of the child. Generally speaking, it can be said that these mechanisms are rarely observed in the pure state, except in certain very well structured neuroses, and that, as a rule, they accompany more or less superficial failures of the ego, which is forced to bring into operation defences whose anachronistic character persists well beyond their immediate function. In neurosis, the conflict between the id and the superego is intensely invested, but the consequences, namely, the symptoms and the defences which are still comprehensible in terms of desire and prohibition, remain confined in a part of the psyche and do not involve a patent regression of the ego. Naturally, this statement has to be qualified when there is a serious neurosis, as can be the case in obsessional neurosis which tends to invalidate the ego, obliging it to multiply its defences indefinitely, and to turn the defences themselves into a symptom that is a source of unconscious *jouissance*, and so on. However, contrary to borderline cases, one does not observe noticeable disorders in the ego's functioning. The pregenital fixations, which induce corresponding regressions, may explain the resistance to recovery in many patients; but I continue to think that there is something to be gained from distinguishing these serious neuroses from non-neurotic structures, as I have shown in *The Work of the Negative*.

Bouvet gave indications, which remain useful, concerning the opposition between genital and pregenital fixations. In the latter, the transference is often stormy; projection is more massive, and aggressivity not infrequently presents a clinical picture which is an obstacle to the emergence of the erotic transference. When this manifests itself, it is often characterized by erotic forms that are barely – or only with difficulty – analysable, resembling the description, already evoked by Freud, of the erotic transference which wants to know nothing of interpretation or which takes the form, as Lacan called it felicitously, of *hainamoration*.[13] These are all disguised forms of the negative therapeutic reaction. On the other hand, some patients seem incapable of understanding the transferential nature of their reactions to the analyst, seeing no relation between the past, which is highly defended, and the present, which is scarcely any less defended. Freud had already observed this phenomenon. These psychic manifestations, resisting analysis, may be said to have lost the character of transitional psychic processes described by Winnicott. In fact we are close here to a 'delusional' mode of thinking which only wants to hear what it itself affirms. This, moreover, is often the case – when there is no associated erotic transference – of many patients who cannot tolerate interpretation and only want to hear from the analyst's mouth a paraphrase recognizing that they are within their rights and authenticating their conscious thoughts as the only ones that are valid. They are in fact unable to abide any variation from the version that their own ego-defences have elaborated. There is only *one true* version of the story they are telling, namely, the one that they have just recounted, which has the value of incontrovertible reality and is thus uninterpretable.

It has already been pointed out that we lack a scale of development concerning the ego comparable to the one that exists for sexuality. Ferenczi's work on the process of gaining access to reality has not been consecrated by the *vox populi* of analysts. As for the descriptions founded on a genetic theoretical basis, starting with child observation, they cannot be made use of for such a conception. Moreover, it may be that more specific concepts need to be introduced here. For instance, in his article 'The Uncanny' (1919), Freud introduces the notion of 'overcoming'. Rather than having repressed unpleasant contents, themes or desires, the ego has not overcome the earlier phases of its development which can, eventually, re-emerge under suitable conditions. No phase that is overcome is ever conquered once and for all! Provided that the conditions lend themselves, as the examples cited in 'The Uncanny' indicate, an earlier phase reappears without disturbing profoundly or in a lasting way the functioning of the ego. It goes without saying that the referents are not the same as for sexuality. They most probably range from omnipotent thinking to a flexible access to reality. There is nothing here, though, to justify an appeal to a dogma concerning reality – quite to the contrary. As Bion maintained, it is rather the *negative capacity*[14] (Keats) which bears witness in such cases to a high level of differentiation. This capacity gives the power to tolerate, without becoming irritated, mysteries, doubts and enigmas, while coexisting with them. It is equally possible to rank humour among these very evolved forms of the ego's functioning, requiring the ability to keep some distance from oneself, to relativize the events which affect psychic life and call for the preservation – come hell or high water – of a benign irony. Ultimately, this capacity to stand back, which is implied both in negative capacity as well as in humour, is the best possible disposition for receiving interpretation. As far as humour is concerned, its relations with the superego, as Freud had already seen, are easily noticeable. Freud himself, of course, the author of the *Witz*, was richly gifted in humour. Is not the famous Jewish humour, of which he was one of the representatives, the response to the sum of misfortunes endured by the people to whom he belonged and in relation to whom he did not cease to show his capacity for self-derision?

To conclude, we now need to consider other mechanisms which I propose to call the *overflows (débordements) of the unconscious*. César and Sára Botella have analysed the function of the hallucinatory in Freud's work. This is marked by two periods. One, at the beginning of his work, immediately attains a function of reference in *The Interpretation of Dreams* (1900). Freud's discovery of the function of hallucinatory activity in dreaming is of cardinal importance. Not only because he had understood that dreams had a meaning – which had been accepted since time immemorial and illustrated differently across the cultures – but also due to the fact that they gave him the possibility of describing the *dream-work*, which was his most decisive contribution. His observation according to which the primary processes tend towards hallucinatory expression is very often forgotten. For my part, I will add, as I have already noted, that the psychical apparatus has an extraordinary capacity for creating a second reality through dreams, a reality in which we believe as much as we do in that of waking life.

> The fact that we create this reality, intermittently, without the aid of any perception of the external world, and that we believe in it as long as we are immersed in it and wake up considering it both from a distance and with an indubitable interest, gives us an idea of the plasticity of our psychical apparatus and its tolerance for our withdrawals from external reality even though it returns to it upon waking and displays an incredible creative capacity extending far beyond the dream phenomenon proper.[15]

Freud subsequently distanced himself from the dream-model which he had discovered in 1900, while retaining interest in the phenomenon, even after he had proposed another model linked to the second topography, that of the instinctual impulse and its action. Nevertheless, at the end of his life he returned to hallucinatory functioning in 'Constructions in Analysis' (1937),[16] where he underlined the interest of hallucinatory manifestations during the session which correspond to a return of the repressed in connection with traumas prior to the age of two – that is to say, before the acquisition of language which allows memories to be fixed as such. It turns out, then, that the famous proposition of the early days – namely, that 'the hysteric is suffering from reminiscences', is not only true of the hysteric, since hallucinatory activity, whose manifestations extend much further, is likened by Freud to a form of reminiscence.

Alongside this 'overflow' through hallucinatory activity, one can describe two other forms, standing in sharp contrast to each other. The first, whose orientation is the most internal and the deepest, is *somatization*. There opens up before us here the vast register of the psychosomatic, in which the descriptions and ideas of Pierre Marty dominate. Even if one cannot always agree with him, one should acknowledge the importance of this work[17] – the only one so far to counter the Lacanian theory with really serious arguments. The limits of the concepts of the signifier, or of the unconscious structured like a language, appear in sharp relief here. The issue is not to side with Marty against Lacan or the contrary, but to show that the field of practice of psychoanalysts today has to include them both. It remains to be said how. The descriptions of the psychosomaticians are impressive. They oblige the psychoanalyst to reflect on the limitations of his theory and its relevance in the face of such phenomena. It pleads in favour of a more elaborate differentiation which assigns a place to each territory, without reciprocal inclusion or exclusion.

Finally, whereas we have just been focusing on what is most internal, that is, on the soma which is situated even *deeper* than the unconscious, in complete conformity with Freud's ideas ('psychical processes are rooted in the somatic and are already part of the psychical in a form that is unknown to us', a formula that we can never remind ourselves of enough), *acting out*, on the contrary, is situated at the most external pole. That is to say, whereas somatization implies a discharge towards the most inaccessible depths, in acting out, the discharge occurs in the direction of the external world, beyond psyche. The Freudian model of discharge, one of the principal characteristics of the drive theory, has been subjected to much criticism. This model has been accused, ironically, of being 'hydraulic'. I have the impression, once again, that facile Freudian criticism is founded on a very reductive psychoanalytic vision, since it calls into question a mechanical model, while thinking of patients who do not clearly show this form of relief and decompression. Is this not to decide that any reflection on the model arising from the classical indications of analysis alone – which, it is true, do not privilege in any obvious way these mechanisms of discharge, and even often present contrary attitudes of inhibition – would be enough to call into question a general vision of the psyche found in Freud's writings? I will make two remarks here. The first is that the concept of discharge, as implied by acting out, is not limited to the case of instinctual discharges and the acts connected with them. Bion had remarked that, in psychotic structures, the model of the act remains prevalent *even where no act is noticeable in the most diverse psychic manifestations*. In these cases, for Bion, phantasy and discourse also conform to the model of the act, on account of their function of evacuation. Bion says that they have a function that is more *expulsive* than *integrative*.

In recent years, psychoanalytic conceptions have proposed the theme of *action schemes* (Widlöcher,[18] M. Perron-Borelli[19]). Although I am not certain of the truth of this position which raises the action scheme to a level of generality claiming to be a substitute for that of the drive, I would like to mention in passing that, for me, the field of the act far exceeds that of realized instances of acting out. Thus, there is obviously discharge in the case of affect (the notion is included in its definition), as well as in the thing-presentation, and even in exercising the function of speech. In every case there is a discharge which consumes energy to a greater or lesser extent, but which nonetheless implies a transformation, a mode, a psychic work which evokes this characteristic.

Recent studies have enriched our knowledge in a remarkable way thanks to certain therapeutic ventures in prisons, where psychotherapies have been attempted with convicted criminals. The observations which have emerged (thanks to C. Balier[20] and his collaborators) emphasize the links between instinctual acting out and depersonalization, coexisting with a characterical attitude akin to paranoia. However much one acknowledges the importance of certain environmental factors (affective and educational deprivation in the parental milieu, life in urban zones more or less outside the law, insufficient schooling, potentialized parental misery and defects, poverty of identifications with parents affected by various scourges such as alchoholism, prostitution, social degeneracy, etc.), the final result, at the individual level, is indeed this traumatic mark of psychic functioning which gives it its specificity. The fundamental motive forces behind the mental functioning of such people deserves to be understood better. Let me say right away that what can be observed does not arise from anxiety but from *a panic fear verging on terror* which obliges the subject to adopt active forms of behaviour to escape the danger of having once gain to suffer and relive the trauma; for very often these criminals have themselves been the victim of other adults when they were young (acts of violence, rape, etc.).

The second observation is the paradox that I have often pointed up between the current opinion of psychoanalysts who are more and more inclined to minimize the value of the concept of the drive and the parallel evolution of a world in which it is evident that instinctual life takes the lion's share (at all levels).

The misunderstanding becomes total. One can no longer see very clearly how a theory which withdraws interest to this point from the environment in order to give precedence to ideas arising from the analytic setting alone, can be worthy of interest in the patrimony of current knowledge. If psychoanalysis makes such a marked dissociation between what it witnesses in the world and the knowledge it gains from within the analytic setting, it becomes literally schizophrenic.

One can understand, then, how these three forms of 'overflow', that is, hallucinatory activity, somatization and acting out can be extrapolated to the point of making us think of the three forms of segregation in social life. Their respective sites are: the psychiatric hospital, the general hospital and the prison. A certain coherence thus enables us to find an element of unity in the study of the psyche, its deviant forms, its overflows, and its destiny.

Notes

1 See A. Green, La sexualité a-t-elle un quelquonque rapport avec la psychanalyse? *Revue française de psychanalyse*, 60, 1996, pp. 840–848. This lecture was first given in London on the occasion of a Sigmund Freud Birthday Lecture. To my great surprise, although I was simply reiterating truths which for me seemed self-evident, the lecture was received as if it comprised important innovations. Later, I had to publish my report which was pre-published at the Barcelona Congress: 'Ouverture à une discussion sur la sexualité dans la psychanalyse contemporaine', *Revue française de psychanalyse*, 61–1997, pp. 225–232. Reprinted in my work *Les chaînes d'Eros. Actualités du sexuel*. Paris: Odile Jacob, 1997. [English edition: *The Chains of Eros*. London: Rebus Press, 2000.]

2 Freud, S. (1940 [1938]). *An Outline of Psychoanalysis*, S.E. XXIII, p. 151.

3 The ideas presented in this chapter comprise no more than the essential points of a more complete exposition which the interested reader will find in my work *The Chains of Eros*. London: Rebus Press, 2000.

4 *The Language of Psychoanalysis* by J. Laplanche and J.-B. Pontalis offers an excellent summary of the issues pertaining to the ego. London: Hogarth Press, 1973. Reprinted by Karnac Books, 1988.

5 Rosenfeld, H. A clinical approach to the psychoanalytic theory of the life and death instincts: An investigation into the aggressive aspects of narcissism. *International Journal of Psychoanalysis*, 52, 1971, pp. 168–178.

6 Green, A. (1983). *Narcissisme de vie, narcissisme de mort*. Paris: Editions de Minuit. [English trans. Andrew Weller, *Life Narcissism, Death Narcissism*. London: Free Association Books, 2001.]

7 Greenson, R. (1967). *The Technique and Practice of Psychoanalysis*. London: Hogarth Press.

8 Green, A. (1993). *Le travail du négatif*. Paris: Editions de Minuit. [English trans. Andrew Weller, *The Work of the Negative*. London: Free Association Books, 1999.]

9 For a thorough and extensive study of the question, see J.-L. Donnet, *Surmoi* (1): Le concept freudien et la règle fondamentale. *Monographies de la Revue française de psychanalyse*. Paris: Presses Universitaires de France, 1995.

10 Green, A. L'analité primaire. In: *La pensée clinique*. Paris: Editions Odile Jacob, 2002,

p. 79 (first published in *Monographies de la Revue française de psychanalyse*: 'La névrose obsessionelle', 1993).

11 See A. Green, 'Masochism(s) and narcissism in analytic failures and the negative therapeutic reaction', ch. 5, *The Work of the Negative*. London: Free Association Books, 1999.

12 Bouvet, M. (1960). Dépersonnalisation et relations d'objet. *La relation d'objet. Oeuvres complètes*, vol. 1. Paris: Payot, 1967.

13 Translator's note: a term forged by Lacan which condenses *la haine* and *l'amour*. It is also homophonically evocative of *énamourer*: to be enamoured with.

14 Jackson, J.E. (2001). Capacité négative. *Souvent dans l'être obscur*. Paris: J. Corti.

15 Green, A. Mythes et réalités sur le processus psychanalytique. De *l'Abrégé de psychanalyse* à la clinique contemporaine, article 2, *Revue française de psychanalyse*, 20/2001.

16 *S.E.* XXIII, 255ff.

17 Marty, P. (1976). *Les mouvements individuels de vie et de mort*, and (1980) *L'ordre psychosomatique*. Paris: Payot.

18 Widlöcher, D. (1996). *Les nouvelles cartes de la psychanalyse*. Paris: Odile Jacob.

19 Perron-Borelli, M. (1997). *Dynamique du fantasme*. Paris: Presses Universitaires de France.

20 Balier, C. (1996). *Psychanalyse des comportements sexuels violent*. Paris: Presses Universitaires de France.

6

PSYCHOANALYSIS (ES) AND PSYCHOTHERAPY (IES)

Modalities and results

That I place psychotherapy alongside and on the same level as psychoanalysis does not mean, however, that I regard them as being part of one and the same vague ensemble. So as not to create any misunderstanding, let me repeat that for me psychoanalysis remains the model; the psychotherapies result essentially from the impossibility of creating a situation which respects the requirements of this model. Psychoanalysis remains in any case the reference. Let us begin, then, with the psychoanalytic treatment. It is perhaps as well to acknowledge right away, though, that the plural is more apposite. The model is the abstraction to which diverse realizations refer.

Psychoanalysis (es)

I do not intend in this chapter to give a detailed description of the process of what, in France, used to be called *la cure type* (classical treatment on the couch), but which is no longer often referred to thus. First, because no description, however precise it may be, can have the ambition of summing up the essential characteristics of a treatment, such is the variety of the polymorphism of the manifestations that can be observed in it; and, above all, because what is expressed there is first and foremost the singularity of an experience specific to a unique subject. Second, because, as Freud pointed out, psychoanalytic treatment is like a game of chess; only the opening and closing moves can be described. As for the rest of the game, that is to say, the main body of the exchanges, no generalization is possible owing to the complexity and the multiplicity of configurations possible. In the 1970s, Viderman subjected the postulates and axioms of the treatment to a close critique, challenging the basic principles of the theory of Freud's technique. Though his ideas made a lot of noise at the time when his principal work, *La construction de l'espace analytique*,[1] was published, it is to be regretted that it did so much to whet our appetite only to leave us unsatisfied when it came to deciding which theory should replace Freud's, regarded as being so insufficient. It seems to me that Viderman encountered insurmountable problems in proposing a coherent and sufficiently complete body of theory to serve as an alternative.

Today, I think it is even doubtful whether the opening and closing moves of the treatment can be the object of a generalization. I will therefore just make a few observations. The idea of the double transference, of which I spoke earlier, can help us advance. By separating *transference on to speech* and *transference on to the object*, I am trying to elucidate a configuration which is not easily apprehended by the idea of an undifferentiated transference, or even differentiated according to its nosographical particularities (transference of genital and pregenital structures: Bouvet). By distinguishing transference on to speech, I am trying to acknowledge the value, in my own way, of the propositions of Lacan, who not only put forward the idea that the unconscious was structured like a language, but also, and first and foremost, laid emphasis on the importance of the relation of the subject to the signifier. However, having given prominence to what is called the *heterogeneity of the signifier* – that is to say, the idea that the psychoanalytic signifier, which is not identical to the signifier of language, comprises genres and types which range from word presentation to the drive (psychical representative of the drive, thing and word presentation, affects, one's own bodily states, acting out, representations of reality, etc.) – I deduce that the possibility of evaluating the analysis depends on the manner in which the subject's discourse circulates between its different levels, from the body to thought, and on the flexibility of the communication between the registers and the indexation value of the discourse. It is quite evident, as other authors have recognized, that the discourse, more or less loaded with affects, assumes a different value from that which is only animated by a rationalizing, intellectual pseudo-coherence excluding any kind of relationship to the body as in certain obsessional and narcissistic caricatural forms. On the other hand, a discourse charged with potentialities for acting out, owing to insufficient holding mechanisms, and thus a lack of elaboration, has the tendency to abort attempts to give meaning and also to schematize the resulting complexity of the interplay of psychic processes.

The other aspect is the *transference on to the object*. Here, it is useful to take up again what has been given abundant treatment in psychoanalytic literature, and developed, as a rule, in the context of object relations. The transference on to the object consists in the projection on to the analyst during the session – an analyst who is supposed to present a relatively neutral surface (we know that this aim is not absolutely realizable, which is not a reason for rejecting it) – of impulses, desires, phantasies, wishes, anxieties, fears and terrors that the transference experience may reactivate or inspire. Repetition of the past? New experience? It is impossible to give a univocal answer. If the transference was not linked, at least in part, with a past experience, more or less restricting and tending to repeat itself more or less massively in the present, it would not have any reason to exist. But, on the other hand, if the past had the possibility of repeating itself as such, without getting mixed up with elements belonging to different, and even newly created periods, the transference would be an automatism and not an original experience. One can already conclude that, the more we are dealing with very regressive forms, the more repetition-compulsion will play an undifferentiated role to the pitch of preventing the emergence of something new and impeding the contribution of interpretation; on the contrary, the more one is dealing with a neurotic experience, the more the structure will be flexible and enriched by the facts of the present and of the external world, and the more it will allow for nuanced and subtle interpretations. For herein lies the misunderstanding. In analytic discussions, analysts throw arguments at each other that are supposed to destroy those of their adversaries; but *they do not see that they are not speaking about the same patients.* Moreover, even when one is speaking of the same patients, this does not prevent different psychoanalytic conceptions from distorting listening and orienting interpretation towards different semantic fields. Recent experience has allowed us to become aware of this. I am referring to the progressive shrinking of the field of sexuality. Not only has its place been reduced by the intervention of other factors (narcissism, destructivity), but even when the sexual material is present and perfectly identifiable, the analyst refuses to accord it importance on the pretext that it is just a defence. I have even heard one of my patients qualify as an *artefact* a dream with perfectly manifest homosexual content.

We must now try and combine transference on to speech and transference on to the object to see if there is a common factor uniting them. For in practice they are always two sides of the same coin. My experience has taught me that what the analyst first has to listen to in the patient's transferential discourse, is the *movement* which animates it. This is just a way of formulating what I was referring to in the description of free associative functioning. For it is this movement that passes from one association to another and progresses or regresses – that is to say, advances in a progressive mode or returns backwards in a retrogressive mode – which defines the course taken by the analysis and gives an idea of the process, in its advances and its returns, depending on the desires that animate it and the resistances it encounters. The importance of listening to the movement is precisely what is often difficult to get across to a young analyst in supervision. But, once the idea has been integrated, it is also what opens up the finest perspectives and allows one to hope for the most promising results, making intelligible that which, at the outset, did not seem to be so.

I have proposed the idea of *tertiary processes* in order to define those processes whose main function is to link up the primary processes and the secondary processes, for it is the interplay between the two that alone makes the fecundity of the psychoanalytic discourse possible. It is clear that these processes have no material existence as such, but are limited to the bindings that can be established between the first and the second in order to give unconscious desire a greater degree of legibility. To Freudian binding and unbinding, may fruitfully be added rebinding.

The evolution of the treatment, whose zigzag profile has been underscored by all authors, makes it possible to observe a tripartite cell, already demonstrated by Bouvet: resistance–transference–interpretation. Simply from the announcement of this triad, it can readily be seen that it is its middle term, the transference, that conditions the two others. In other words, resistance is, above all, a resistance to the transference; interpretation is aimed at the transference insofar as it gathers together, in the present, the elements of the conflict. Nevertheless, the question of the exclusivity of the transference interpretations is not self-evident. With regard to this, one might recall Freud's initial distinctions in his analysis of the case of Dora, which he subsequently abandoned, perhaps mistakenly. That is to say, he opposed *transferences* and *the* transference, maintaining in short that transferences permanently punctuate the psychoanalytic discourse, and that their principal figure, *the* transference, appears in the course of things and in a dominant fashion, in a way that is at once more meaningful and more condensed. This situation is not peculiar to the transference. It would seem to me that we are justified in inferring a general rule here – namely, that within a general context, a particular element can take on the role of representative for the whole.

I am now going to give an example from outside the frontiers of psychoanalysis. The mythologists of ancient Greece are astonished that psychoanalysts give a privileged status to the myth of Oedipus, when the latter is only one among many others in a burgeoning production of myths. They question, then, the legitimacy of the importance psychoanalysts accord to it, accusing them of making use of mythology for partisan purposes, unfaithful to its spirit. Apart from the fact that the study of the Oedipus myth presents singularities justifying the particular interest which psychoanalysts devote to it, one can also consider that it occupies the position of an element representing the anthropological dimension of the others. It is as if an abundant mythical production had been necessary for one myth to succeed in expressing the essence of human subjectivity. An analogous line of reasoning perhaps induces us to defend the distinction between transferences and the transference. But here again there is no uniformity of transference. The ideal transference is like 'the rose that is absent from every bouquet' (Angelus Silesius). In effect, there is no ideal transference; and if someone were to take it into his head to describe one, he would have to be suspected of a certain degree of blindness. Every transference is more or less impure, containing within it elements which distort its function. Nevertheless, it is very true that the modalities of the transference depend on the suitability of the psychopathological structures for the setting. Here we come up against the *limits of what is analysable*, which modern praxis is continually trying to define. The limit or border, as epistemologists have rightly acknowledged, is a concept that allows one to describe what falls short of it and what lies beyond it (or, if one prefers, within a territory defined as its interior inside the limit or its exterior outside the limit). But, when one situates oneself on the limit, it is also what allows one to see on both sides of the frontier that it represents. Let us note in passing, as I have already pointed out elsewhere, just how present the concept of limit[2] is in Freud, since he sets up demarcations between the agencies. Freud adds that one should not expect to encounter features similar to those that demarcate countries on geographical maps; but, on the contrary, buffer zones with a transitional role. Even at the heart of the foundations of psychoanalytic theory, the limit is present in the definition of the drive (a limit/border concept between psychic and somatic). This means that the decision to opt for or against undertaking a psychoanalytic treatment or to establish an indication for psychotherapy remains aleatory and subject to the analyst's appreciation. Aside from so-called objective considerations, the analyst's evaluation of the patient's capacities to deal with the foreseeable perils of the undertaking enters the equation here. Be that as it may, and to return to the classical treatment, the latter will be marked, session after session, by the actualization of the patient's conflicts.

It is very difficult to provide detailed indications on the art of interpreting and on what justifies interpretation. Formerly, it was customary to assert that the transference should only be interpreted when it became a resistance. This kind of assertion can be challenged today. I do not think that there is any other indication for interpretation than the sense that it comes at an optimal moment; i.e. when the configuration of the elements of the material is sufficiently intelligible and calls for the analyst's intervention as if the latter made it possible to gather up, in a significant moment, elements that had previously been dispersed – elements, moreover, that will continue their more or less fragmentary course after the interpretation. The interpretation should not be expected to produce effects of illumination along the lines of Eureka! and it is often the case that, even when unacknowledged, it acts on the material in an underground way, leading to a silent integration. The merits of mutative interpretation have frequently been praised (Strachey). I must confess that I have rarely had occasion to observe it. But it is not recommended to bombard the patient with interpretations which merely result in solidifying and bolstering his resistances. What seems to be essential, since Winnicott, is that interpretation retains its transitional value, as if it should be formulated in such a way that it implies what it does not say (indexation) in the form, 'It could be that . . . *or,* Perhaps it is that . . . *or,* One could think that . . .'. I know that some will reproach these formulas for not directly addressing the analysand's unconscious. The necessity for the analyst to be subjectively committed, especially in difficult treatments, must never veer towards dogmatic assertion. The latter, even when it seems to be accepted by the patient, can only further the setting up of masochistic defences and a state of dependence on the analyst's words. Conversely, excessive silence abandons the patient to dereliction, which is not the worst that can happen to him. Worse still would be if the patient's 'organization' were to respond to the analyst's silence by a sort of narcissistic indifference in which he puts himself out of reach. But let me repeat that it is not acceptable for the analyst to expect the patient to supply the interpreter with the response that he wants to hear. This would be a case of transference collusion, denounced by Winnicott long ago. Nevertheless, the analyst knows very well that an analysis unfolds and progresses over a long period, albeit step by step, and with much back-pedalling, before the most fundamental conflicts are approached. When the transference analysis has reached an advanced stage, the moment arrives when the analyst can envisage the possibility of ending the analysis. This occurrence, which today is not always the most frequent or the most evident, still remains an eventuality that the analyst must not lose sight of. In all other cases the analyst will have to ask himself:

1 If something has not escaped him during the analysis which was perhaps already present when it was indicated?
2 If some sort of variation would not have been desirable; and if so, of what kind, and for how long?
3 If it would not have been better to indicate psychotherapy from the outset? In certain cases, the analyst is led to propose the continuation and the end of the treatment in the face-to-face position.

If, once the analysis is finished, the analysand comes back to see the analyst owing to the reappearance of some of his old symptoms or the emergence of new ones, the analyst will have to decide: (a) if it is appropriate to follow up his request by accepting to continue the work already begun; or if it is better to refer the patient to another analyst; (b) if it is preferable to continue in the previous mode (a new stretch of analysis) or if it would not be better to adopt another therapeutic modality (face to face with the same or with another therapist, or even another therapy such as group psychoanalysis or psychodrama).

The psychoanalytic space is first and foremost one of freedom. What luck! one might think. Yes, when this fact is considered from the outside, in relation to what can be imagined about the benefits that could result from it. But, in fact, such liberty causes the analysand anxiety; and he is all the more afraid if he is lacking assurance in its structural stability. The more the neurosis is decipherable in terms of the Oedipal configuration, the greater is the freedom, and the more the analysis is enriching, opening the way to a psychic creativity with remarkable effects. On the other hand, the more the subject moves away from the Oedipal configuration and approaches pregenital structures, borderline structures or narcissistic organizations – roughly speaking, non-neurotic structures – the more the danger of regression will be feared and the more a lifting of defensive control will be difficult to obtain. For, here, it is no longer only the dynamic regression of sexuality which constitutes the threat, but rather the danger, following the regression, of ego disorganization. When one is clearly approaching the confines of psychosis, then the regression can take on an alarming nature – often more alarming for the patient than for the analyst. The analysis frequently comes up against a wall here, as the analysand is unable to have confidence in the analyst's capacity to hold the analytic situation which gives him the possibility of facing a regression that could not run its full course in the past (Winnicott: fear of breakdown[3]). It is often in these difficult moments that the question arises of adopting, more or less temporarily, a variation (switching from the couch to the chair; increasing the frequency of sessions; or extending their duration). As regards the variation, I feel in agreement above all with Bouvet, C. Parat, and Winnicott: the aim of variations is to favour the efflorescence, interpretation and (eventual) resolution of the transference neurosis. Along with Winnicott, I consider that the variation must depend on the level of regression. Already, in 1954, well in advance of his time, he had already tackled this phenomenon.[4] As far as I am concerned, when I think it is necessary to initiate a variation (a variation, it is surely not), with a view to inflecting the relation towards a psychotherapeutic orientation, it is because the relation has reached an impasse. It is not a question, then, of proposing the adoption of measures aimed at giving positive reassurance or support, any more than of advocating some kind of departure from neutrality in order to give the patient the impression that he is loved or accepted. The justification for such measures is the attempt to find ways of saving a process that is blocked. It is not that I consider these attitudes to be negligible; it is simply that I do not really believe that the analyst's 'kindness' (Nacht) is really enough to overcome the testing situation. On the other hand, sustained attention, the maintaining of interest in the patient, the analyst's concern to remain firm in the face of the tests with which he is confronted, a nuanced interpretative attitude, and, above all, unfailing availability, seem to me to be the most favourable factors for giving the patient the feeling that he is accepted, even in a regression that is difficult to tolerate. It has to be recognized that, owing to the anxieties and dangers he senses, the patient will seek, via irreversible acting out, to kill the process, either as a consequence of his own actions (with the external intervention of the family, for instance), or by provoking a violent countertransference reaction from the analyst. Let us be honest, this last eventuality is not always avoidable, for it is important to recognize that, however well analysed the analyst is, he is nonetheless limited in his capacity for tolerance. What is important, in this case, is that he manages to acknowledge in front of the patient that he has reached his limits and no longer feels capable of conducting the analytic work properly.

In this way, instead of having to face a divorce for misconduct, the situation is more one of divorce for shared misdemeanours. At any rate, all psychoanalysts know that, without excluding empathy, which in itself is not enough, it is the attitude of impassivity or remaining unruffled (Bouvet) that should be preserved. However, let it be added that such impassivity does not signify indifference, which would be the worst fault of all. Impassivity means that the analyst is sufficiently confident in his method to face the tempests by manoeuvring against the storms, the roaring forties, the currents and the ground swells. In such a situation, one has to rely on the qualities of the method (Donnet) and those of the pilot. It is vain to pretend that the situation is always under control; one still has to be careful not to capsize and founder.

We now have to envisage the case where, from the first, the indications for analysis suggest that tolerance for the setting will be so limited that the analyst's margin for manoeuvre will be very reduced. This is because the patient has little or chronic tolerance for the application of the method of treatment. Among the requirements of the method, it is difficult for the subject to tolerate the conjunction of the analyst's invisibility and his silence, which condemn him to a state which cannot be better described than as the revival in adulthood of infantile distress (*Hilflosigkeit*). In these conditions the analyst must renounce letting the patient go through experiences which would end up being more sterile than fruitful, with the analysis becoming chronically traumatic. It is in these cases that what has been called, rather felicitously (Nacht and Viderman), the analyst's 'presence', takes on its full meaning. Instead of favouring the state of absence, which is supposed to lead to the emergence of desire, here the state of absence, a variant of which I have described as *psychic desertification*,[5] leads the analyst to take a gamble. For it is at this moment that the problem is posed either of going for broke, as it were, in maintaining the analytic situation or of abandoning it in favour of another solution. Here there is no recipe indicating the path to follow; and it is up to the analyst, each time, to adopt a stance and to choose the solution that seems to him to be the best. To put it in another way, he either has to change the setting or modify it. What does this modification consist of? Some will say that they change the orientation of their armchair in such a way that the patient, without having to turn round, can assure himself of the analyst's presence by simply glancing sideways. In this way the patient can see the analyst if he feels the need to. But it is not always necessary to shift the armchair. In other cases, the analyst will above all make sure that silence does not become a source of too much anxiety. His interventions will punctuate the patient's discourse, echoing it, and, eventually, he will comment on it by giving the hypothetical preconscious meaning that can plausibly be conferred on it. In these conditions, interpretations of the unconscious, concerning both the patient's object relations and the transference, will be distilled with great prudence, progressively, and always in such a way that they never take on an authoritarian form. The interpretations will often seem like commentaries, and the analyst will try to give them this transitional dimension that the patient is incapable of giving them. He will give up the status of the interpreter who hammers out an intangible truth as if he were an oracle, and instead present his interpretation as a proposition which can be called into doubt. Moreover, when it is a question of interpretations which seem to arouse a sharp movement of rejection from the analysand, it is always worth remembering that this is the analyst's own way of seeing things; it is possible that his viewpoint is mistaken and nothing obliges the patient to adhere to it. Some even add: 'Maybe this will become clearer for you later on.'

Psychotherapy (ies)

The foregoing observations have prepared the ground well for approaching the psychotherapies. The indication for psychotherapy results from the analyst's estimation that the patient will not be able to tolerate the constraints of the setting and that, accordingly, it is better from the outset to envisage another mode of working. The option of switching to a classical setting at some later point remains open, but only after a certain period of time. I have described elsewhere[6] the particularities and even, one could say, the metapsychology underlying the face-to-face psychotherapeutic relationship. However, it is in these moments of tension that one realizes to what extent this perception of the therapist is misleading; that is to say, on these occasions the patient makes a massive projection of his emotions on to the analyst. Here, patients rely on the analyst's visibility and, above all, on his facial expressions reflecting approval or disapproval, satisfaction or irritation, etc. I have shown, moreover, that with these patients, what was unconscious was not related to a primary experience of satisfaction, but was marked by an internal experience of fright, whence the necessity of a perception that counter-invests the return.

We can see that what normally guarantees the function of dreaming – that is, the role of an internal view of the psychic processes whose existence is translated by the dream process – is lacking. Let me say right away that there is no means of contradicting these projections or correcting these erroneous perceptions. Though perception of the analyst is indispensable for the unfolding of a therapeutic process, it does not mean that this perception guarantees any sort of access to reality. It is understandable that here perception plays the role that representation cannot play for analysis. In other words, it is easier to call into question a representation in that it is necessarily subjective. One cannot do it for a perception that is supposed to perceive reality. All that one can hope for is that in the long term the patient is able to ask himself questions about what he perceives. In my article 'Analité primaire',[7] I have described behaviours involving a massive projection on to a persecutory object at the centre of an anal and narcissistic conflict. It is striking to see a surge of destructivity invading the patient who starts trampling on the object-analyst and tearing him to pieces, on the pretext, of course, that the latter is indifferent to his suffering, that he takes pleasure in his anxieties, is incapable of helping him, is spiteful, hostile, and so forth. What these patients want, above all, is for the analyst to act. It is patently obvious for them that words are powerless to provide a remedy for their condition, and that the analyst should therefore accept to drop his reserve (Ferenczi's O! Manes) by taking them in his arms, consoling them, caressing them, cuddling them, and so forth, without their being the slightest thought in the back of their minds of a sexual relationship. This is simply the analyst's phantasy, something the patient cannot even imagine, and the interpretation of which he can accept even less. In fact, to the extent that, in all these situations, it is perception that dominates, what we see occurring here, behind the projection which can often assume a quasi-hallucinatory character, is *negative hallucination*. A negative hallucination of what is perceived of the analyst and covered over by projections serving as a negative hallucination of the patient's own emotions and affects or even thoughts.

Generally speaking, psychotherapies are often marked by repetition-compulsion. A real work of Penelope can be witnessed – going well beyond its manifestations in analysis – where each interval between the sessions is used to undo what has been woven with difficulty during it. The analyst has no choice but to come to terms with the situation, for he has to suffer, endure and survive the patient's destructivity while continuing the work with him, that is, continuing to think. Winnicott shed a great deal of light on this situation in his article on the use of the object.[8] It is evident, then, that the transference presents itself in a form that is difficult to interpret or even to tolerate. It is either so massive that the patient is unaware of the value of repetition which impregnates its manifestations or, on the contrary, it is systematically occulted because the patient is totally absorbed by the extreme situations which he is speaking about, and through which he continues to live out scenes with important figures from his childhood who have not been relegated over the course of time to the place that belongs to them – namely, as dramas of the past. Thus the family, and especially the mother, play an important part in the subject's torments and misadventures. It is not so much a question of recognizing the objectivity of the complaints expressed by the patient as of noticing the extent to which these complaints continue to preoccupy the subject's mind to the point of preventing him from experiencing satisfactions in the present. It would seem that the sense of not having been loved by his mother as he would have wished remains a wound that has not healed and is always prompt to open up again when the slightest event takes him back to the situation of childhood. Needless to say, here, the Oedipus complex is vague, poorly structured, not easily identifiable, and largely infiltrated by pregenital fixations.

When they are not proposed as a rapid resolution of a conflict that has not yet become too organized and is not too far from consciousness, and when they make it possible to avoid the constraints of an analytic process – in other words, when they are due neither to material conditions which make analysis impracticable, nor to an easily surmountable conflictual problem – psychotherapies are a long-term undertaking, much longer on average than psychoanalysis. They go through interminable periods of stagnation, resistance, incessant returns of disorganizing masochistic behaviours, allowing for almost no insight. Is the game really worth the candle? My answer is yes! For when one shows patience, tolerance, tenacity, confidence in the method, and when one is moved by a genuine interest for one's patients, modifications eventually occur which indicate that 'something' of this psychoanalytic relationship has been integrated. The subject begins to understand that, whatever external factors may have had a bearing on the destiny (character and structure of the parents, general or personal historical circumstances, a more or less unfavourable environment), the question is really about the *subject*, not only the part that he may have played in the organization of his own unhappiness, but also because everything that he has experienced as coming from the outside world has necessarily been remodelled internally by himself; and thus *belongs to him by right and only belongs to him*. It is undoubtedly the most difficult thing to acknowledge for those subjects who have really been victims of circumstances or vicissitudes stemming from the environment. In the end, after a long period of analytic work, the subject accepts the fact that the objects of the environment simply did what they could, being themselves victims of their own conflicts. Moreover, as I have already said elsewhere: '*Everything that is in me is part of me. Everything that has been put into me has been reappropriated by me. Everything that is in me is ultimately mine – that is to say, a possession of my ego and not a graft or a parasite of an organism extraneous to me.*'

Assessments of the results

When psychoanalytic experiences, with or without variations, or psychotherapeutic experiences, can be brought to an end by common agreement between patient and analyst, the results compared with those of other techniques have to be nuanced. Let me say right away that, in treatments where there is a high potential for regression, once the situation is well under way and the transference has been established with sufficient reliability, whatever circumstantial vicissitudes the patient may experience, he settles into the therapeutic situation and often finds it so satisfying owing to the fact that it is such a new experience for him to be listened to, understood, not disapproved of (or approved of either) and helped to understand what is happening to him that, after a while, one notices that his fear of progressing is related to the fear that progress will lead to his being abandoned by the analyst. He fears the analyst will seek to get rid of him by using the improvement as a pretext and inviting him to stand on his own two feet. The patient thus navigates between two stumbling blocks. He fears being abandoned if he no longer feels loved by the analyst on account of his lack of progress; and he equally fears being abandoned if the analyst thinks that his progress means that he is able to get by without him. Certain symptoms are thus maintained so as to justify continuing the treatment, and to retain the analyst's interest and solicitude. The analyst must avoid this trap by letting the patient know that he does not need to continue to be ill to have the right to continue his psychotherapy in order to become better acquainted with his conflicts. For, as a matter of fact, even in normality there are many reasons for having blockages and for encountering limitations, inhibitions and residual conflicts that need to be analysed. It is plain that the state of illness in no way constitutes a sufficient justification for an analyst, whose judgement reaches beyond its frontiers and into the heart of 'normality'.

Nevertheless, what has given impetus to the upsurge of psychotherapies and led to an extension of the indications for them is not only that the latter seem less restrictive than those of the psychoanalytic setting. In the long run, the question has also arisen of the relation between the demands of the setting and the quality of the results of psychoanalysis. We have already seen how the intersubjectivist movement in the United States provides an answer to this situation, even though it can scarcely be said to be satisfying. But the lid has been removed, and, at last, tongues untied. Analysts have spoken of their own assessment of their results.

I have always thought that the question of the evaluation of the results of analysis could not be based on a so-called objective survey whose parameters risked distorting the conclusions. On the other hand, I also think that a survey ought to make it possible to obtain the opinions of psychoanalysts themselves who could provide precious indications concerning their results, under the cover of anonymity. I have already pointed out that a large proportion of psychotherapies was constituted by the failures, or semi-successes, of psychoanalytic treatments. Today, I think that there is an urgent need for psychoanalysts to speak about their results which are correlated with other factors such as the exclusive or partial character of the therapist's psychoanalytic practice; the length of time he has been practising his profession; the patient's structure, and so on. It is no longer possible to rely solely on the character of the patient's tolerance or intolerance for the analytic setting, *a posteriori*, i.e. after the attempt to put it into operation has failed. Naturally, this problem is discussed in all the psychoanalytic associations, but not on the basis of common criteria. Constant reflection is necessary if it is to be resolved, not by establishing grids or scales, but by a self-critical effort to harmonize the modes of psychoanalytic thinking.

The situation seemed sufficiently worrying to the International Psychoanalytic Association for the former president, Otto Kernberg, to propose a thorough reflection on the relations between psychoanalysis, psychoanalytic psychotherapy and supportive psychotherapy,[9] and for a commission to be given the task of examining the question in detail. From the initial investigations, observations have emerged that are very much worthy of our interest – namely, that analysts have long observed a sort of conspiracy of silence (the word is not too strong; we are paying the price for it today) with regard to the results of psychoanalysis, the idealization of which has been underlined retrospectively. In fact, a few authors came clean on this issue a long time ago. I think that Winnicott played this courageous role in denouncing, almost 50 years ago, collusion in the transference, drawing attention to the analytic non-lieux which made it possible to continue certain experiences to the point where analyst and analysand decided to separate in a context of explicit – or frequently tacit – dissatisfaction.

The widespread practice of 'successive' analyses, where an analysand considers that he has not reached the end of his possibilities in the analysis and decides to continue either with the same analyst or with another is familiar to us. What is not known is the proportion of patients who have recourse to further periods of analysis with the same or another analyst, and what the final result is. In my experience, I have been greatly struck by the fact that analysts have come to me for analytic help, considering that they still needed to work with an analyst, proposing to come and see me at variable, but very loose intervals, and refusing firmly the suggestion that they undertake a further period of analysis with me or someone else. In many cases it seemed to me that I was dealing with a dissociation between the analyst and the analysis. The analysand had a very good memory of the analyst, although the experience had often not been very positive, and had been of little help to him. The situation here, as one may imagine, is somewhat surprising. It would be desirable to be able to harmonize the feelings towards the transference-object and the analysis of it – in other words, to achieve a coherent evaluation of the analysis according to the classical – or modified – analytic setting.

In view of the line of reasoning I have pursued, it will be understood that I have been led to defend the need to train analysts in psychoanalytic psychotherapy. It seems to me that it is a means of extending the field of psychoanalysis. Needless to say, the issue is one of training analysts, and only analysts, to practise a psychotherapy that is as close as possible to analysis, and whose aims are not very different from those of analysis; only the means employed have been modified. Otherwise, two dangers menace psychoanalysis. The first is that of seeing requests for analysis shrinking away for reasons that reside both in the constraints involved and in the restrictions of the indications for which success can reasonably be hoped for. The other danger would be of abandoning the field of psychotherapies to non-analysts who practise their activity according to principles which are not those of analysts but which may offer more attractive conditions for patients, even if they compromise the results. And the last possibility would be a situation where psychoanalysts accept to take on these psychotherapeutic treatments without being properly trained for this work. They would thus divide their activity between the pure gold of analysis and the basest metal (baser than copper or lead), authorizing themselves to do more or less anything whatsoever since rigour is no longer the order of the day and, in any case, these patients. . . . There was a time when it was considered – it was Lacan who said so – that, in psychotherapy, 'anything goes'. Today, I do not think this is the case, and what I notice is that, for the Lacanians, anything does go, even in the exercise of psychoanalysis (short sessions, manipulation of the transference, violence towards patients, blackmail, intimidation, etc.). All this in spite of protests which do not shrink from dissimulation in order to save their practice. Is this the cynical remains of a revolutionary ethic which does not have to give an account of itself to bourgeois morality? Can the analytic ethic be equated with a bourgeois moral code? Does Lacanian practice claim to have its roots in a revolutionary ethic? Our ex-Maoists will surely not be long in providing us with a dialectically structured response.[10]

Notes

1 Viderman, S. (1970). *La construction de l'espace analytique*. Paris: Denoël, coll. 'La psychanalyse dans le monde contemporain.'
2 Green, A. (1976). Le concept de limite. *La folie privée*. Paris: Gallimard. [English trans. The borderline concept. *On Private Madness*. London: Hogarth Press, 1986.]
3 Winnicott, D.W. The fear of breakdown. *International Journal of Psychoanalysis*, 1974.
4 Winnicott, D.W. (1954). Metapsychological and clinical aspects of regression within the psycho-analytical set-up. *Collected Papers: Through Paediatrics to Psychoanalysis*. London: Tavistock, 1958.
5 Green, A. (2002). Le syndrome de désertification psychique, François Richard et al., *Le travail du psychanalyste en psychothérapie*. Paris: Dunod.
6 Green, A. L'analité primaire dans la relation anale, In: *La pensée clinique*, Editions Odile Jacob, 2002.
7 Ibid.
8 Winnicott, D.W. (1971). The use of an object and relating through identifications. In: *Playing and Reality*. London: Tavistock.
9 Kernberg, O. Psychanalyse, psychothérapie psychanalytique et psychothérapie de soutien: controverses contemporaines. In *Revue française de psychanalyse*, special edition: 'Courants de la psychanalyse contemporaine' under the direction of André Green, 2001, pp 15–36.
10 I have expressed myself at length in two articles published in the *Revue française de psychosomatique* in 2001: 'Mythes et réalités sur le processus psychanalytique'. What I maintain there is basically that the whole current situation can be traced back further than one thinks, i.e. to the years around 1920–1923, when Freud decided to change the model of the first topography in favour of the second. This means that the keys of the problem can only be found at a theoretical and practical level.

PART TWO

Theory

7

FREUD'S EPISTEMOLOGICAL
BREAKS

In order to have an exact idea of Freudian theory, it is indispensable to recognize several epistemological breaks – to use the now consecrated expression – in its evolution. In general, psychoanalysts know their history quite well, but they are often content to advance facts without justifying the arguments which induced Freud to modify his opinion. I shall retrace the principal stages of this evolution, laying particular emphasis on the well-known and decisive mutation called the 'turning-point' of 1920. It is necessary to show how this turning-point was prepared and how it plays the role of an essential cornerstone for understanding Freud's thought once the latter had reached its term. It can be said, in a general manner, that the ground covered by Freud constitutes in itself a summary of the ground covered by psychoanalysis as a whole.

At the outset, as we know, Freud tried to apply the hypnocathartic method. The justifications for doing so are familiar to us: the role of trauma, strangled affects, the removal of the obstacle by means of hypnotic suggestion and the resolution of the trauma through catharsis. This introductory and relatively brief phase was followed in 1897 by the abandonment of the theory of seduction. As I have already pointed out, Freud's positions apropos of seduction are not always as clear as they might be. Until the end, Freud continued to refer to trauma. Moreover, trauma was to reappear in a modified form in Ferenczi's writings, enriched with new traits. Be that as it may, if the theory of phantasy supplanted the theory of seduction, it was because of its general value – that is to say, though not all patients have been seduced by a perverse parent or adult, all of them, whether they have actually been seduced or not, have set up a conscious and unconscious phantasy organization whose presence can be found in all of them. If the analyst cannot demonstrate this, it means he is in the presence of an exceptionally powerful repression, or even a foreclosure, and it cannot, then, be an argument in favour of normality. Subsequently, the theory of phantasy eventuated in the first topography. Many analysts who are connoisseurs of Freud's work will have no difficulty in acknowledging that his principal work – it is with regard to it, above all, that an epistemological break is referred to – is *The Interpretation of Dreams* (1900). It is indeed in this work that one witnesses the real birth both of psychoanalytic thought proper and of the first topography. It was now that the three agencies of the psychical apparatus, conscious, preconscious, and unconscious, were defined with all the requisite rigour. During more than 20 years, this theory served as a reference for the comprehension of the normal and pathological psyche. So much so that when Freud decided to abandon this conception in favour of the so-called second topography, many analysts continued to refer to the earlier theory which, they thought, could not be rendered completely obsolete. Though certain analysts, including myself, consider that the second topography represents decisive progress in relation to the first, many others consider that it is necessary to retain both topographies, using now one, now the other, according to the circumstances. Even though I, too, recognize the usefulness of the first topography, I want to show how the second conception of the psychical apparatus is more in line with the evolution of clinical evidence.

In the first topography, it is naturally important to note the difference between the preconscious and the unconscious. According to Freud, this difference resides in the fact that the preconscious is that part of the unconscious which is susceptible of becoming conscious, whereas the unconscious cannot do so. It manifests itself through its temporary activations producing unconscious formations which, once analysed, reveal its existence or make it possible to deduce its characteristics (slips of the tongue, parapraxes, acts of forgetting, dreams, phantasies, symptoms, transference, etc.). But let me repeat, for the risk of misunderstanding is great, that the unconscious can only be deduced, hypothesized, but never revealed by observation, as a careful examination of Freud's writings shows. What is more, one can only speak about it *après coup*, after the event; that is to say, when it is possible to think, *a posteriori*, that a given phenomenon is in fact explicable by an activation of the unconscious. On the other hand, the preconscious represents the part of the unconscious in proximity to the conscious, capable of crossing the barrier of repression and presenting itself to consciousness in a more or less disguised form. From this arises the affirmation according to which the preconscious is part of the *Cs.-Pcs.*, whereas the *Ucs.* forms a separate domain.

Here two opposing conceptions divide psychoanalysts. For the French, the separation between preconscious and unconscious is not open to discussion. There exists a real break, a change of regime separating the two agencies which differ in numerous characteristics. For the Americans, on the contrary (Wallerstein), this scission is too radical and must be replaced by the idea of a *continuum* which extends from the conscious to the unconscious, without a hiatus. In my opinion, this last point of view, which supposes gradual stages towards the unconscious, has the drawback of dissolving the originality of Freud's theory and would be much more appropriate for characterizing the relations between the conscious and the preconscious. I have challenged this idea of a *continuum*.[1] Let us turn now to another theorization which carries out an abusive unification founded on different theoretical bases. When one considers the preconscious, one notices that Freud was ready to recognize its intrinsically contradictory nature. He writes in the *Outline*:

> The inside of the ego, which comprises above all the thought-processes, has the quality of being preconscious. This is a characteristic of the ego and belongs to it alone. It would not be correct, however, to think that connection with the mnemic residues of speech is a necessary precondition of the preconscious state. On the contrary, that state is independent of a connection with them, though the presence of that connection makes it safe to infer the preconscious nature of a process.[2]

It can be seen that these lines contradict the idea put forward by Lacan that the unconscious is structured like a language and even more that it *is* language. In other words, inclusion within the system of speech is not a condition of the preconscious state, defined in a different way, even though one can identify the process conditioned by speech as preconscious. What Freud is trying to tell us, constantly and vigorously, is that the unconscious can only be constituted *by a psyche which eludes the structuring of language*, it is constituted essentially of thing-presentations, 'the first and true object-cathexes'.[3]

The question of affect is more difficult to settle: there is still an ongoing discussion as to whether it is legitimate to speak of unconscious affect. I will deal with this point later on, but for the moment I will acknowledge that the unconscious is essentially constituted of thing-presentations and affects in variable proportions depending on the case.

These clarifications allow us to understand several of Freud's implicit axioms. The system unconscious is made up of representations which exclude the sphere of word-presentations, or of ideas and judgements representing reality (material). Representations and affects are governed by the characteristics that Freud was to go into in detail in the article on the unconscious in the *Papers on Metapsychology*: (1) absence of negation and contradiction; (2) absence of doubt or degree in certitude; (3) ignorance of the passage of time; (4) mobility of the intensity of cathexes; (5) prevalence of mechanisms of condensation and displacement, together defining the primary processes. On the other hand, all these characteristics, qualified negatively here, are present and make it possible to recognize the secondary process.

Freud's description constituted, at that moment, a strong theory in full assurance of its legitimacy. The unconscious comprises a triple dimension, in conformity with the *Papers on Metapsychology*: economic, topographical and dynamic. Moreover, one can also note a categorial dimension, concerning negation, contradiction and time, having a philosophical value. This constituted an advance of considerable importance since Kant. But that is not all. In examining the formulations closely, one notices that Freud, in the course of the text, sometimes speaks of representations as forming the material of the unconscious, and sometimes of instinctual impulses which are assumed to be underlying them. This hesitation may be considered to be revealing in the measure that Freud alludes either to the world of representations with its diverse varieties, or to that of affects, closer to the instinctual impulses. It still remains that one can think that the worm is already in the fruit. To speak more clearly, the reference, already present in the *Papers on Metapsychology*, to the instinctual impulses, already indicates the orientation which was to guide later Freudian thought. I would say that, since 1900, like the *Interpretation of Dreams* which privileges the work on representations compared with that which concerns affects, the evolution of clinical evidence and practice led to a certain reserve with regard to representation and to a validation of the dynamic element (affective) characteristic of the drive and its most primitive expression, the instinctual impulse.

The first topography, as we have seen, is centred on the notion of consciousness. This is the common factor uniting the three agencies which are defined by their relation to it. Whether it is a case of postulating a more or less absolute non-conscious (the unconscious), or a relative non-conscious (capable of becoming conscious [the preconscious]), consciousness is the pivotal point around which reflection revolves. In other words, Freud still needed the model of consciousness to define his own thinking. When he came to propose a new conception, in 1923, he did so on the basis of theoretical, clinical and technical arguments. With regard to theory, Freud emphasized the difficulty of postulating the unconscious of an unconscious, itself the unconscious of another unconscious, ad infinitum, that is to say, the intervention at each stage of another mode of consciousness. Clinically, he found support in the existence of clinical structures in which representations do not play such an important role as in the neuroses.

This was an old problem which had already led in the past to the isolation of the transference psychoneuroses in relation to the actual neuroses and the narcissistic neuroses. One only has to read attentively 'Mourning and Melancholia' to see that, already in the *Papers on Metapsychology*, Freud differentiates, in the pathology of mourning, between the object-presentations and the object-cathexes. In this affection the object, moves up, so to speak, to the front line. It is not the object-*presentations* which constitute the specificity of melancholia, but the fate of the object-*cathexes*. The loss of the object and the sacrifice of a part of the ego to replace it are in the foreground. And finally, economically, the quantitative factor of transformation seems to play a much more important role than in the economy relative to the representations. One of the proofs of it is the frequency with which one encounters the compulsion to repeat and the negative therapeutic reaction in non-neurotic structures. Of course, the link between the proposition of the last drive theory (1920) and the invention of the second topography (1923) deserves to be examined in detail. It is as though Freud was proceeding in two stages. In the first stage, he recasts his theory of the drives, first by gathering together under the same heading all the erotic drives, also called the love or life instincts (self-preservative drives, narcissism, object-related drives, etc.), and second by creating the new category of the so-called death or destructive drives (oriented internally, responsible for primary masochism, or externally, by deflecting the destructivity mobilized in the aggressive processes directed towards the object). Then, having modified this pedestal of psychic activity, he constructed a new psychical apparatus characterized by the id, the ego and the superego.

The id

The id includes the drives of the two major groups (Eros and destruction) *inside* the psychical apparatus. This point has not been given sufficient attention for, in the first topography, the drives, as such, are *outside* the apparatus; only their representatives are allowed to be part of it. Now, the drive belongs by right to the psychical world and is no longer situated outside it.

The definition of the id includes many points already used to define the unconscious. But though the similarities must be noted, it is still more important to point out the differences. One notes, in fact, at the level of the id, *the absence of any reference to representation.* The id is made up of contradictory tensions seeking release. This absence of reference to representation is a real indication that Freud has finished, once and for all, with referring to consciousness and its satellites in the different kinds of representation. This suggests that the old model of representation (unconscious, preconscious, conscious) has been replaced by a new model which, via discharge, is based on the act. In short, the most primitive aim of the psyche is indeed the instinctual satisfaction involved in the *act* (internal or external) and the energetic *discharge.* The principal fact that emerges from a comparison of the two topographies seems to me to be *the change of paradigmatic reference from representation to instinctual impulse.* Nevertheless, it is less a question here of the act as action than of primitive acts that have been internalized and are often confined to discharge into the body. This being so, the change can be explained by the discovery of the *com*-pulsion to repeat in *Beyond the Pleasure Principle*, *com*-pulsion forming the nucleus of the drive (its imperious tendency to discharge) and repeating itself blindly, in the best of cases in the quest for pleasure, or less happily, indifferent to pleasure, and worse still attracted by unpleasure and pain. One cannot stress enough the extent to which the discovery of the compulsion to repeat, first in 1914, and then in 1920, in *Beyond the Pleasure Principle*, turned the Freudian system completely upside down.

101

Freud did not abandon the unconscious, but its status was profoundly modified. In fact, Freud now relegated the old agencies, conscious – preconscious – unconscious, to the rank of *psychic qualities*. Their significance was thereby clearly limited. *Nevertheless, as the term unconscious has such a strong resonance, and as the term id is rather difficult to handle owing to its very opacity, it has remained customary to continue to refer to it, and to continue to call unconscious that which is now defined in quite a different way from the characteristics enumerated by Freud apropos of the id.* For it should be pointed out that we speak of desire in patients in respect of whom it is legitimate to ask oneself if this category is really present, to the extent that its raw, and barely nuanced forms, expressions of imperious instinctual demands, throw a doubt over the relevance of this qualification. It would be much better to characterize them by other denominations. I am, of course, alluding to patients with non-neurotic structures.

The ego

Another new finding: the ego. We have already seen just to what extent this concept is open to diverse interpretations and how much its academic, ante-Freudian use always had the tendency to return to the foreground, notwithstanding Freud's warnings. In the second topography, he introduced an absolutely decisive modification to it. Whereas, previously, he had always spoken of the ego as the psychoanalyst's ally in overcoming the neurosis, now he affirmed that a large part of the ego and, he adds, 'Heaven knows how important a part', was unconscious. *This idea of an unconscious ego bears witness to a modification of the status of the unconscious; it now ceases to be limited to the contents of the repressed and concerns its structure.* Admitting that a large part of the ego is unconscious means recognizing at the same time the limitation of the analyst's power, for unconsciousness here takes the form of the ego's unconsciousness of its own resistances.

What is the unconsciousness of the ego and what is implied by the observation that the ego is unconscious of its own resistances and defences? To elucidate this point, one must recall a certain number of notions connected with it. From the beginning, Freud considered the ego as a representative of rationality, unlike the id which knows no other logic than that of the instinctual impulses which animate it. But to say of the ego that it is the agent of rationality and that it refuses to recognize its defences and resistances, signifies, in fact, that the ego is essentially divided. However, though it is usual to recall that the ego is the result of a modification of the id under the influence of the external world, I do not think today that external reality alone plays a role in this transformation. I conceive of the ego more as a sort of interface between excitations related to the experiences of the internal world (affects, representations, etc.) and those coming from the external world (sensations, perceptions), where the importance of everything related to the object must be given particular emphasis. Finally, going beyond this dichotomy, I think that the ego plays an essential role in establishing transitional phenomena. Furthermore, alongside the receptive agency for registering and elaborating excitations, both external and internal – which means perceptions as well as representations and affects – can be differentiated, by means of a phenomenon of fundamental division, a function of *reflexive self-observation*. As the latter is capable of maintaining a certain distance, it is in a position to judge the quality, utility or dangerousness of what constitutes experience, and establishes processes of judgement, in the light of which it will have to decide what to do with these excitations. In this respect, Freud's article of 1925 on negation[4] is of crucial importance. It follows from the observation I have just made that the ego registers, observes, judges, decides while remaining under the triple influence of the id, the superego, and reality, and, above all, of everything that is related to the object. As for the relation to the external world, accessible via perception, it is governed by the reality principle and the choice, either to obey it, or to transform it, insofar as it can. Freud came to doubt the reliability of perception – thus the apparatuses of the ego – by discovering the disavowal in fetishism (1927e). The ego was from thereon considered as a double agent and nothing was assured any longer. But as far as internal excitations were concerned, and particularly those related to instinctual life and the two main groups of drives (Eros and destruction), the ego has to carry out its tasks by elaborating defences against anxiety arising from instinctual activation and various sorts of disapproval of which it has cognizance through the affects (condemnation from the superego, remonstrance from the object, dissuasion from reality, because it involves a threat of disorganization). While elaborating its defences, the ego retains the capacity to evaluate their function, their range, their efficiency, etc. However, as I have already said and often repeated, this last sector of self-observation has lost the notion of its original defensive value which, while keeping dangers at bay, can also prove, under certain circumstances, to be useless, anachronistic, and thus restrictive. Having lost this capacity, the subject is left to maintain and repeat defences which once had their use, at the moment when they were set up, but no longer do so in adulthood. In order to abandon these defences which have become more troublesome than useful, it is necessary to have retained a form of minimal consciousness, in order to be able to identify them and recognize them. Beforehand, as Bion says, the psyche has to accept to elaborate frustration rather than simply evacuating it. That is, to be more precise, the subject has to effect an instinctual introjection (J.-L. Donnet). The ego also has to recognize the existence of the drive by taking note of the excitation it produces and identifying the internal origin of the excitation. As Freud stipulated, as early as 1926, the solution does not consist in repressing the representatives of the drive but, on the contrary, in recognizing those which can be useful in nourishing the ego, in acknowledging the demands for satisfaction that are capable of being satisfied and in repressing those which, at a certain point in development, become useless, or even harmful and dangerous for the ego.

Thus pregenital impulses do not disappear so much as they become integrated in genitality more or less harmoniously, finding a latitude of expression in the form of a 'certain abnormality' (J. McDougall).[5] It is clear that, here, a certain amount of splitting is not only acceptable but desirable between the ego of experience and the ego which recognizes this experience. On the other hand, when the ego can tolerate neither the drive nor any of the manifestations which accompany it and which challenge the ego owing to their rather uncontrollable character, it finds itself obliged, in order to relieve tension, to evacuate the anxiety-producing excitations on account of their excessive erotic charge or their destructive potential. To achieve this, the ego engages in excessive projective identification which impoverishes it through the process of 'emptying' that it entails, leaving it, to use Bion's expression, with *denuded* object relations.

We are indebted to Bion for an impressive description of the manifestations linked to the factor −K (negative knowledge). This description gives a very vivid idea of the processes of denial which have the inevitable effect of extenuating the ego in psychosis. Conversely, in the interplay between internal and external reality, the ego can succeed in creating a special category of objects and phenomena, that is, *transitional objects and phenomena* (Winnicott),[6] which play a particularly important role in play and cultural experience and represent a form of sublimation whose enriching effects on the psyche are indisputable. What I am saying here with a view to elucidating the notion of the unconsciousness of the ego clearly goes far beyond the question of the unconsciousness of the defences. For it implies taking into consideration the awakening of instinctual life, the acceptance of it, the recognition of its manifestations, the conservation and introduction of what is attached to it, the sorting out according to their qualities, among the erotic and destructive aspects, of those which respect the major prohibitions and conserve the ego's vitality, without any risk of disorganization and without the contrary danger of sterilization. As I have said elsewhere, *the ego navigates between chaos and sclerosis.* It is hardly necessary to point out that I am in agreement with Winnicott when he states that it is better to have a patient who has retained certain symptoms at the same time as preserving or increasing his creative vitality and his spontaneity, than a patient completely free of his symptoms and psychically neutralized, that is to say, psychically dead.

At all events, when Freud feels the need to give prominence, in the second topography, to this characteristic of the unconsciousness of the ego, it must be understood that he is killing two birds with one stone. On the one hand, he now sees the ego as being to a large extent unconscious of itself, even in normality. In his own way, Lacan is saying nothing different when he underscores the role of *méconnaissance*[7] from a perspective inspired by Hegel. But, on the other hand, Freud is seeking to define the state of certain structures where the pathology is no longer limited to disorders in the sphere of the instinctual drives, but affects the ego itself. The unconsciousness of the ego is no longer, then, a matter of coming up against a limit present in each of us; it is an intrinsic opaqueness to itself. In certain cases, this leads to an extreme state of blindness that is accompanied, moreover, by other manifestations in which one can detect a certain weakness of representative elaboration and a deficiency of the possibilities of holding which characterize it, opening the way to regressions back to a stage prior to representations, namely, *hallucinatory activity, somatization and acting out*. One can understand, then, that the operations of expulsion into the soma or into action, that is, burrowing into what is most internal or discharging into what is most external, occur as if there had been a lack of what I call *intermediary formations* – precisely those in which unconscious wishes can find a singular form of expression (dreams, phantasy, bungled actions, slips of the tongue, etc.). In all these cases the ego appears to be almost blind to itself, becoming blind when it is carrying out these operations. The analyst then has the impression that he is addressing a patient who is in a state of permanent somnambulism, wandering like a shadow in full daylight.

This, I think, is the lesson to be drawn from the transition to the second topography and its dominant trait, the consequence, no doubt, of the modifications I described when accounting for the replacement of the unconscious by the id or for the particularities of the organization of the superego. At each stage of my reflection, the second topography shows us that the psychic domain appears to be caught between the demands of the instinctual impulses, anchored in the somatic, and reality, against which there stands out the figure of the Other (Lacan), arising from culture, a source of demands that are no less restricting. Between the two there is the psyche, structured in my view by the world of representations, which I will consider in detail at a later point. These representations are bound on the one hand to the drive and, on the other, via language, to thought, that is to say, also to the cultural tradition and to its productions laid down as a 'treasure of the signifier' (Lacan) structured by the order of signs. That it has been possible to see in the reference to the Other one of the expressions which marks the place of the third comes as no surprise. It is up to us to make the best use of it, that is, to refuse to ignore it, as is the case in certain theories (Kleinian, for example), and to resist the temptation to make a fetish of this dimension. This inclination led Lacan and his followers, in the long term, to underestimate, and even, in some cases, to deny the transcendence of the drives.

If the ego cannot realize, by virtue of the analyst's interpretations, that it sets up resistances to avoid seeing *its* truth, then the analyst is reduced to resorting to techniques which correspond, more or less, to the old and disowned methods of suggestion – methods he thought he had got rid of once and for all thanks to analysis. What is in question is a technique of interpretation whose aim is to lead the ego to recognize, *volens nolens*, the way it sets up defences in order to avoid insight. This would make us run the risk of falling back into the erring ways of forcing techniques and of resorting to authoritarian arguments which only have an immediate, ephemeral, and superficial effect. It is clear that here the opaqueness of the unconscious is based on what has to be called the obstinate blindness of the ego defending its narcissistic foundations.

The superego

The second topography saw the creation of the superego, without an equivalent in the first topography. Admittedly, when Freud introduced narcissism (1914), he was already speaking, with regard to the delusion of being observed, found in certain psychotics, of an internal division with the constitution of a critical agency keeping watch over another part of the ego. Likewise, when turning to the problem of melancholia ('Mourning and Melancholia'), he treated of the division of the ego, one part of which aims to replace the lost object, thus creating a highly conflictual situation, and another part which will be decimated by the criticisms it addresses to itself. This ego, part of which behaves with cruelty towards the other part, reproduces an earlier primitive relation in which the ego addressed its criticisms to the object (1917e). It is worth noting that delusions of being observed or attacks of melancholia were considered at the time to belong to the category of the narcissistic neuroses, and concerned the narcissistic foundations of the ego. But it was clearly with the elaboration of the second topography, and after Freud had devoted all his attention to the study of group psychology and the analysis of the ego by observing the phenomena of iden-tification (1921) that the conception of the superego emerged into broad daylight. On this point I would refer the reader to the study carried out by Jean-Luc Donnet.[8]

It is important, however, to recognize the double nature of the superego. On the one hand, it has its roots in the id, that is to say, its most primitive source is connected with the sphere of the instinctual drives and its degree of tolerance or cruelty will depend, from one case to another, on the predominance of the erotic (or life) drives or the destructive (or death) drives. And, on the other hand, its constitution depends on the division of the ego into an observing, critical, judging part, and another part that is under the examination of the former. Which amounts to saying that, here too, the instinctual base extends its influence. Nothing in the psychical apparatus can escape it, and whatever the degree of differentiation of the elements arising from this basis, its original label 'Made in Id' will never disappear.

Nevertheless, if I had to characterize with one stroke, and one stroke only, the novelty of this second topography in relation to the first, I would do so, without hesitation, by referring to the *unconsciousness of the ego*. For this whole construction merely served to provide Freud with an explanation for the all too frequent breakdowns, or worse still, in certain cases, the complete collapse, of the analysis. The analyst's collaboration with the ego is found, under these circumstances, to be deficient. His interpretations only reach the patient superficially. Their impact is ephemeral. Once the session is over, what has been said is forgotten, repressed, subjected to amnesia. The ramifications of the interpretation in the unconscious do not create new links; nor do they liberate investments. In the words of the proverb cited by Freud, 'Soon got, soon gone'.[9] Or, on the contrary, the instantaneous dramatic effect of the session occurs and exhausts itself on the spot. Many other situations can arise which cannot all be fully enumerated, but they all have the same meaning. Their purpose is to make it understood that something in the patient resists becoming engaged in the analysis, resists investing the analysand's discourse sufficiently or the analyst's listening, along the lines of, 'Why not . . . and so what?!' In other words, an essential split occurs which affects the interpretations of the analysis of two movements which mutually cancel each other out: one seems to be willing to recognize the exactness of these interpretations and the other is unwilling to let go of its belief that it is necessary to sustain its misrecognition (*méconnaissance*) at all costs. There is an evasion of what one had originally perceived as a wish to get better. It is in such cases that the treatment can go on and on for ever. A negative therapeutic reaction leads it into an impasse. It is quite remarkable that, in such circumstances, it is not the patient who takes the initiative to break off the analytic relationship. As a rule, it is the analyst who throws in the towel, having no strength left. The patient finds this very difficult to tolerate, being deprived of the sadistic and masochistic satisfactions derived from the analysis and experiencing this abandonment as an unacceptable rejection. Though it is impossible to deny the character of the rejection, what needs to be noted above all is that the analyst's decision is motivated by the persistent sterility of the exchanges in a parasitic relationship, just as Bion theorized it. Apologizing is a way of admitting one's guilt.

I have accorded considerable importance to this mutation concerning the ego; it was a real turning-point in Freudian theory, occurring in the middle of its development, around 1920, and it was maintained till the end. Did the process of constant renewal come to a standstill because Freud, with advancing years, no longer had the same creative resources at his disposal or was it because he sensed that he had reached the finishing straight? It is no doubt difficult to decide on this definitively. However, it is important to recall certain mutative developments, after 1924, which, though they did not have the same importance as those of the turning-point of 1920, nevertheless had a bearing on the orientation of Freudian thought. Here are a few of them.

From 1924 onwards, 'The Economic Problem of Masochism'[10] forcefully marked the position of *original primary masochism*. Freud emphasized strongly that masochism could no longer be considered solely from its secondary angle, nor in terms of the interpretations that he had given of it previously – and which are very much in vogue today ('A Child is Being Beaten' is a must among the studies on masochism). Along with primal masochism, another question of upmost importance to be studied was libidinal co-excitation and the primary masochistic organization of the ego. Meanwhile, Freud had introduced the notion of bisexuality. But it has been pointed out (F. Guignard)[11] that he made use of examples taken from masochism in men to support the thesis of masochism in women. What seems important here is not so much the question of the feminine, in other respects fundamental, but the increasingly marked tendency in Freud's work to bring into play, in combination, two major theoretical axes: bisexuality and the opposition between Eros and the destructive drives. This line of inspiration extends right up to 'Analysis Terminable and Interminable'.

In 1924, there also appeared the two articles on the relations between neurosis and psychosis. From then on, Freud, who had been interested from the start by the relations of neurosis with perversion, sought rather to situate neurosis in relation to psychosis. As he had not written much on psychosis – his principal work on President Schreber's *Memoirs* being no substitute for a case history – it was as if the articles of 1924 were supposed to correct a certain deviation, whose relations, moreover, would be clarified at a later point. It is clear that this orientation arose from the application of the new topography (neurosis: result of the opposition id vs. ego; psychosis: id and ego allied vs. external world: introduction of the repression of reality).

Three years after, in 1927, there appeared the major description of a new mode of defence, *splitting,* accompanied by *disavowal* in 'Fetishism'. It is there that it is possible to speak of an articulation between perversion and psychosis; for Freud unquestionably counted fetishism among the perversions. Nevertheless, the disavowal of an external perception can be conceived as a form of repression of reality. Moreover, when Freud took up the question again in *An Outline of Psychoanalysis,* he linked the fragmentation of the ego with widespread and generalized splitting. In short, it is as though what appears to be limited in fetishism (the splitting off of a sector of reality) presents itself in psychosis in a form in which the perversion is no longer recognizable as such in the psychotic fragmentation affecting the ego. The discovery of splitting is of an importance that should not be underestimated.[12] Nonetheless, one should distinguish between the sense that Freud gave to splitting and the senses that his successors were to give to it subsequently, in particular Melanie Klein and her pupils. Kleinian splitting is defined as a *schize,* a dissociation, a more radical separation than that carried out by repression. In Kleinian thought, one has the impression that the result of splitting entails unconsciousness more than repression, but can one go any further? It is necessary, then, to complete the notion with projective identification. In this context, it is difficult to apply Freud's definition to the letter. For Freud, splitting always comprises a positive aspect, that of the recognition (*reconnaissance*) of the truth, counterbalanced by the corresponding part of misrecognition (*méconnaissance*), which annihilates any possibility of making the reality principle effective. In short we are faced here with situations of stalemate. To put it another way, the game is declared null, without either the pleasure principle or the reality principle prevailing.

Freud closed his work by reconsidering the question of this defence of the ego in which he thought, not without hesitation, that he could see a major discovery. The future would confirm that he was right, in a way that went far beyond the use made of it by Kleinian authors. Yet what more was Freud doing than contributing fresh material for reflection on the unconsciousness of the ego? We are thus going to have to identify the *permanent dialectic between mis-recognition and recognition in psychic work*. The place accorded to misrecognition is not only the result of an extended clinical investigation in time and space; it touches upon the essence of man, who, in order to construct an acceptable image of himself, is obliged to deny or misrecognize the essential aspects of it via a process of occultation with a view to avoiding anxiety. Here, as we can see, the frontiers between the different sectors of pathology are erased, as are the frontiers between the normal and the pathological, the divine and the infernal.

Freud's work closes, then, with this fundamental couple, constantly at work throughout life. The last writings seek to clarify the internal axes of clinical work and theory. It was Freud's ambition to push these views as far as possible, as he does in *Moses and Monotheism*, by placing parricide at the centre of culture. This opinion was to become the object of one of the most radical forms of misrecognition on the part of psychoanalysts and investigators from other disciplines.

And yet, the immense Freudian construction is no longer enough to satisfy us today. I shall not speak of the criticisms that have been directed at this or that postulate or axiom. Nor shall I make my own the objections against the concept of the drive or the reductionist character of his so-called hydraulic model. In their broad outlines, many of Freud's postulates do not arouse a need on my part to criticize them, or to replace them with others; at the most, a need to reformulate and recontextualize them. Nevertheless, there remains a critique which is still valid in my view. The question, moreover, is to know whether this critique is to be taken literally or whether it calls for a reinterpretation of Freud's work. It is, as we know, and I have already stated it many times, the absence of a sufficient reference to the response of the object in the structuring of the psyche. This is what has motivated the defence of relational theories (object relations, intersubjectivity), and there can be no doubt that the relational point of view gains by being reinforced in Freud's theoretical framework. At any rate, the place, the role, the functions and the dynamic of the object are well worth updating, theoretically, clinically and technically. I shall not shrink from daring to envisage the interest of a third topography. Already in 1975, in my London Report, I indicated that this seemed to me to be an emerging possibility.[13] Today, I think it is a done thing, but it still remains to clarify the lines of force and to articulate the relations between the terms and the concepts that make it possible to understand them. This is what I intend to do.

Notes

1 Green, A., and Wallerstein, R. in *Clinical and Observational Psychoanalytic Research*, Monograph Series of the Psychoanalysis Unit, University College London, and the Anna Freud Centre Monograph, no. 5.

2 Freud, S. (1938). *An Outline of Psychoanalysis, S.E.* XXIII, 162.

3 Freud, S. (1915). *Papers on Metapsychology, S.E.* XIV, 201.

4 Freud, S. (1925). Negation, *S.E.* XIX.

5 McDougall (1978). *Plaidoyer pour une certaine anormalité.* Paris: Gallimard. [English edition: *A Plea for a Measure of Abnormality.* New York: International Universities Press, 1980.]

6 Winnicott, D.W. (1971). *Playing and Reality.* London: Tavistock. Reprinted by Routledge, 1989.

7 Translator's note: a central Lacanian concept closely related to knowledge (*connaissance*), borrowed from Hegel: the sense is of a failure to recognize, a misappraisal, an ignorance of consciousness about itself.

8 Donnet, J.-L. (1995). 'Monographies de la Revue française de psychanalyse', *Le surmoi*, vol. 1. Paris: Presses Universitaires de France.

9 Freud, S. (1937). Analysis terminable and interminable, *S.E.* XXIII, 241.

10 Freud, S. (1924c). 'The Economic Problem of Masochism', *S.E.* XIX, 155–170.

11 Guignard, F. Le sourire du chat. Réflexions sur le féminin à partir de la pratique analytique quotidien. In: *Bulletin de la Société psychanalytique de Paris*, 1986, no. 9, pp. 3–18.

12 Bayle, G. Des espaces et des temps pour l'objet (clivage structurel et clivage fonctionnel). In *Revue française de psychanalyse*, 1989, vol. 53, no. 4, pp. 1055–1067.

13 Green, A. (1975). L'analyste, la symbolisation et l'absence dans le cadre analytique. Reprinted in *La folie privée.* Paris: Gallimard, 1990. [English edition: The analyst, symbolization and absence in the analytic setting, trans. Lewison and Pines. In: *On Private Madness.* London: Hogarth, 1986.]

8

OPENING THE WAY FOR A RENEWAL OF THE THEORY

Subject line and object line

I have endeavoured to show the full measure of the coherence of the Freudian development and to emphasize the decisive contribution of the second topography. Unfortunately, what, to me, appears to be a considerable enrichment of the theoretical corpus of Freud has not always had the desired effects. Two facts should be noted. The first is that this new distribution of the agencies in the second topography gave rise to schematizing distortions of Freud's thought. What I am referring to here are, of course, the reinterpretations envisaged from the angle of *ego psychology*. But in any case, it would be dishonest to say that Hartmann, Kris and Loewenstein invented ego psychology. They simplified, schematized and largely reinterpreted, not to say distorted, Freud's thought. It is true, though, that they did not do this, so to speak, from zero, and that a certain reading of Freud was compatible with the interpretation that they promoted and which has enjoyed such success, especially in the United States. I have shown that the principal trait of the innovation of 1923 should be looked for in the accentuation of the unconsciousness of the ego. In my opinion, this meant that, from thereon, Freud denounced the ego, hitherto considered as an ally, and unmasked its duplicity and inclination less for curing than for ignoring the causes of its suffering, often with the purpose of sustaining it, contrary to what he had believed. In point of fact, it seems undeniable that, from 1923 on, both with regard to masochism and splitting, it was the ego's responsibility to which Freud wanted to draw attention, as if he wanted to warn analysts that they not only had to deal with a terrible adversary that was unknown to them, the death drive, but, in addition to that, the agency which they thought was on their side in the cure, was nothing other than a double agent. I know that elsewhere, in 1926, Freud adopted a more nuanced position with regard to the ego, halfway between the excess of confidence that was felt initially and the total mistrust that was now being manifested. The general tendency is as follows: Freud's work closes on the essential role of splitting as a process of defence. It is evident that here we are at the opposite pole from the positions that Hartmann was to defend – namely, free energy, autonomous ego, etc. We find ourselves faced with the necessity of examining the currents that traverse Freud's work internally and those that were to emerge in the history of psychoanalysis after his death.

This brings me to my second observation. Whatever one does to rehabilitate Freudian thought which has been somewhat tarnished, one cannot deny that the community of analysts has recognized, almost unanimously, the insufficiency of the Freudian position regarding the very restricted place it accords to the object. It was logical that, in building the pedestal of his conception on the instinctual drives, Freud made the major share of the weight of the theory rest on them, and equally logical that he insisted on the pre-eminence of instinctual life, more influential by far than that of the object. Moreover, in this respect, a contradiction should be noted to which I have drawn attention on many occasions. The object is often conceived of theoretically from the angle of the drive organization (it is then a highly substitutable element of it, and thus almost contingent). To this object of the drive organization corresponds the object in reality and the object of the earliest period. One again encounters here the model linked to representation referring to the relation of the image to the object. Nevertheless, in 'Mourning and Melancholia', in respect of the primitive forms of the psyche, the object is unique, indispensable and irreplaceable, to such an extent that the lost object of melancholia cannot be replaced by another, as it can be at the end of a normal situation of mourning. In order to deal with this loss, the subject has to get the ego to split itself so that a part of it is sacrificed, mutilated, as it were, so as to take the place of the lost object.

After Freud, it is quite clear that it was this second conception, coupled with the 'genetic' developments of *Inhibitions, Symptoms and Anxiety*, which prevailed in the large part of the analytic community. At any rate, from then on it became necessary to take account of a conception which left more room for the object. Fairbairn,[1] who was the initiator of it, was to be largely supplanted by Melanie Klein who gave a highly personal interpretation of it. She postulated the existence of an ego and an object that are separate, each playing their role from the moment of birth. This conception of object relations, it must be emphasized, was followed by many authors who, even without adhering to Kleinism, retained Fairbairn's original idea. I will mention, for memory's sake, the conceptions of Edith Jacobson, which created a considerable stir in the United States, well beyond the allegiance of their author to Hartmann's ego psychology, and, in France those of Maurice Bouvet, which do not owe much either to Melanie Klein or to Edith Jacobson, but which are concerned with a psychoanalytic clinical theory of pregenital and genital relations. As for Lacan, although his theory was above all centred on the subject, he also wanted to make the object play a more important role by inventing the concept of the object a^2 (object of desire, part object of the drive)[3] and, in complete contrast with it, the big Other, as a locus of truth. What is remarkable, in any case, is the refusal to accept the existence of a total object like that of Melanie Klein, any idea of totalization, whether it be of the ego or of the object, necessarily being, in his view, misleading.

The position I have taken consists of recognizing the observation of the deficiency of the response of the object in Freudian theory; but I have not accepted, however, that this be taken as a pretext to get rid of the irreplaceable theory of the drives. I have, accordingly, proposed that the fundamental cell of the theory be constituted by the *drive–object couple*.[4] Having developed my ideas under the joint influence of clinical evidence and theoretical reflection, I am now ready to propose my solution.

Included in it we shall find a familiar line of thought, that of the subject–object relation whose constancy can be very widely identified, beyond the frontiers of psychoanalysis. From the perspective I am adopting, the issue is not to oppose the subject and the object, but to inscribe each of these terms at the centre of a line. In other words, as I see it, in the current state of our knowledge and existing theories, it is not possible to bring together under one heading the subject and the object in psychoanalysis. There are two currents, at once independent of each other and richly interconnected, in which subjective formations and object formations are linked together. Each current possesses a unity, but can be broken down into diverse entities. With each problem, it is a matter of looking for the entity most concerned.

Thus I group together psychic life into two major polarities. Far from rejecting it, I consider that Freud's work has been undeniably useful to us in understanding what the *subject line*[5] is. It is worth noting here that the whole of post-Freudian psychoanalysis was, for a very long time, dominated by considerations of the object, without the question even being asked as to *what* the object was related *to*. Object relations were talked about without anyone saying *what* stood in relation to the object. I will be told that the answer was self-evident: the ego. But why was there a readiness to use the expression object relations without saying what stood into relation to what? It was perhaps because a certain difficulty had already become manifest – namely, that the reference to the ego seemed insufficient and questionable, in any case, unsatisfying. We know that it was not long before there appeared what I could call the ego's satellites. That is to say, all the notions which claimed to complete Freud's theory of the ego. We thus saw the genesis of the Self with Hartmann, Edith Jacobson, and later with Melanie Klein and even Winnicott, as well as the emergence of references to the I (Piera Aulagnier). Racamier added to this the person (or the *persona*, the mask) and finally we had long been familiar with the centrality of the subject in Lacan's work. Later, the subjective returned in another mode in the theory of intersubjectivity, without any original definition emerging however. Here, two attitudes are possible. The first is to choose a central reference in relation to which the others would be but products. This attitude does not seem to me to be able to sustain its claims. Lacan, who thought he held the right position by referring to the subject, could not cover, with this concept alone, the whole clinical field. For a certain time, I myself referred to the concept of ego-subject to emphasize both the gap that separated the two notions and the necessity of coupling them. Today, I would not defend this idea any longer, preferring instead that of the *subject line*. What I want to say is that the attitude, which at present seems to me to be the right one, is to inscribe within the subject line most of the propositions which have been made one after the other (Subject, I, Self, etc.), while assigning to each one definitions which account for its field of action. Thus the Freudian ego will retain its specificity and its limits; the Self will be conceived essentially as the phenomenological unity of the person; the I will correspond to definitions given by Piera Aulagnier which, moreover, seem to me to be legitimate in the measure that they imply its relation to the other.

We thus have a *subject line* – the term subject seeming to me to be the most apt for characterizing the series from the perspective of a subject and object opposition. But what I am proposing which is new is that we consider the *drive as matrix of the subject*. In point of fact it is absolutely impossible to attempt to conceive of the foundations of the subject without seeing the work of the drive in operation. An 'I', or a subject with its instinctual dimension amputated, is an inanimate, mechanical, operative and, if you wish, cognitive entity. What defines the drive is, on the one hand, as Freud indicated, that it is a limit or border concept between the psychic and the somatic which grafts the psyche definitively on to the body. And, on the other hand, that it is the demand of the body made on the mind – 'the demand for work' – so that the mind finds solutions that make it possible to overcome the situation of lack. It demands an end to the tensions that inhabit it and cries out for satisfaction. In other words, the development of the psyche is less dependent on its relation with reality than on the necessity of dealing with internal constraints, pushing the mind to search for solutions in order to obtain the satisfactions that it is lacking. Here we find again the qualification 'hedonist', which Edelman saw at the basis of the system of the self.[6] It can be seen there that the structure of the human order makes it possible to free ourselves from the model of the instinct, in order to see the drive as the general animator of psychic life, and to see what it is in the subject that gives him the feeling that life is worth living. Blocking out the pleasure in all this can only be the work of humans shut away in their ivory tower, ignorant of life and ignorant of themselves, failing to recognize the characteristics of which their being is made. By proposing the notion of subject line I am, then, proposing a range of notions which is rooted in bodily states and branches out into the deployment of thought. I do not wish to deny in any way that subjectivity, starting from desire, culminates in the intellect and in thinking. Aristotle had already seen this clearly more than 24 centuries ago (see below). It is more difficult on the other hand to understand how this trajectory is formed, what its dynamics are, what aim it tends towards, and what tasks it accomplishes. In the criticisms which I sometimes make of cognitivism (with the backing of Gérald Edelman), the issue is not to deny the virtues of the intellect, but to ask oneself if they can be considered as being independent or 'autonomous', or if one should not always recognize the necessity of placing intellect and cognition at the heart of a theory of the psyche linking them to the body.

One can understand, then, that the reference to a range or a spectrum makes it possible, depending on the problem being considered, to give a role to this or that aspect without laying any claims to a unification which would end up feeling artificial. Let us take an example. When we are speaking of a borderline case, we cannot avoid giving prominence to the notion of the ego: its limits, its defences, its object choices, its relation to repetition-compulsion, etc. In such a case, it would seem to me wrong to put the chief accent on the subject, not because the latter does not exist, but because he is not the cornerstone of the conflictual situation. On the other hand, when we are speaking about a neurotic case, the reference to the subject seems more pertinent than simply referring to the ego, which would seem to be somewhat reductive and incapable of accounting for the symbolic richness of the manifestations. And if we consider now a patient suffering from psychosomatic disturbances, it will be seen that it is necessary to take into consideration a factor situated at the level of the instinctual or affective sphere, which has not been able to organize itself at this level, and which has shaken the foundations of the psyche. At bottom, I am doing nothing more than recalling Freud's quasi-Heraclitean aphorism: *Wo Es war soll Ich werden*, for which rival translations do not cease to abound. And yet the idea in question is clearly expressed: 'Where id was (the id and not it), there ego shall be (and not, there I shall be)'. As for knowing if one should say the ego or the subject, without pretending to be able to decide in domains in which I am not competent, it would seem to me that reference to the theory requires that we refer to the terminology that it uses referentially – in other words, the id and the ego. It is not by complicating the vocabulary and the syntax that one succeeds in modifying the semantics of the proposition.

It remains that an approach is lacking that is capable of gathering together, and even of giving a meaning to, that which might appear somewhat nebulous with functions that are very difficult to grasp. This is what was being attempted by proposing the notion of the *process of subjectivation* (R. Cahn[7] followed by S. Weinrib and F. Richard[8]). Although this notion has not acquired as much clarity as one would like, it can be assumed that the process of subjectivation is a new perspective making it possible to think about psychic evolution from the standpoint of a *subjective appropriation*. This does not simply transcend past stages, but integrates them in the name of a subjectivity in process, encountering many perils which compromise its acquisitions, and navigating at the risk of running into inclement weather of psychotic nature, especially in adolescence. There is nothing to be gained from concealing the pitfalls of theoretical exposition which, on the one hand, runs the risk of falling into phenomenological description, and, on the other, of representing a new version of a normative genetic vision. It is nonetheless true that the perils of subjectivation offer an interesting way of understanding adolescent pathology.

I am more and more persuaded that psychoanalysis would benefit from adopting a *theory of gradients* which, along each line, is obliged to decide which aspect is most concerned in the problem under consideration. I am quite certain that the idea of considering the drive as the matrix of the subject will give rise to many objections. A careful re-reading of Freud will show that he does not say anything different. What is the compulsion to repeat? The 'instinct of the instinct', as Pasche used to say; the essence of the drive, as I would say today; or again, a subjectivity in action which is unaware of itself, a force, a will, which, after an evolution and sufficient maturity, will take the form of a desire, rationalized for consciousness. What does the fabric of history or the fabric of our present consist of, if not a confluence of instinctual vicissitudes?

Let us return once more to the *Outline*. In the chapter on the theory of the instincts, we can read, immediately after the term is mentioned for the first time in the work: 'Though they are the ultimate cause of all activity, they are of a conservative nature.'[9] These exigencies which, at the outset, were of a somatic order and represent in the psyche 'the imperious needs of the id', will remain, over the course of time, and against all the odds, 'the ultimate cause of all activity' – the more things change, the more things are the same. This cause has to be sought for in the foundations of experience and it also has to be understood that it is little suited to changes, marked as it is by obstinate conservatism. Does this not amount to saying that the id is linked to the oldest and the most reactionary sources of our existence?

Opposite, is the *object line*. For this we have less help from the Freudian elaboration than for the subject line, for, though he spoke about it, and not-withstanding some observations of great interest, Freud has been recognized as being guilty of not having defined its place sufficiently. In the post-Freudian literature and already in Freud's lifetime, with Abraham, the place of the object has constantly grown and been embellished to the point of suffocating the representatives of the subject line, reducing them to the meanest share. In the limited confines of this study, I cannot develop all the aspects related to it in an exhaustive manner.[10] When one reflects on the question of the object, one sees that the conception that analysts give of it depends largely on the context in which they situate themselves (Melanie Klein, Winnicott, Lacan). Accordingly, it is always a matter of referring to a particular concept, whether it has been treated by Freud or not, in its own theoretical space. We know that it is the space which creates the object, whereas the object can only suggest by its immediate environment the space in which it is situated. Nevertheless, a consideration of the question enables us to reach important observations or conclusions.[11] I shall recall them here. The object can be broken down as follows:

1 A part, assimilable by the ego, received by transmission and deposit, of the product of the exchanges between the drives and the object. The identifiable part can be detected through identifications.
2 A part defined as the *property of the ego*, and different from it. Its essential aim is to ward off the strangeness of the object and includes the potentiality to burden it with hate owing to its difference, to its resistance, its independence. Its essential vicissitude is loss.
3 A *desired* part which the ego wishes to appropriate. Conceived of as being external to it, it is expected to become a party to desire. It has to face up to what is impossible and what is prohibited as well as to their consequences.
4 A *transformable* part, either by the appearance of new satisfactions, or to satisfy substitutive desires for those that have not been realized, or to ward off the vicissitudes of non-realization.
5 A part serving as a support for the *creativity* of new objects or of new functions which will be able to receive the status of objects secondarily.
6 A part that is *irreducible to any form of appropriation by the ego* which calls for the recognition of difference and alterity.

It can be seen that we are dealing here with different ideas that are met with constantly in different contexts: those of multiplicity, heterogeneity, and the impossibility of arriving at a unified concept. Here the example of language has a conceptual referential value, but refers to its partial equivalence in the psyche. We must accept that a homogenizing unity has to be renounced. The object line is thus at once similar and different to the precedent line. It differs from it in that it opposes only two terms: object (*objectal*) and objective.[12] In the theory, before envisaging the multiplicity of the aspects in which the object intervenes, its function should be clarified: phantasy object, real object, object of the id, object of the ego, etc.

I have attempted to establish the *co-determinants* of the object: that is to say, the function of what I now define as forming part of the subject line (ego, drives, etc). As far as the drive is concerned, I have examined in detail the way in which the object reveals the drive, the latter appealing to the object for its satisfaction. The numerous studies which have referred to the object relation have taken the transference as their point of departure: that is to say, in psychoanalytic practice, the object manifests itself primarily as a transference object. It can be said that the transference takes its object as its starting-point and constructs itself around it, just as, conversely, the object is constructed by the transference.

It is this reference to the transference which has brought about a progressive retreat of psychoanalytic theory into clinical practice, while keeping its distance from applied psychoanalysis, a cause of numerous disappointments on the part of specialists in the disciplines concerned. Freud had had the sad experience of this (kite taken for a vulture in Leonardo, questionable speculations on the murder of Moses, etc.). Henceforth, by basing themselves on clinical practice alone, psychoanalysts do not run the risk of suffering fresh rebuffs and unnecessary humiliations by arguments that are often more clever than convincing (think of Vernant crushing Anzieu). As far as I am concerned, and although the present work makes no reference to it (like the *Outline*), I think I have contributed to demonstrating the fruitfulness of such an approach. I even think that the absence of any perspective of applied psychoanalysis tends to shrink the vision of the so-called 'pure' psychoanalyst.

As I have emphasized, at each stage, the absence of homogenization, I am going to pursue this direction, by considering the functions of the object. In order to define the 'physiology' of the object, I have proposed 12 functions.[13] Here I will just cite the chapter headings with a minimum of explanation:

1 Function of investment.
2 Function of reflection: the invested object sends back the investment to the source from which it comes, after transformation.
3 Function of arousal and framing: the object stimulates instinctual life. Framing is the trace of its mark outside the experiences of satisfaction.
4 Function of perceptibility: perception attests to the presence of the object. Outside it, there is the field of representation and, beyond it, the representations of relations (thought).
5 Function of acceptability: it brings into play the capacity of the ego which, by accepting this function, allows the ego to find itself again in the object as the cause of its pleasure while waiting for reciprocity
6 Function of illusion: upholds the idea of a mutually unique and irreplaceable relationship.
7 Function of attraction: at the origin of the decentring of the subject towards the object.
8 Function of satisfaction: always partial and temporary. It contributes to the development of the means for increasing the capacity for integrating the destructive drives. When direct satisfaction is lacking, the function exerts a valorizing action due to the resistance to satisfaction.
9 Function of substitution: replacement of one object by another, one aim by another, one investment by another, while guaranteeing the continuity of the pole from which the investments originate.
10 Function of releasing anxiety as a danger signal.
11 Function of induction in order to establish the modalities of reunion and separation.
12 Function of creation: creation of new objects, new activities and new fields capable of becoming objects in their turn (objectalizing function).

This description often blends properties attributable to the ego. But when included in this ensemble, the dominant note remains on the side of the object. After Marjorie Brierley, Lebovici wrote: 'The object is invested before it is perceived.'[14] The study of these 12 functions is far from exhaustive. The list could be extended; perhaps one could also achieve a greater condensation.

When one speaks of the primary object relations, what is being referred to? On the one hand the reference is to a force of attraction on the part of the object (J.-B. Pontalis)[15] and, on the other, via the relationship, to the establishment of a fundamental magnetization. Nevertheless, it remains useful to distinguish between attraction, giving rise to desire and thus mobilizing the subject, and attachment, which is a more basic process, of a quasi-ethological nature.

The most striking point in my study is the description of what I have called the *objectalizing function*, and its antithesis, the *disobjectalizing function*. Their origin can be traced back to the final theory of the drives, but one can describe their principal mechanisms by drawing on concepts less ideologically loaded than Eros and the destructive drives, using the terms *binding* and *unbinding* as equivalents at the level of the basic modes of functioning of instinctual activity. Binding and unbinding should be conceived of from the double angle of the bindings within the ego and internal objects, and of those which unite the ego with external objects. Without knowing it, Freud gave an illustration of the objectalizing function in the theory of melancholy, where the ego divides itself in order to deal with the loss of the object, one part of it identifying with the lost object. This sacrificial mode maintains the cannibalistic oral relationship. But the objectalizing function can also manifest itself during sublimation or in the production of transitional objects emerging from the intermediary space (Winnicott). The object of sublimation is not the book, but reading. One can see, in fact, that what is involved is a metafunction, the product of the super-cession of the functions described above, which form the starting platform. If incorporation and introjection are the post primitive modes of relating to the object (coupled, of course, with excorporation and projective identification), it is possible to imagine that these continue, throughout the whole of life, beyond the period when they represent the general model of psychic activity. This is what is at stake in internalization and identification. However, the appropriation of the ego is not limited to a process which makes the object 'travel' from the outside towards the inside. The ego is not content with transforming the status of the objects with which it enters into relationship; it *creates* objects out of instinctual activity, when the latter, by transforming itself, becomes an object. Thus psychic functions assume the status of objects. The limit of the process of transformation of the objectalizing function is that beyond which this process cannot be pursued.

During all these changes, it is essential that the *significant investment* referring to what is full of meaning and important is maintained. It can be seen that psychic life continually creates object forms which nourish psychic life. What

119

can perhaps be understood here is that, for the psyche, the issue is one of ensuring, by means of multiple, constantly renewed and nourished moorings, that the necessary detachment from primary objects has been compensated for without too much damage by virtue of a substitution (metaphorizing, in some cases). This process endows the ego with internal possessions by tearing it away from the grip of a narcissism that is running in neutral, as it were. Thus the limits or the failures that can be encountered in the quest for satisfaction are part of the general equilibrium in which what is lost on one side can be compensated by what is gained on the other. But of course, this economic perspective cannot help the subject surmount the loss of objects considered as unique and irreplaceable, such as the primary object. I think that even if one recognizes the most elementary instinctual bases of the concept of the object, it must, in contradistinction to what Lacan claims, culminate in a relative formal unity (or at least be on the way to totalization: Melanie Klein), as clinical work shows. On the other hand, I would say that the whole object is not the crowning achievement of the object's path. Just as, in Freudian theory, the Oedipus complex continues with the superego, in contemporary theory recognition must be given, in accordance with Lacan, to the big Other. Of course, I am quite aware that the problem deserves more than a passing reference. It nonetheless seems futile to attempt to win acceptance for the conception of the object in order to do without that of the other (the Other), or the contrary.

As is often the case, once I have concluded a study, a citation of Freud[16] comes back to my memory: in the posthumous notes that he left, dated 12 July 1938, he wrote:

> 'Having' and 'being' in children. Children like expressing an object-relation by an identification: 'I am the object.' 'Having' is the later of the two; after loss of the object it relapses into 'being'. Example: the breast. 'The breast is a part of me, I am the breast.' Only later: 'I have it' – that is, 'I am not it' . . .

As is often the case, Freud's lucidity is a few lengths ahead of our theorizations. How can one express oneself more clearly? Object relation and identification are linked. Having is not conceivable without being. The loss of having makes one relapse into being. Many polemics would be avoided if only analysts would be a little more attentive in their reading of Freud.

I shall round off this chapter by referring to a function that is complementary to the one before, which I have called the *disobjectalizing function*. It is immediately clear that, while the objectalizing function appears to be an interesting elaboration of what Freud calls Eros, the disobjectalizing function is connected, on the contrary, with the difficult question of the drives of destruction. It will be understood that in the disobjectalizing function, it is not only the relation to the object that comes under attack, but also all its substitutes and, in the long term, the ego itself. Ultimately, it is *investment, inasmuch as it has undergone the process of objectalization*, which is at stake. The manifestation which seems to me to specifically characterize the destructivity of the death drive is *disinvestment*. Among the important contributions of Melanie Klein for our understanding of psychosis is her reference to the paranoid-schizoid position which speaks more of the paranoid component than of the schizoid component (that of the 'schize'). This means, in fact, that this complex process couples *paranoid investment with schizoid disinvestment*. Paradoxically, in the case of mourning, the disobjectalizing function, far from coinciding with it, is the most radical procedure for resisting the work which should lead to its resolution. Similarly, I have linked the disobjectalizing function to the activity of a *negative narcissism*, thereby arriving at a dual conception of narcissism to which I have already referred. In short, this duality opposes positive narcissism or the narcissism of the One, where the psyche aspires for ego unity by concealing, in its own interest, object investments which are maintained but not lost, and, negative narcissism, an aspiration for a zero level of investments which have suffered the fate of loss, and where it is the investment of the ego itself that finally succumbs to this deadly form of subjective disinvestment.[17] An entire sector of pathology can be seen under a new light when these considerations are taken into account – namely, disorders of the elementary functions of incorporation and introjection (anorexia, and even certain forms of depression in which *essential depression* [P. Marty] plays a prominent part).

This disobjectalizing function can be related to concepts presented by other authors (Bion's 'attacks on linking', Lacan's 'foreclosure'). Generally speaking, it is clear that what is involved are operations of radical negativity (excessive projective identification, or the refusal of 'wanting to know nothing about it'). Underlying these operations is the illusion of freeing the psyche of conflicts which it cannot resolve, without realizing however that, at the same time, it empties the psychic apparatus and bleeds it white.

By giving a place to the two main categories of the objectalizing and disobjectalizing function, one obtains a rich range of combinations of the type that Freud had already proposed with fusion and defusion. Since we are touching here on the idea of the relations between binding and unbinding, I want to suggest the following formulation: if it is fair to consider that the pathology connected with Eros consists of a dialectical play in which binding and unbinding alternate and are combined (which means in short that, owing to fusion, the process of unbinding has in a way been partially integrated, if not tamed), on the other hand I think that the effects of the destructive drive, insofar as it tends towards defusion, without being counterbalanced by an interplay with Eros, should lead us to make the hypothesis, in the most extreme cases, and the most radically destructive situations, of mechanisms almost exclusively characterized by destructivity.

Conclusion

It can be seen that, in accordance with my hypotheses, I am endeavouring to bring together the heterogeneous constituents of the major modalities of functioning. These groupings will serve to define synergetic or antagonistic modes of functioning. We thus arrive at a theory which is less concerned with describing singular entities than with attempting to reinsert these unities within a dynamic spectrum or within a range of states which are in a permanent state of potential transformation. I have, accordingly, constituted separately the subject and object lines, by proposing to consider, each time, which element of a given line is involved and by envisaging the relations which may exist between the element within its line and the element, or corresponding elements, in the complementary line. I propose to designate this way of seeing things as a *theory of gradients*. In meteorology, a gradient is the variation of atmospheric pressure evaluated in millimetres and by geographical degrees between a given point and the closest centre of cyclones or anticyclones. Without claiming that a correspondence exists point for point, it can be seen that I am more sensitive to the variation of pressure than to the definition of a delimited zone, and that I link this variation to a centre (in fact to two: cyclone and anticyclone governed by a relation of opposition). In short, my theoretical exposition relates the elements of the line, both the subject line and the object line, to the cyclone and anticyclone of the groups characterized by the drives of destruction and of Eros. This not only means that one swallow does not make a summer, but also that the atmosphere is always more or less agitated, undergoing the effect of contrary currents, except in the ephemeral happiness of the state of shared love.

In so doing, it seems to me that we are fulfilling a double aim. The first is to envisage Freudian theory within a new context; and the second is to remedy the deficiency denounced by the majority of authors who have reproached Freud for not having given sufficient consideration to the role of the object and its response to the desires and demands of the subject. I am not be satisfied with acknowledging the validity of this reproach without proposing to formulate it slightly differently with a view to understanding it. Though it is true that the role of the object does not occupy a sufficient place in Freud's work, it still needs to be understood that ultimately, *what the analyst is dealing with is a subject who is the product of his exchanges*; but, insofar as he has constituted himself through them, he can now only be envisaged *on the basis of his own structure as a subject*. This argument, without clearing Freud, throws some light on his theoretical position. If I hesitate to push this thesis further, it is because in practice, in the analytic situation, such an argument can too easily be used for turning analysts into emulators of Pontius Pilate. As for what unfolds in the treatment and in the transference, those who have adopted this role claim to have no responsibility for it. It is the patient's affair. Let him get by as best he can with his Other. I mean the other who is in him; for the other outside him simply reflects the image that the analysand has of it. This attitude can often be recognized in Lacanian practices. And yet experience shows that what is involved here is a point of view *ad usum delphini*, which puts the analyst, in all circumstances, beyond any possibility of reproach, whatever he says or does not say, whatever he does himself or allows to happen. Here fortunately, other examples than those linked with Lacan come to our rescue, giving us a more exact appreciation of the analytic situation. We can think, for instance, of Bion and Winnicott, without however claiming that they resolve all the problems. They nonetheless lead us to think about how the analyst, who is massively involved in a heavily charged situation, has to be able to respond to it without satisfying the patient's demand, while remaining firmly on course and lucid in his interpretations. There are many Lacanians, I am sure – and they are not alone – who think that this is a reprehensible deviation.[18] As we know from Freud, 'The Book tells us it is no sin to limp.'[19]

Notes

1 Fairbairn, W.R. (1952). *Psychoanalytic Studies of the Personality*. London: Tavistock Publications.

2 See Green, A. L'objet a de J. Lacan, sa logique et la théorie freudienne, *Cahiers pour l'analyse*, 1966; reprinted in *Propédeutique*, ch. 6. Paris: Champ Vallon.

3 Green, A. *Propédeutique*, ibid.

4 Ibid.

5 The note in French here is: I prefer *subjectal* to *subjectif*, on account of its symmetry with *objectal*.

6 Edelman, G. (1992). *Bright Air, Brilliant Fire. On the Matter of Mind*. New York: Basic Books.

7 Cahn, R. (1991). *L'adolescent dans la psychanalyse. L'aventure de la subjectivation*. Paris: Presses Universitaires de France.

8 Richard, F. (2001). *Le processus de subjectivation à l'adolescence*. Paris: Dunod.

9 Freud, S. (1938). *An Outline of Psychoanalysis, S.E.* XXIII, 148.

10 I refer the interested reader to the third part of my work *Propédeutique. La métapsychology revisitée*, Paris: Champ Vallon, 1995, which comprises four studies: chapter VI: 'L'objet *a* de J. Lacan'; chapter VII: 'La psychanalyse, son objet, son avenir'; chapter VIII: 'De l'objet non unifiable à la fonction objectalisante'; chapter IX: 'L'objet et la fonction objectalisante'.

11 Green, A. ibid., p. 221.

12 What is designated in French here, quite clearly, although *objectal* is not used much in non-specialized vocabularies, has no equivalent, it should be noted, in English. '*Objectal*' does not exist; only 'objective' bears a relation to its French homologue. What is used, then, is 'object' as in object relationship.

13 I refer the reader to my work: De l'objet non unifiable à la fonction objectalisante. In: *Propédeutique*. Paris: Champ Vallon.

14 Lebovici, S. La relation objectale chez l'enfant. In: *La psychiatrie de l'enfant*, 1961, III, part I.

15 Pontalis, J.-B. (1999). *La force d'attraction*. Paris: Le Seuil.
16 Freud, S. (1941[1938]). Findings, Ideas, Problems, *S.E.* XXIII, 299.
17 Elsewhere (*The Work of the Negative*, pp. 148, 149, 156), I have called this 'the *subjectal* disengagement of the Ego'.
18 Which will not prevent them, in private, from conducting highly transgressive practices. By way of illustration, see the article – not read enough – by Helena Schulz-Keil entitled 'A Trip to Lacania', *Hystoria*, Special Issue 6–9, published by the New York Lacan Study Group, NY, 1988, pp. 226–245. One could also profitably read by the same Helena Schulz-Keil, 'Lacan in the English Language', in the same issue, particularly pp. 202–203.
19 Freud, S. *Beyond the Pleasure Principle, S.E.* XVIII, 64.

9

THE ANALYSIS OF THE MATERIAL INTO ITS COMPONENT PARTS

Representations

It is difficult, in a work of this kind, to avoid repetition. The way it is divided up leads one to touch upon the same problem several times owing to the different angles from which it presents itself. If I had, at all costs, to characterize the essential paradigm of psychoanalysis, I would situate it, without hesitation, on the side of representation. When one speaks of the world of representation in psychoanalysis, one confines oneself in general to the canonical couple thing-presentation–word-presentation. There is no denying that such a couple is at the heart of the Freudian problematic of representation. Every connoisseur of Freud's work will recall Appendix C of the *Standard Edition* for the paper on 'The Unconscious' in the *Papers on Metapsychology*, where Strachey traces the ideas put forward by Freud in 1915 back to his much earlier monograph on aphasia in 1891.[1] This often happens when a powerful idea emerges in Freud's work; not infrequently the roots of it can be traced back to a much earlier time, in this case 24 years before. Even though the intuition of 1891 emerged from reflecting on the physiology of the brain, it anticipated future approaches to the psyche. It culminated in the clear distinction between the system of word-presentations, comprised of elements of language formed of exclusive and limited unities (*Project*) forming a closed ensemble, and the system of thing-presentations, described as a multiple system made up of memory traces belonging to different senses and open. It should be noted that the word-presentation is not linked to the object-presentation by all its constituents, but only by its sound-image – visual associations being for the object what the sound-image is for the word. At any rate, Freud's inventiveness in approaching this problem from the neuro-logical angle would be pursued and enriched when he was led to distinguish the system preconscious-conscious in which word-presentations are associated with thing-presentations, whereas the system unconscious is formed only of thing- or object-presentations, which Freud qualifies as the 'only true object-cathexes'.

I have insisted in many of my writings on the necessity of conceiving of a theory of representation which covers a more comprehensive field. In my opinion, a distinction must be made between the ideational representative of the drive and what Freud calls the psychical representative of the drive. Many differences allow us to understand the interest of distinguishing them. When Freud speaks of the ideational representative (*Vorstellungsrepräsentanz*), he has in mind the part which concerns representation in repression insofar as it is opposed to affect. Let us recall here the important distinction to the effect that representations are memory traces, whereas affects are processes of discharge. This element of the psyche is linked to a model in which representation is the image that refers to an object situated outside the psyche, in external reality, through perception. Here we are in the context of the optical model and in the extension of the psychical apparatus of *The Interpretation of Dreams*, the source of the first topography, based on the model of the telescope. On the other hand, when Freud speaks of the psychical representative of the drive (*psychische Repräsentanz*), he is referring to the way in which instinctual excitation, of endosomatic origin, reaches the psyche and manifests itself at the level of the body – for example, thirst, translating itself into a tickling sensation of dryness of the mucous membrane of the pharynx (*Papers on Metapsychology*). Let us note in passing that Freud scarcely makes any distinction between need and desire, a distinction hypostasized by Lacan. But the essential point is to understand that the psychical representative of the drive is a manifestation of the delegation of the demands of the body to the psyche. There is, moreover, matter for thought here, since the drive, according to Freud's definition, *is* the psychic representative of stimuli arising from within the organism; and Freud also says that the drive *has* psychic representatives. The drive as such is unknowable. Only its representatives are knowable, in the first rank of which must be placed the psychical representative of the drive. The drive is theoretically a phenomenon on the boundary between the psychic and the somatic. It has its roots in the soma and, in this form, it is scarcely knowable; whereas its psychical representative can be known, since it manifests itself through an alteration of the state of the body in need of satisfaction, which is felt by the subject. The drive, as a demand of the body, is waiting for satisfaction, but this satisfaction is not always in the service of adaptation. A glass of water relieves thirst, but the thirst can become the sign of an alcoholic addiction. Likewise, during a prolonged stay in the desert, quenching one's thirst immediately without an appropriate intake of salt can worsen the somatic condition and result in harmful consequences. What we have to understand here is that the optical model is no longer appropriate. There is no connection between the tickling sensation in the throat, which the psyche associates with thirst, and the dehydrated state of the organism, which translates itself in biological terms by haemoconcentration among other things. The model in question in this last case is that of the somato-psychic relation where the psychic is conceived of as a delegation of the body. One could conceive, at the unconscious level, of an appeal aroused by a need requiring satisfaction which is manifested by the emanation of a psychical representative, the psychical representative calling to its aid the vestiges of an earlier experience of satisfaction deposited in the form of mnemic traces of the ideational representative of the drive (thirst + imagination of the thirst-quenching drink). Thus the two models require each other to produce the elaborated instinctual excitation, that is to say, accompanied by the representation of the object of satisfaction (thirst + breast).

I know that this explanation raises many difficulties. Freud explains that it is the failure of this solution which, entailing persistent or even increasing dissatisfaction, leads to a state of motor agitation in the child expressing his unease and his expectation of a more efficacious response – a state of agitation that is deciphered and understood by the mother who then provides the desired satisfaction. The objection has been made that it is difficult to understand why the child does not exhaust itself through hallucinatory wish fulfilment (Laplanche). To be honest, I do not find this argument very convincing. It seems admissible that the child resorts to hallucination in the hope that a lure will bring the same relief as the object; then, noticing that nothing has changed, and even that everything is getting worse, he expresses greater signs of distress which are perceived, understood (that is, a meaning is given to them, an interpretative violence [P. Aulagnier]) and calmed by the mother. In reality, this critical position translates the desire to introduce the object at a very early point in the relation of distress while reducing the margin of manoeuvre of intrapsychic trans-formations due to the drive. Now, in my view, the conceptions of anaclisis, clearly identified in Freud's text by Laplanche, seem to me to be very useful for underlining the autonomization of desire in contrast to need. Furthermore, psychical elaboration based in the drives seems to me to be of cardinal importance for mental functioning, in that it gives birth to hallucinatory wish fulfilment. It places strong emphasis on the subject's omnipotence, on the illusory effect of personal psychic constructions; similarly, it helps us to understand the role of primitive narcissism constructing its world by making use of the object (internal) as it wishes. Naturally this is only possible, as Freud had already pointed out, if the system of maternal care does not allow the subject to decline into impotence.

I have already defined three modes of representatives: (1) the psychical representative of the drive, closest to the body; (2) the ideational representative, that is, representation in the form of the memory-trace of an object situated outside the psyche; and (3) the word-presentation, a system constituted via derivations uniting concretely and abstractly the subject, the object and the referent. This system arises from a work on the thing-presentation. But that is not all. In 1924, in the first of the two articles on the relations between neurosis and psychosis, 'The Loss of Reality in Neurosis and Psychosis', Freud was led to clarify the nature of the transformation of reality in psychosis which is carried out upon ideas derived from former relations to it, that is, 'upon the memory-traces, ideas and judgements which have been previously derived from reality and by which reality was represented in the mind'.[2] We understand here that the conception of reality in Freud is by no means simple; nor, in spite of appearances, is it something purely given. Though in the definition I have selected there is a clear reference to memory traces, the reference to ideas and judgements shows that Freud has the necessary distinctions present in his mind. It is the function of judgement that is involved here. Freud wrote this sentence a year before tackling the problem of negation, which he was to treat in an original manner by bringing into play successively the means of the judgement of attribution and the judgement of existence. His master stroke was to put the judgement of attribution first (chronologically) and, the judgement of existence second. Such is the coherence of psychoanalytic thought which sees, in the work of the psychical apparatus, first the distinction between good (that which can be incorporated) and bad (that which can be expelled), according to purely internal criteria.[3] It is only later that it is decided if the objects thus classed are the pure product of its functioning or if they also exist in reality.

We are now in possession of a complete system which starts with the psychical representative of the drive, closely linked to the body, opens out into thing- or object-presentations (unconscious and conscious), links up in consciousness with word-presentations, and finally joins the representatives of reality in the ego, implying relations with thought. My theory of gradients is once again confirmed as necessary for a fruitful interpretation of Freudian theory.

My reason for stating, at the beginning of this series of reflections, that I would situate without hesitation the paradigm of psychoanalytic theory on the side of representations, seems to me to be justified due to the fact that the essence of psychoanalytic experience, insofar as the classical treatment is concerned, depends on the very fact of the analyst's presence–absence (that is, his invisibility), on psychical activity inducing representation and exciting the patient's earlier memory traces which are here put to the test in the transference. The spectrum of modes of representation that we have defined merely corresponds to the range of psychic manifestations that are connected, on the one hand, with the body, and, on the other with reality and thinking. Going even further, one could conceive of the whole psyche as an *intermediate formation* between soma and thinking (Figure 9.1).

The relation defined by the interaction between an organismic soma and its environment in reality is the one we use most of the time for apprehending animal life. Accordingly, in man it is the high consistency, range and complexity of the processes of this intermediate formation which constitute its richness. It must also be added that it is here, in a manner in which Freud, as we know, did not fully explore, that the role of reality comes into play, the locus of the other,

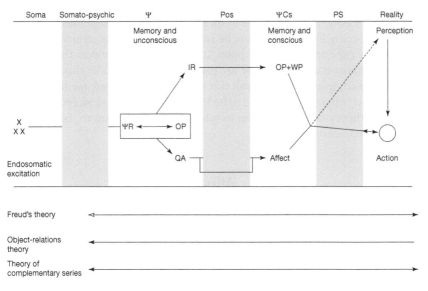

Figure 9.1 It is easy to transform this schema which refers to the first topography into the terms of the second topography: Id, anchored in the somatic, devoid of representations; Ego, unconscious and conscious; Superego, anchored in the Id, covering the territories of the unconscious and conscious Ego, crowning the whole. *Schema of the four territories: soma, unconscious, conscious, reality.* It will be seen that the field of relations between the subject and the world is divided into four territories: the *soma* proper, in which the drive is anchored in a hypothetical psychic form; the unconscious, the locus for the constitution of the basic cell psychical representative of the drive and object representation (subdivided into ideational representative and quantum of affect which will seek to enter consciousness); the conscious, where bindings are formed between the corresponding object (or thing) presentations and word presentations and qualitative affect; reality, the locus where the external object is linked with the precedent through perception and action. Three zones of transition: between *soma* and unconscious: the somato-psychic barrier; between the unconscious and the conscious: the preconscious; between the conscious and reality: the protective shield. This schema can be transformed from the first to the second topography and according to object-relations theory.

ψR = psychical representative of the drive
IR = ideational representative
QA = quantum of affect
OP = thing or object presentation (conscious or unconscious)
WP = word presentation
O = object

The dotted lines represent respectively:
– the somato-psychic limit (in short ψ *Ucs*)
– the barrier of the preconscious (*Pcs*) and the representative
– which is coextensive with it
– the protective shield (P.S.)

the *similar other*, I would say, and then the Other, a more general category which can only be defined in relation to a subject. *There is no subject except for another.* We are leaving behind us here the individual representations of which we have just been speaking in order to add to them those which emerge for us through cultural experience. For could there be an Other which is not an elaboration of this cultural experience? On this point, it is necessary to compare the conceptions of Winnicott and Lacan. For my part, although I consider that these two theories are complementary, I admit that my own journey took me from Lacan to Winnicott, whose work seemed to be less ideologically marked. From it there emerges a theory of symbolization to which I feel closer than to the Lacanian theory of symbolism.

Affects

When analysing the Freudian conception of representations, I used to wonder if it was not possible to speak of an affect representative of the drive. This seems to me to be both possible and debatable. The argument that can be raised against such a solution is the opposition, in Freud's thought, between ideas as memory traces and affects as processes of discharge. The difference stands out immediately. The traces, owing to the fact that they are not discharged, are retained in the psychical apparatus and form part of the memory system. By contrast, affective discharge cannot be bound because it is liquidated each time it is invested. And yet, how can one contest that there is an affective memory? How can one deny that the discharges leave traces of the experiences which have pushed towards the discharge and 'memorize' the discharge itself. There is thus justification for thinking that it is less a question of an absolute opposition than of two different modalities, one of which inscribes the traces with a very reduced quantity of psychic energy, the essential portion being affected to the binding of ideas; and the other, which, consuming more psychic energy, liquidates itself in part through discharge but also leaves, in its own manner, traces which can be reawakened (see anxiety). Today I would say that, metapsychologically, if one takes into account the product of the division of the psychical representative into ideational representative and affect representative,[4] it is not illegitimate to see in affect a derived form of the instinctual representative – one, precisely, which cannot be accounted for by the links between the ideational representatives. However, if one wants to stick to the Freudian distinction, then affect will be excluded from the system of representative memory traces. Clearly, both conceptions can be defended and, as far as I am concerned, I would be more in favour of placing affect at the heart of the general system of representation, acknowledging its specific and particular traits. Such a preamble is, I think, necessary before engaging in a reflection on this problem of the *Papers on Metapsychology*, which remains one of the most difficult to resolve. It seems to me indispensable to recall that the links between affect and the body have always been recognized as essential. This is borne out by the different theories of the emotions. They differ on whether the participation of the body should be given first or second place. Between my first theoretical exposition of this question (1970–1973) and the most recent (1999),[5] I have become increasingly aware in my thinking of the complexity of the problem. I want to return here to two ideas. The first concerns the integration of affect in the chain of the discourse, accentuating or colouring qualitatively this or that part of it; or, on the contrary, the case where one witnesses the unfurling of affective forces, overwhelming the concatenation of the discourse. I will take the liberty of citing from my own work from 1970–1973:

> The affect appears to be taking the place of representation. The process of linkage is a linkage of cathexes in which the affect has an ambiguous structure. Insofar as it appears as an element of discourse, it is subjected to that chain, includes itself in it as it attaches itself to the other elements of discourse. But insofar as it breaks with representations, it is the element of discourse that refuses to let itself be linked by representation and takes its place. A certain quantity of attacked cathexis is accompanied by a qualitative mutation; the affect may then snap the chain of discourse, which then sinks into discursivity, the unsayable. The affect is then identified with the torrential cathexis that breaks down the dikes of repression, submerges the abilities of linkage and self-control. It becomes a deaf and blind passion, but ruinous for the psychical organisation. The affect of pure violence acts out this violence by reducing the ego to hopelessness, forcing it to cede to its force, subjugating it by the fascination of its power. The affect is caught between its linkage in discourse and the breaking of the chain, which gives back to the id its original power.[6]

The second idea that needs to be recognized, it seems to me, is that representation and affect appear to differ essentially with regard to their mode of binding. Whereas representations are bound together via concatenation, the mode of binding specific to affect is that of diffusion. It is indeed the danger of the spreading of an uncontrolled diffusion which creates the danger of affect overwhelming the chain of representations; affective diffusion can take over the entire body and dominate psychic life as a whole. In other words, affect, much more than representation, refers to forces which traverse, animate, or may even destroy the psyche.

This observation justifies the classical French perspective concerning the distinction between affective registers. It is in fact recognized that it is useful to classify the manifestations of affective life into feelings, emotions and passions.[7] A fourth field would be that of the humours, colouring affective life in general. Nevertheless, this classical psychological viewpoint becomes somewhat more complicated when one considers it from the standpoint of psychoanalysis.

Melanie Klein describes *memories in feeling*,[8] that is, recollections in the form of feelings. Generally speaking, though French psychoanalysis, with Lacan, is very faithful to the traditions of the intellectualizing thought of our language (with certain exceptions: Bouvet, C. Parat), English authors have a tendency, on the contrary, to give prominence to emotional experience as the fundamental paradigm of psychic life (W. R. Bion; D. W. Winnicott).

The mere statement of these different forms shows that the accent can be placed either on the representations, or on a more or less paroxysmal state, or on a relation which monopolizes psychical life and orients it as a whole towards realizing the aims of passion.[9] One notices immediately that the range of affects cannot be entirely dissolved into that of representations. Without being overly schematic, one can contrast a relative unity of affective life with the diversity of the functioning of the modalities of representation. Let us note here, however, something that has not been sufficiently observed by those authors who have explored the problem of affect: in his last theory of anxiety, divided into signal anxiety and automatic anxiety, Freud in fact developed a theory in which the affect of anxiety can assume the functions of a signal and thus forms part of the series signal − sign − signifier.[10] Thus, to the attempt to distinguish and categorize the events of psychical life corresponds the idea of a bridge between certain forms and others.

However, alongside the conception of the field of affect extending from the body to language (by the mediation of the voice, notably), the question which still remains problematic is that of the conscious or unconscious nature of affect. From this point of view, one of Freud's definitions (*Introductory Lectures on Psychoanalysis*) is marked by great clarity. Acknowledging the complex nature of affect, Freud detects two sorts of manifestations of it: (1) processes related to discharge; (2) the perception of these actions (motor) and the direct sensations of pleasure and unpleasure. Without any shadow of doubt it is the latter which are the most striking and which make a great richness of expression of affective manifestations possible. Freud's definition, as can be seen, tends to divide the phenomenon into three elements: (1) *discharge* is, in effect, a bodily process verging on the physiological; (2) the *perception of the discharge* is the translation of the bodily movement into that which manifests itself at the psychical level; the body is moved, because affected;[11] (3) finally, this perception of the movement is accompanied by an experience of specific quality, as has been pointed out, moreover, by Edelman. Here again, the work of a *process of 'affectation'* (M. de M'Uzan) may be noted, extending from the body to consciousness. As I have written:

> The endeavour to define affect is based on an indefinite use of the term: sometimes it designates a dynamic process whose fundamental characteristic is that it unfolds in a temporo-spatial sequence affecting, during one of these phases, the body beyond the ego; and, sometimes it designates the state proper

to a given moment or to a stage of this process, noticeable by its quality perceived by the ego.[12]

This definition which distinguishes between the dynamic process and one of its sequences seems to me to permeate the problematic of affect caught between diffusion and specific quality.

We still have to consider the problem of unconscious affect, which continues to divide authors. Logically, if one follows Freud, the characteristics of the conscious affect (the *qualia*) cannot exist at an unconscious level, which is completely reduced to processes. However, just as unconscious ideas are not devoid of content, it is necessary to conceive of an equivalent form for the qualities, notably of pleasure and unpleasure, without their qualitative features being present as such. We know that Freud tried to do this – not without difficulties – seeking initially to establish a correspondence between unpleasure and tension, and pleasure and relaxation. He was obliged to acknowledge subsequently, in 'The Economic Problem of Masochism' (1924), that there exist agreeable states of tension and also states of relaxation which generate unpleasure. In fact, the discussion of this problem has advanced since Edith Jacobson's contribution. She helped us to see that states of pleasure and unpleasure vary in respect of an axis of situations of tension and relaxation which can give rise to one or the other. Moreover, if one reads Freud closely, one realizes that he had come very close to this solution in *Beyond the Pleasure Principle*, when speaking of the necessity of taking into consideration *the modification of the quantity of cathexis or its oscillations in the unity of time*. At any rate, affect has the merit, by means of notions such as rhythm or continuity, of making us sensitive to certain primitive forms of the experience of time (Anne Denis). All the preceding remarks lead us to acknowledge what could be called the calibration and modulation of the affect depending on the agencies which take charge of it or on which it leaves its mark. The more we think about the bodily pole, the closer we come to the determinations of the id. The more we consider the affects, which can assume many shades, even to the point of functioning as a signal, the more we envisage the incidence of the ego. Finally, the more we refer to internal tensions, whose content is often imprecise, the more we see the mark of the superego. Nevertheless, in all these cases, the affective reference makes affect a fundamental internal phenomenon. It can be provoked, either by an excitation arising from the inside or from the outside, or by a reaction to another person's affective state. *It remains that the affective topography is an internal topography and that its investments are oriented from the inside towards the periphery of the body.* I have proposed to consider the affective process as an anticipation of the encounter of the subject's body with another body (the body of the other, imaginary or present).[13] Furthermore, I have pointed out for a long time now that the psyche may be conceived of as *the relation between two bodies, one of which is absent*. Let me say in passing that, in my view, the position which consists in preferring, where the question of affect in particular is concerned, the theory of object relations over Freud's metapsychology in no way resolves the problem of the unconscious affect. It is not clear how referring to the object relation which, from a psychoanalytic perspective, consists essentially in demonstrating its unconscious modalities, would allow us to advance an inch. But the lure of the object relation often lies, in fact, in the idea of describing a conscious or preconscious relation and making it pass for an unconscious one. This position has been defended by minds more concerned with appearing fashionable than rigorous.

In my Santiago report, I pointed out that none of the *alternative solutions of contemporary psychoanalysis has provided an answer to the questions posed by Freud: the relations between the somatic and the psychic; the relationship at the heart of the psyche between the derivatives of bodily demands owing to prematurity and those arising from contact with external objects possessing the capacity to respond to them; the specific work and mode of transition from representation of the world of things to the world of words; links between external objects and their forms in the internal world; the difference between representations and investments; the opposition between psychic reality and external reality; modes of transcending object-losses, etc.*[14]

Nevertheless, although these questions still remain in abeyance, clinical experience since Freud's death has faced us with new problems. I am thinking of states in which it is difficult to make a distinction between representation and affect. As a rule, such states can be recognized in patients who are often profoundly regressed and belong, in general, to non-neurotic structures. They have been given various labels by different authors (fear of annihilation, M. Klein; nameless anxiety, W. Bion; tormenting anxiety, D. Winnicott; essential depression, P. Marty; reduction of the double limit, A. Green, etc.). Fresh elements observable in the psyche of such patients have led to the creation of notions such as *ideographs* (Bion 1963); *pictograms* (Castoriadis-Aulagnier 1975); *composites of representation and affect* (Green 1973). What one is seeking to delineate here is modes of thinking that are archaic or more attached to psychic representatives of the drive as inchoate forms than as differentiated products.[15] In these affective configurations, one is often dealing, not only with the unsayable but with the irrepresentable.

If one takes the psyche en masse, one notices the absence of intermediate formations, that is to say, formations of the unconscious proper. The id dominates. It is not easy to characterize the defences of these subjects. Processes of evacuation through action or expulsion into the somatic predominate (Green 1975). One is struck by the poverty of phantasy life, as if the psyche were continually caught up in the actual, referring to the raw state connected with the events of life. Often, instead of taking the form of dreaming, hallucinatory activity is here experienced in waking life (hallucinatory presence felt without hallucinated content of the primary object). In any case, identification on a more or less kaleidoscopic level is present. It is easy to understand that acting out and/or somatization are commonplace. As for affective life proper, certain singular characteristics are striking. For instance, the sense of there being an *overflow* (*débordement*) of affect, which seems to drown the psyche. Likewise, variations in bodily perception, ranging from fusional proximity to varying degrees of distance including the abstraction and discarnation of bodily experience, show the importance of phenomena which have to overcome the danger of confrontation. As for the status of the object, transitionality is frequently lacking. The object undergoes transformations which make it pass from the state of being an omnipotent agency to a denial of its existence. Generally speaking, the psyche lives on a war footing, carrying out mutilating defences, such as the phenomena of negative hallucination, which often open the way for an invasion by the irrepresentable and for the manifestations of a tyrannical, arbitrary and demented superego.

These states give rise to a rich reflection on their origin as well as the functioning of the subjects in whom they are observed. One can exhaust oneself trying to construct genetic hypotheses – from the observation of development. Rightly or wrongly, I will not refer to them because I do not have the feeling that they really shed light on the problem. I shall even go as far as to assert that in fact they obscure it, while claiming to offer ideas which make it possible to simplify the conception of it improperly.

To conclude, we are reduced here to speculations drawn, on the one hand, from the very development of psychoanalytical thought, from Freud up to the present day and, on the other, from various fields of knowledge which have dealt with the problem of affect. I will not expand much on the contribution of phenomenology which often boils down to the formulation of paraphrases, without enabling us to get a better insight into the workings of the complex of affect. Let me emphasize, once again, the functionally inoperative character of intermediate formations: *that is, of psychic productions organized by primary processes involving a relative work of differentiation between affect and representation.*[16]

In other words, the psyche has an indispensable need for affect insofar as it is actively involved in the psychic processes. But any excessive dimension – and this is the moment to underline the considerable importance of the quantitative and, more generally, the economic point of view in affective life – disturbs the work of representation extending into the realm of thought. It will be seen, then, that for me, the primary process plays the role of an essential regulator at the origin of the formations of the unconscious.

One can hardly insist enough on the role of affects in the exchange between the mother and the child, and, more indirectly, of the child's relation to the father via the mediation of the mother's thinking. It can be said that one of the most successful forms of psychical activity in relation with affect is the genesis, differentiation and consolidation of the processes of *play*. Herein lies the considerable contribution of Winnicott, to which must be added his clarifications on the relations between instinctual activity (which destroys the capacity to play) and playful activity which extends far into the psyche and even involves highly abstract forms of functioning.

Before bringing this chapter to a close I want to speak of the important source of stimulation that I have received from certain contemporary thinkers whom I have cited en route. Let me recall the influence that the ideas of René Thom have had on me concerning the concept of *prégnance*, containing an explicit allusion to a model of affectivity (connected with the process of continuity) opposed to that of *saillance* (on which discontinuity is based). It is comforting to note that Thom proposed this theoretical statement during a period dominated by structuralism, which tended to deny the role of affect (one remembers with sadness the elaborations of Cl. Lévi-Strauss linking it with lactic acid!). On the side of neurobiology, here more than ever, I want to pay tribute to Gérald Edelman and his conception of the system of the Self, constituted by the relations between the *hedonist* (limbic) system and the thalamo-cortical system, whereas the system of relations with others is above all marked by its cortical networks. In short, the kernel of the Self, the most intimate part of ourselves, is marked by the categorization which gives prominence to the pleasure–unpleasure principle. These are simply orientations which cannot claim today to resolve decisively the problem of affect. Nevertheless, I find it very satisfying to note the agreement of psychoanalysis with certain theoretical conceptions of major interest that have emerged in recent decades. We are thus brought back to what is essential, namely, affective life, which is so deeply rooted in our body, as well as to its arborescent forms, in which the Other plays a decisive role, from the primary object to the Other of divine transcendence and concerning which the psychoanalyst can read, without being astonished, modern studies which do not hesitate to link up the productions of the great mystics (St Teresa of Avila, St John of the Cross) with the most fundamental erotic and sexual relations.

Character

Psychoanalysis was confronted with a problem which often caused authors difficulty, without their realizing the origin of what was embarrassing them. I am thinking to begin with of Freud himself, and then of some of his successors. Freud, as we have seen, chose a clinical model of reference, that of the transference psycho-neuroses. He was led to define *neurosis as the negative of perversion*. It seems to me that it can be legitimately claimed that, as time passed, and especially after 1924, it was no longer perversion that he wanted to set in opposition to neurosis, but psychosis. There is a significant deviation here. Subsequently the contrast in psychoanalysis between neurosis and borderline (a very imprecise and vague entity) was emphasized increasingly, resulting in the need to differentiate *neurotic structures and non-neurotic structures*. In due course, the development of certain theories led to another basis of comparison being proposed, for example, that of patients presenting somatic disorders. To the extent that neurosis today can no longer claim to play the role as a centre of reference in psychoanalytic practice, a certain disarray can be observed. Clinical thinking has become disoriented and is condemned now to content itself with juxtapositions, without our knowing yet which clinical entity is serving as a descriptive basis. I will be told that there is no need to have recourse to a central clinical entity and that it is enough to refer to psychic mechanisms that are sufficiently general to guide our thinking (the unconscious, repression, the Oedipus complex, etc.). I am afraid, though, that the facts resist such a suggestion more than one thinks. For one only has to take each of the elements selected for such a configuration to see that the transformations which they undergo in some patients scarcely allow us any longer to consider them as references that are sufficiently consensual. In 1975, in my report to the London Congress: 'The Analyst, Symbolization and Absence in the Analytic Setting',[17] I proposed a model for borderline cases, with a view to distinguishing the structure of borderline cases from that of neurosis. But soon, the convenient schematization of the two models was more or less called into question with the appearance of new ideas elaborated on the basis of other clinical structures. I am thinking particularly of theorizations concerning patients presenting somatic symptoms, a domain dominated by the conceptions of Pierre Marty in France.[18] Moreover, most theorists were not satisfied with a simple opposition between neurosis and psychosis. Very often, they added perversion or depression. The observation of these different difficulties has led me to undertake an important revision of the question and to propose another choice.

It seems to me that this idea of a revision followed the internal discussions which took place within psychoanalysis on the necessity of revising the concept of the drive. Several alternatives have been proposed. One should cite, first of all, the important current of object relations, illustrated in the most dazzling manner by the school of Melanie Klein; and then, under other skies, the defence by Kohut of a psychology of the self. I have shown, in the previous chapters, how there is a counterbalancing movement from one pole of the pendulum to the other. At one extreme, there is the object; at the other, the self and narcissism, leading to intersubjectivity. One cannot fail to be struck by the general movement which induced analysts to turn away from Freud's hypotheses and to widely reject the theory of the drives. It is not difficult to see that the arguments raised are based on Freud's negligence concerning the object (or the other subject of intersubjectivity) due to what has appeared, over the course of time, as the mark of an excessive and frankly, arbitrary biologism – a consequence of having never freed himself from his original training. One felt authorized, in the name of this anti-biologism, which quickly confused drive with instinct, to propose versions which, in many cases, reflected an open (ego or self psychology) or camouflaged psychologizing position. The question of the relations between instinct and drive undoubtedly deserves a scrupulous and detailed examination.

Few authors have attempted it. Laplanche is an exception, but I am not sure I agree with his conclusions. Even in the case where it is recognized that Freud's writings allow for a distinction between instinct and drive, there is still too much endogeneity in this vision. However, it seems to me that this same endogeneity can cover two different conceptions. On the one hand, as the references to instinct indicate, this idea is linked to an innatism which is out of season, now that no one any longer denies the role of *epigenesis*. On the other hand, endogeneity would have to be conceived as *that which maintains itself as a hard core across the variations of structure*. This is the signification that I am adopting and which can, perhaps, be found in a concept such as *self-organization*. I shall be dwelling at greater length on this problem which is the object of a fresh re-evaluation.

In any case, one is almost constantly encountering a reference to the archaic. Without speaking of the almost inevitable tendency to trace back the level of fixations to an earlier point in the antagonism, there exists a quasi-mystical propensity for attempting to have a direct connection with the archaic. We know that there exists, in Kleinian circles, a belief that phenomena linked to the very earliest phases of development re-emerge in the treatment and are thus accessible – in a scarcely modified form – in the *here and now* of the session. Now, in my opinion, it is important never to lose sight of the fact that the archaic is always *après coup*, apprehended retrospectively, and that it concerns *principles* of organization of the psyche. I have referred to the fruitful opposition established by G. Dumézil between *prima* (the first) and *summa* (the most important).[19] If we look in the clinical field for what corresponds to such a definition, it seems to me that we can approach the notion of self-organization by turning towards the elaborations inaugurated by Freud in the psychoanalytic conception of character. If one thinks, in fact, of all the clinical entities that we have been considering, the psychopathological processes that are discovered in them undoubtedly vary from one category to another. But all of them, without exception, come into operation around a personality organization which, clinically, can be defined as *character*.

Character made a decisive entry with Freud's article 'Character and Anal Eroticism' in 1908.[20] There then appeared, with Reich, the notion of *character neurosis*, and then *neurotic character*, *pathological character*, and so on.[21] I am less inclined to follow the peripeteia that have marked this notion than to try and clarify the reasons why I think that the model of character can serve as a basis for contemporary clinical description.

Let us turn first to what is known by way of common knowledge. In the various uses of character, the quality underlined is that which consists in having character, that is, in showing energy, determination and even resistance so as not to submit blindly to the wishes of those who are more powerful than oneself. Having character also means making one's mark, possessing a style, exhibiting a strong moral physiognomy. One speaks of '*having* character', but one can also speak of *being* a character. The difference is often slight between having character and having a bad character. I will not expand on the various linguistic nuances, preferring to accentuate that which, starting with the common ground of all men or, in a more restricted manner, of a social ensemble, constitutes the basis of the community which unites them (national character), allowing for mutual identifications in the community, but forming part of the singularity of each individual. What is the reason for choosing such a criterion? If I turn towards clinical psychoanalysis, I observe that it rests, on the one hand, on an organization of symptoms which differs according to the various sectors under considera- tion (neurosis, psychosis, perversion, etc); and, on the other, on a set of general, metapsychologically defined theorems (castration complex, pregenitality and genitality, Oedipus complex, etc.). Now, this conjunction was the source of fruitful questioning. Freud started out from a selective core (as we saw earlier, he chose the transference psycho-neuroses and excluded actual neuroses and narcissistic neuroses). Even though he made this choice himself, it was not respected in the long term. The article 'Psycho-Analysis' in the *Encyclopaedia Britannica* of 1926 adds to hysteria, obsessional neurosis and the phobias: inhibitions, character anomalies, sexual perversions and the difficulties of love life. It even includes organic illnesses. It is clear that the initial coherence is some- what disrupted here. By centring the indications on symptomatic organizations, one encounters affirmations contrary to the principle one began with. If we analyse this enumeration we are bound to recognize multiple forms of anxiety, various sorts of defence, different types of transference, which are difficult to place under a single heading – without forgetting the libidinal stages taken as a descriptive basis for character types. In 'Analysis Terminable and Interminable' (1937c), Freud, carrying out as thorough an examination as possible, ventures to give a general answer which distinguishes three types of factors: trauma, constitution and the structure of the ego. 'Constructions in Analysis' (1937d), a later offshoot of the earlier text, draws attention to the role of hallucination. I do not think it is an exaggeration to say that, from the standpoint I am adopting, Freud does not arrive at a satisfying conclusion.

After Freud, analysts would in turn propose their miracle solution for getting out of the impasse. Melanie Klein said: 'We have to go deeper and go back to the very beginning.' Hartmann, Kris and Loewenstein said: 'Since we do not know the id and have no means of knowing it, we need to analyse the ego more deeply.' After Hartmann, Kohut said: 'Neither the drive nor the ego hold the solution to the problem; it is the self that has to be analysed.' After Kohut, the intersubjectivists (Greenberg and Mitchell, O. Renik) contended: 'You are not going far enough; only intersubjectivity will provide a way out.' Elsewhere, and under other skies, Bion saw the solution in analysing the *alpha function.* Winnicott *invented the transitional dimension* and Lacan closed the process with *the signifier.* As the Swiss say, it looks rather untidy! Of course I, in turn, am in danger of passing for a new Archimedes who is proposing his discovery while crying out: Eureka!

In recent years there has appeared the idea that, contrary to what was believed hitherto, the pathological cannot serve to help us understand normal development. This position is often advanced by those claiming allegiance to cognitivism. At any rate, the initial choice of the transference psychoneurosis certainly entailed, *nolens volens*, a deviation towards psychosis and an implicit change of paradigm (psychosis in the place of perversion). An interesting metaphor used by Freud comes to mind here. He points out that when crystal breaks (as a result of a shock, of a trauma I would say), it does not break haphazardly, but along the lines of force which form its structure. By the same token, Lacan liked to cite the saying of Goya: 'The sleep of reason engenders monsters.' The sleep of reason does not engender just anything whatsoever; monsters are only what reason attempts to put to sleep, and which wake up during sleep. It is clear that the multiplicity of the lines of fracture of crystal prompts us to look for another model.

At the outset of psychoanalysis, normality and neurosis were opposed. Today, the position has changed and neurotics and normal (*neurotico-normal*) people are grouped together and contrasted with non-neurotic structures. It is less a question of seeking out normality than of identifying what its least ideologically marked general traits are. *I propose to isolate the elements of this generality in the psychoanalytic conception of character.* I say *character* and not character neurosis or neurotic character, which appear to me to be singularities situated outside the general features that I am looking for. I will content myself, then, with describing character as the *stable part of psychic organization on to which the effects of several types of organization belonging to pathology are grafted.* I obviously recognize, moreover, that there is an intrinsic pathology of character which is open to being understood in different ways, starting with the initial contributions of W. Reich which have been theorized, particularly in French psychoanalysis, under the denominations of pathological character (F. Pasche), narcissistic character defences (E. Kestemberg), and envisaged in an original way from the angle of the relations between character and behaviour (P. Marty). I thus propose to consider a common core of psychic personality, namely, character. In this respect, character can be subject to the vicissitudes of an intrinsic pathology or an associated symptomatic pathology. My purpose, then, is to ground clinical reflection in a common source. I am thus trying to go beyond the dichotomy symptom/character; just as I wish to transcend the quarrel brought against the drive by the partisans of the object or the self. I recall how surprised I was on hearing one of my teachers, then at an advanced age, proclaim out loud his new credo: 'I do not believe in the drive any more.' The problem is that I am unable to believe in what he believed at that moment.

Let us turn now to the psychoanalytic conception of character. When one considers the problematic of character according to Freud, two lines of thinking are possible: the first is that of a closure, namely, of a circumscription within the psychical apparatus under the auspices of the ego; and the second, opposed to the first, consists in envisaging the leaks which do not allow themselves to be confined within the closure and enter into relation with other parts of the psyche. These factors and the problems they raise in Freud's work, are multiple. Outside psychoanalysis, character is often linked to heredity. The latter is sometimes contrasted with what is acquired or accidental, and sometimes conceived as a component of a much broader picture (the innate and the acquired). The concept of personality is criticized by Freud himself; it is too marked by its associations with superficial psychology (in contrast with the depth psychology which is what psychoanalysis is supposed to be). It would seem that character allows of a more rigorous delimitation than personality. Furthermore, in the psychoanalytic conception, character is opposed to the symptom; it is related to the libidinal types (see Freud's article on this subject); it gives rise to a more or less appropriate psychoanalytic characterology; and, finally, it arises from a mixture. It is formed by impressions unified by the action of the ego. The mixture makes it possible to attach these constituent features sometimes to what Freud calls defences, sometimes to perversion, and sometimes to neurosis. In any case, character is the object of two formulations: the first, short but decisive, is dated 1908 ('Character and Anal Erotism'); and the second is later. The entry of character into the theory occurred in a sensational mode. When one thinks of the few pages which paint a picture of it in 'Character and Anal Erotism' (1908), one cannot fail to be impressed by the lucidity and acuity of Freud's vision. No doubt it can be said that Freud was himself an anal character, which merely reinforces our sense of admiration, for it is easier to observe what one wants to describe in others than in oneself! The concept of character appears in psychoanalysis as a reject, an offcut, a product of afterthought. The fact that it entered the field of psychoanalysis via anality cannot make us overlook the fact that, almost at the same time, Freud had embarked on the even more ambitious project of writing up the analysis of the Rat Man (1909d). Moreover, this article preceded another, more complete, and with important repercussions: 'The Disposition to Obsessional Neurosis' (1913i),[22] for which it could serve as an introduction. One can follow this trajectory and link it up with the analysis of the Wolf Man which gives anal erotism pride of place, and, roughly at the same period, with another very important article, 'Transformations of Instinct as Exemplified in Anal Erotism' (1917c). Thus the two components of the article of 1908, namely, character and anal erotism, are closely bound together. The problem of the solidarity of the notions uniting character and anal erotism would remain an issue for a long time. There will be no difficulty in accepting that the most convincing description of a characterological structure can be made in respect of anal erotism, which is not contingent. The analytic characterology which followed from it would have more difficulty in imposing itself than that suggested by the description of 1908. What is more, such a general characterology lends itself to a nosographical deviation that is often more descriptive and, ultimately, normative, than metapsychologically convincing. Let us examine things a little more closely.

To begin with Freud related character trait with bodily experience, thus referring to the instinctual sphere. This was a discovery of analysis, which was not preceded by any preconception. The impact of the bodily functions (and the organs concerned) immediately involves, in the case under consideration, i.e. anality, the ego. For otherwise how are we to understand the reference to orderliness alongside thrift and obstinacy? Though thrift can be linked with retention, and obstinacy with opposition to the object owing to instinctual fixation, it is easy to link retention with the ego. In the article of 1908, Freud writes [referring to the *Three Essays*]: 'I there attempted to show that the sexual instinct of man is highly complex and is put together from contributions made by numerous constituents and component instincts.'[23] No concession, then, to a schematizing simplicity; the elementary is already complex. Is there not a convergence here with the theories of emergence? In point of fact, Freud, dissects, that is to say, analyses, and thereby discovers, behind the action of the ego, something which has its origin in the instinct, in the form of fixations or reaction-formations. In fact, when one takes the trouble to go back three years earlier to the *Three Essays on the Theory of Sexuality*, one finds in the final chapter, 'Summary', in the section 'Sublimation', the description of mechanisms which would crop up again in the study of character: notably, reaction-formation. Freud writes:

> What we describe as a person's 'character' is built up to a considerable extent from the material of sexual excitations and is composed of instincts that have been fixed since childhood, of constructions achieved by means of sublimation, and of other constructions, employed for effectively holding in check perverse impulses which have been recognized as being unutilizable.[24]

It would be wrong to see in character an organization of the psyche that is more 'normal' than that of neurosis. The decompensations of character are numerous. They can range from the sexualization of social ties (with all its consequences for homosexuality and paranoia) to the impregnation of the libidinal constituents by narcissism, vulnerability to depression, sensibility to intrusion as well as the risk of somatization or a typical organization of behavioural neurosis. On the other hand, character can open itself to sublimation, as Freud realized.

In short the character trait is a complex, in the real sense of the term, comprised of a sexual instinctual part, added to which there is another part, distinct from it, which has undergone the vicissitude of sublimation; and, finally, an anti-instinctual defence mechanism, reaction-formation. *The complex is thus composed of direct instinct, sublimated instinct, and anti-instinct.* All this is in relation to an object of demand (that of sphincter training). This trinity is in itself more than significant. However, the fact that anality serves as a case of reference must also be related to its specificity, namely, the relation container–contained (mucous membranes and faeces); the contradictory desire between retaining and expelling, the status of internal (proper to oneself)/external (proper to the other), the existence of an object with two aspects to it (the object of anal production and the object which requires its release, the dialectic of possessing and of giving, the attraction to dirtiness and the reaction-formation of cleanliness, the tendency to sadism and the repression of aggressivity, etc. All this forms a coherent picture and one which does justice to the situation. Such a constellation shows the participation of the instinct, the ego and the object, and also designates the place of the other prefiguring a future character complex during the phallic phase. We can understand then the value of an emblematic formula which defines character in the following terms: 'The permanent character-traits are either unchanged prolongations of the original instincts, or sublimations of those instincts, or reaction-formations against them.'[25]

Freud's second series of reflections would have to wait until the *New Introductory Lectures*, in 1933. In fact, since the formulation of the second topography and even a bit before that, in 'Group Psychology and the Analysis of the Ego' (1921c), Freud had developed and theorized the role of identification, a concept that he was to take up again in *The Ego and the Id* (1923b). Already, in the Minutes of the Vienna Psychoanalytic Society of 6 November 1907, he had emphasized the coexistence of opposites, adjoining to it 'the active tendency to the unification of what is known as character'. But in 1933, he came back to the question:

> You yourselves have no doubt assumed that what is known as 'character', a thing so hard to define, is to be ascribed entirely to the ego. We have already made out a little of what it is that creates character. First and foremost there is the incorporation of the former parental agency as a super-ego, which is no doubt its most important and decisive portion, and, further, identifications with the two parents of the later period and with other influential figures, and similar identifications formed as precipitates of abandoned object-relations. And we may now add as contributions to the construction of character which are never absent the reaction-formations which the ego acquires – to begin with in making its repressions and later, by a more normal method, when it rejects unwished-for instinctual impulses.[26]

One can see the path he was taking. Freud was now linking character closely to the ego. Far from trying to go back to the beginnings he takes into account the incorporation of the super-ego which he does not shrink from designating as 'the most important and decisive portion'. To this he adds the role of external identifications with influential figures but whose importance is less decisive. He describes the 'precipitates of abandoned object-relations' and finally appreciates the contributions of reaction-formations under the influence of repression or 'by a more normal method'. The difference with the article of 1908 is palpable. In 1908 the reflection as a whole revolved around the drive alone.

By underscoring the role of identification in 1933, Freud brought into play the function of the object, an object thought of as having no direct instinctual contact, for we know that the child's superego is modelled on the superego (and not the ego) of the parents (indirect relation). Here we have the germ of a synthetic conception of the instinctual drive, the indirect role of the object, the vicissitude of abandoned objects, and the unifying tendency of the ego. I have no hesitation in comparing this late formulation with Winnicott's conception of the creation of the psyche in the proximity of the object, aroused by the latter's imaginary or real response. It seems to me that this is a privileged path for identification. Let us conclude provisionally by summarizing Freud's approach:

1   At the beginning of the theory, we have the symptom.
2   In second place, there is an opposition between character and symptom, as well as the relation of the symptom to other symptoms.
3   Character is then identified as a locus of resistance, referring to the analysis of narcissistic defences. Narcissism is identified with: id, that is me. I am (like) id.

In this examination, I am leaving aside problems related to masochism, destructivity and the harassment of the ego. These remarks appear to be in line, yet again, with the very rich and condensed posthumous notes. The first of them, written on 16 June 1938, says this:

> It is interesting that in connection with early experiences, as contrasted with later experiences, all the various reactions to them survive, of course including contradictory ones. Instead of a decision, which would have been the outcome later. Explanation: weakness of the power of synthesis, retention of the characteristic of primary processes.[27]

I consider this note to be of cardinal importance. It informs us, in a definitive manner, that in going back to the earliest experiences, one finds oneself faced with a complex ensemble, comprising the various reactions *which have all survived, i.e. the positive reactions as well as the contradictory ones, 'of course'*. In other words, the weakness of the synthesis – that is to say of the ego's activity – allows for the survival of the primary processes, which can only reflect a contradictory ensemble composed of the positive reactions and the contradictory reactions that they provoke. This amounts to saying, in short, that there is no order of succession between the drive and the defence, but something which for me is evocative of *simultaneity*.

I will now say a word about post-Freudian contributions. What authors have been struck by is the translation of the defensive conflict into character traits rather than symptoms. It is true that pathological organizations of character perhaps have less flexibility for tolerating the appearance of symptoms and can present a psychic rigidity to analysis. In any case, after Freud had developed it in various writings that I will not be dwelling on, character returned to the forefront of the scene with the studies of Abraham and Reich, the latter emphasizing the pathological and resistant aspects. The notion was to surface again later with Glover, and then in France with H. Sauguet, E. Kestemberg, and D. Lagache. It is noteworthy that the interest it raised gradually faded as interest in borderline cases developed. But its resurrection in the writings of the psychosomaticians is significant since it is often a sign that the psychic organization is associated with psychosomatosis. In this respect the clinical work of Pierre Marty is very precious. It is notable that this psychic part, thus organized, becomes dissociated from its bodily, and even more, its somatic roots, the psychosomatic unity postulated in normality giving rise here to two divergent directions: character organization, on the one hand, and somatic disorganization on the other.

The reasons why I am proposing to return to the model of character as the basic clinical model rather than any other reside in two particularities: (a) character (and not character neurosis) *is the constant core present in every psychopathological organization*. It is like the earth in which various cultures grow (neurosis, psychosis, perversion, psychosomatosis); and (b) the basic cell which allows us to understand it implies a triple combination which seems to me to be fundamental, associating the direct derivatives of the drive, the result of sublimations and the defences of reaction-formation type. This tripartite cell seems exemplary in its coherence. The posthumous note referred to earlier, taken from 'Findings, Ideas, Problems', shows us that it is pointless to look for an original fixation without understanding that it is attached on the one hand to the direction imposed on it by sublimation and, on the other, to the 'contradictory reaction' of the anti-instinctual defences. This model – for it is one – should, it seems to me, be taken generally without there being an obligation to grant too important a place to the application of the theory culminating in a psychoanalytic characterology. Such a characterology rests, in effect, on the theory of stages, which we regard today in a slightly less schematic way than was once the case: the libidinal stages must now be envisaged more in relation with other constituents of the psyche.

The great interest of such a model is that it can be understood as a combined effect of different parts of the psychical apparatus. The reference to the drives refers to the id, underlining the 'partial nature' of the instinctual fixations. The ego's involvement is present in the tendency to unification and in the orientation towards sublimation. As for the superego, its impact is twofold: at an elementary level, via the reference to reaction-formations; and, at a more general level, by drawing on the role of the mechanisms of identification and, in this latter case, of identification with the parents' superego. Thus, starting with a simple notion, the whole complexity and heterogeneity of the psychical apparatus sees these processes forming into what appears to be a mark of individuality. It would be necessary, of course, to take into consideration the role played by the ideology of a certain culture – the cultural superego – in encouraging or reproving certain character traits. But that is another story.

Inhibitions and compulsions

After the problems relative to representations and affects, which constitute the central axis of the main psychical organizations of psychoanalysis, I will now move on to questions which put us, perhaps, more directly in contact with instinctual drive functioning, its inhibition or, on the contrary, its irrepressible discharge via activation. It seems logical to place inhibitions and compulsions under a common heading. This chapter will doubtless be unevenly distributed for, notwithstanding its importance, Freud only came to the study of inhibition at a very late stage: a short chapter of *Inhibitions, Symptoms and Anxiety*[28] was devoted to it in 1926. Inhibition is only conceived in its relation to symptoms and anxiety. This distinction is itself criticized by Freud. In fact, he points out that an inhibition is not necessarily pathological whereas this is always true of a symptom. However, inhibition can reach a degree at which it becomes a symptom. What is essential, in fact, is to define inhibition in relation to functions, which can be more or less affected depending on the affections involved. The first series of inhibitions that Freud takes into consideration is constituted, as one might expect, by the widespread inhibitions of the sexual function. Let me point out in passing, however, that these inhibitions were much more frequent in feminine than masculine sexuality, at least until recently. On this occasion, Freud noted the close link between inhibition and anxiety, inhibition being a preventative measure to prevent the appearance of anxiety.

Inhibitions and phobias have traditionally been grouped together from this perspective. There is no other way of specifying the function of sexual inhibitions when we consider the different ways in which sexuality can be disturbed. I will not be entering into the detail of these descriptions.

Though sexual inhibitions are the daily bread of analysis, which offers more or less complete solutions for them, today, inhibitions of the nutritional function occupy a much more extensive field than was recognized by Freud in 1926. In recent decades, an enormous literature has dealt with the problem of the anorexias. But it is revealing that here inhibition *and* compulsion often go together, given the connection which is frequently shown to exist in practice between anorexia and bulimia. It is not possible here to give these affections the detailed analysis they deserve. The pathology of anorexia is very difficult to understand, in the measure that the inhibition disguises the problems and covers anxieties which are not always perceptible. The patient simply says that he or she does not feel like . . . or rationalizes his/her behaviour by saying he or she is afraid of putting on weight. Nevertheless, the scope and depth of the conflicts involved – where the relationship with the mother is in the foreground – indicate that the unconscious structure is complex. In fact, it is extremely difficult to see how a function as natural as appetite can be the seat of a paralysis which can lead to death from cachexia. There are multiple ways of approaching anorexia therapeutically, inspired sometimes by conditioning, sometimes by analysing relations within the family, and sometimes by a strictly individual approach. But, as a rule, it is necessary to accompany this treatment by removing the subject from the family milieu and placing him in an institution. Analysing the relationship with the mother proves to be extremely fruitful. In fact, even a superficial examination indicates that it is difficult to isolate nutritional behaviour from sexual behaviour. The young girl who ceases to feed herself is trying to prevent the appearance in her of signs of post-pubertal maturity. She rejects her sexual body: her forms, her breasts and her buttocks become the object of a persecutory relationship, the patient waging war against them mercilessly in order to stop their development. Moreover, by the same stroke, sexuality is inhibited, and it is not difficult to see that, ultimately, the issue is one of an internal struggle against a potential maternity. Furthermore, it is customary to assert that accepting a pregnancy which has reached its term is the real sign of recovery from anorexia. Fixation to the mother is in full evidence – ambivalent dependence consisting of dependency and the struggle against dependency. What the anorexic subject is complaining of is either not being understood by the mother at all or not being able to emerge from the childhood relation with her. Under these conditions, Oedipal rivalry has a lot of difficulty in manifesting itself. Colette Combe has just made a decisive contribution to anorexia,[29] which illuminates the various aspects of this illness – psychosomatic, par excellence. She illustrates brilliantly the position I have adopted which seeks to moderate the place of biology in its relations with the psyche. It is neither a question of an arbitrary and groundless petition of principle, nor of a utopia which has nothing to support it.

If one now envisages the contrary face of anorexia, i.e. bulimia, things do not look any simpler. Perhaps the dimension of camouflage of what is undeniably a symptom is more apparent. For it is indeed anxiety which constitutes the major trait of this clinical picture. Anxiety, here, is not related to a drive, but to its contrary – namely, the void. The subject seeks desperately to fill himself up, in the most disorderly fashion and with contempt for the most elementary taste, with everything that falls within his reach, mixing foods in a way that will arouse disgust in anyone whose appetite is not deregulated. It is, moreover, a frightening spectacle to witness an attack of bulimia in which the unbridled instinctual drive is completely uninhibited and knows no obstacle, there being no remedy for the struggle against the internal sense of emptiness. It is difficult to describe this emptiness; for, behind the impression of being physically empty, it is from a psychic emptiness that the patient suffers, as if he were totally devoid of internal objects and needed at all costs to compensate for this lack by ingesting undifferentiated external objects. Here the dialectic of the drive and the object is particularly sensitive. Whereas the external object appears in the foreground, it is in fact the object of the drive and its repercussions at the level of the ego which are in question. Unlike anorexia, which often takes a critical turn calling for interventions such as hospitalization, bulimia can be both more chronic and more insidious. It can go unnoticed, except by those who live under the same roof as the patient. It is customary to stress the role of the provoked alternations between bulimia and vomiting, which accomplish a mixed state between bulimic fantasies and anorexic fantasies. A comparison comes to mind linking the couple anorexia/bulimia with a symmetrical couple depression/mania. The comparison is not without substance but, once again, what is in question here is a behavioural disturbance which touches upon the sphere of the instincts even more than that of the drives. To be honest, when one reaches these extremes, the difference between instinct and drive is very difficult to establish.

As for compulsions, it is necessary to go beyond nutritional behaviour. Here we are in the presence of disturbances which have their roots in consumption. This introduces us to the subject of addictions of all kinds: from the most ordinary such as alcoholism or smoking to the most dangerous forms of drug addiction, endangering the subject's life. The problem of drug addictions has opened up a new field of exploration that is very large and obscure. It is essential to point out the extent to which addictive forms of behaviour can raise the question of the death drive. But here again, I am tempted to establish a link between the addictions and what Joyce McDougall has described as the *neosexuality of addictive sexual behaviours*, whose function in fact concerns more the ego than sexuality.

Other inhibitions can affect the basic bodily relations linked with relations with the outside world. Hence the inhibition of locomotion cited by Freud in 1926. We are familiar with the existence of the motor paralyses in hysteria and we know how phobias can take over motor activity or become prey to obsessional rituals. It seems that Freud's hypothesis that a function can be eroticized excessively, already defended in 1910 in respect of psychogenic disturbances of vision (hysterical blindness), can be invoked here once again. Very remarkable are inhibitions about leaving certain places in order to go somewhere else, involving a displacement of separation anxieties on to the inanimate (see below). I would like to cite a disturbance that I have frequently observed, but which is rarely described in the literature: the inhibition of sensibility to pain. With these patients, whose disturbances are manifested less by symptoms than by behavioural characteristics, one witnesses a reduction of sensibility, to a greater or lesser degree, to the point even, in certain cases, of being insensible to pain. For instance, when the patient has presented a fracture, which in principle is very painful, and has never complained of the suffering that it causes. Let me add that in certain cases one is surprised to see that the modification of behaviour in the direction of a general improvement is accompanied by the fresh appearance of a sensibility to pain. One then understands retrospectively that it is as though the patient had succeeded in reorganizing himself at a level that could be characterized as *neither pleasure – nor pain.* The reappearance of pain not infrequently goes together with the rediscovery of states of pleasure and wishful phantasies.

One understands, then, the interest of studying inhibitions and compulsions in that they put us in the presence of organizations that are psychically less structured, like representations and affects.

It is easy to describe other inhibitions, often of an obscure character, such as the inhibition of work (especially intellectual). This field of pathology is very wide in scope and concerns an important part of the disturbances of adolescence, which often manifest themselves by an inhibition in the realm of academic activities. These intellectual inhibitions can affect the functions associated with them such as writing and reading. This can even involve an inhibition of personal communication in a sort of paralysis of the exchange or exposition of facts related to oral personal intimacy. These inhibitions are difficult to treat and require much time. As in other cases, one can point to the role of an excessive erotization of these activities, which Freud had already referred to in 1926. A parallel can be drawn between these inhibitions in work with their adverse form which modern pathology has been obliged to take into consideration and which has been characterized by the neologism *workaholics.* These addicts of professional work have been considered by Michel de M'Uzan as the slaves of quantity, and designated by Gérard Szwec as *willing (galley) slaves. Willing?* Displacements are certainly involved, but the term is open to discussion in that this particular displacement has little relation with those to which we are accustomed and which are observable in dreams and neurotic symptoms. Here we are dealing with genuine displacements of instinctual functions. The psychosomaticians define them as *self-calming techniques,* situated at the opposite extreme of auto-erotism.

Anxieties of separation, of being abandoned, object loss, mournings and psychic pains

In this section, I will be discussing forms of anxiety which cannot be qualified either as signal anxiety or as automatic anxiety. I have deliberately chosen to regroup them because it seems to me there is a link between them that justifies this.

Separation anxiety

Separation anxiety is by far the best known or at least the most frequently cited. Notwithstanding its apparent clarity, it conceals more mystery than is often recognized. Considered as a relatively recent discovery linked to the developmental phases of the child (M. Mahler's separation anxieties–individuation), its real origin can be found in Freud's work of 1926. He gives a very striking description of it there which I do not think was taken up and endorsed thereafter. For him, separation anxiety is rooted in the baby's feeling that, by losing his object, he would be losing the person who is capable of providing the satisfaction of his needs and desires. Modern studies insist more on the object relation proper with the mother and one can see here an application of Fairbairn's postulate that the libido is *object seeking*. By the same token, one can invoke Bowlby's attachment theory, revised by Fonagy.[30] It is clear that the early object relationship is very much in question. Perhaps, when one goes back to these periods of development, one should consider that the child's relation to its object is not so clearly differentiated as in the adult. What I mean, in short, is that the bond uniting the subject with his object is as much narcissistic as object related in nature. The object is a narcissistic extension of the child; so much so that any fracture or rupture of the links with it is also a narcissistic tear. If it is contended that, in separation, the object carries away with it a part of the subject, this is what is meant. To be honest, for my part I can only conceive of the subject–object relationship from a complex point of view which leads us to understand that an object can exist from the beginning, as M. Klein claims. This, however, does not mean that there is a clear distinction between the subject and the object, the latter being considered as a projected part of the subject, in continuity with him, without any real separation. The distinction, as many authors think, including Winnicott and the non-Kleinians, only occurs very gradually. Winnicott even thinks that it is only with the intervention of the father – Lacan thinks the same – that a separation is completed, even though it is initiated well before. At any rate, separation anxiety, when it is severe, is a recognized state in all non-neurotic structures. It is very interesting to note that, over the course of the years, separations during the therapeutic relationship (circumstantial interruptions, vacations, etc.) are at first experienced in a dramatic way, sometimes involving abrupt regressions which are noisy but temporary; then, as the transference relationship evolves, they are tolerated with increasing ease. One of the characteristics of the decompensations of such states is the patient's incapacity to phantasize or to form a picture of the analyst in his absence. Whereas a neurotic will have no great difficulty in conjuring up a psychic reality in which he replaces the analyst by imagining him as he wishes, the non-neurotic subject finds he is paralysed in such an activity. The non-neurotic patient's need to see the object-analyst in the session may be compared with the need he feels to know, by having explicit information, where the analyst is and what he is doing during the interruption. Such 'surveillance', doubled by such a ban on fantasizing, can no doubt be elucidated by unconscious phantasies of the primitive scene, which are anxiety producing to the highest degree, in the measure that they combine a pronounced feeling of dereliction with unbridled projective instinctual activity (Melanie Klein's notion of the phantasy of the combined parent figure).

Abandonment

Abandonment neurosis, once described by Germaine Guex, is no longer often evoked in this form, but the symptom of experiencing abandonment and the related structure remain an observable reality on a grand scale. It is easy to connect this symptom of feeling abandoned with a premature separation and insufficient assurance of being reunited with the maternal object. Here again, it is as though the dimension of absence, so essential to the psyche for its growing complexity and progress, was turned against the psychical apparatus, paralysing its functioning, filling it with destructive phantasies or simply being content with blocking all thought processes. To speak of absence is to speak of the threat of being abandoned. To speak of abandonment is to speak of the possibility of really losing the object, leaving the subject's narcissism in a state of helplessness and condemning him to distress. It often takes a long time to get the subject to accept that the experience of being abandoned can be linked with his sense of wrongdoing and guilt for having desired something prohibited or with the idea that he is being punished on account of the excessive and alienating character of his dependence, or again on account of his phantasies of destroying the object.

Object loss

I have just alluded to the fact that the danger of object loss is a permanent one. In Freud's description of 1926, there exists a gradation: the danger of losing the love of the object can go as far as to include the danger of losing the object. One can easily see both the connection between the two states and their difference. Once again, object loss, which Freud recognized in 'Mourning and Melancholia', is a common and repeated vicissitude of existence (the loss can concern objects that are easily replaced or, on the contrary, ones that are irreplaceable), but its consequences will depend on the narcissistic coefficient affecting the object relationship. The more narcissistic the charge is, the more difficult it will be to consolidate the loss. And this is why, in melancholy, the narcissistic relationship to the object is a fundamental fact. Moreover, mourning is only surmountable to the extent that this relationship permits it to be surmounted.

151

Mourning

All this has resulted in according fresh and increasing importance to the role of states of mourning and overcoming them. Jean Cournut has emphasized the role of failed processes of mourning and of unacknowledged or unrecognized deaths in a certain number of patients, where one is astonished, after a long period of analysis, by how the psychoanalytic process is stagnating.[31] It is true that, in non-neurotic structures, one is often dealing with situations characterized by a sort of interminable torpid mourning, the subject having never succeeded in accepting and overcoming this or that loss, which is not always related to the death of an object, but frequently with the loss of a special relationship with it. The most ordinary example is that of the loss of love experienced after the birth of a younger sibling. I have also described, under the name of the *dead mother complex*, a structure which has certain similarities with what I have just described.[32] I refer the interested reader to it.

Pain

Renewed interest has been taken in recent years on the role of pain in psychoanalytic treatment. Litza Guttières-Green has clarified its modalities and given prominence to what she has called *painful transferences*. Briefly, it concerns subjects marked by important childhood traumas which have left behind them very sensitive traces. The transference analysis never allows one to approach them, provoking, as soon as an attempt is made to examine them, a painful affect which bears witness to the continuing acute sensibility of the traumatized zones of the psyche and, at the same time, to the protective value of these defences, in that they guard the access to this unapproachable sanctuary.

Intrusion anxiety, implosion, fragmentation

Intrusion anxiety

In a manner that is complementary and antagonistic to the preceding series, I shall give a brief description of intrusion anxiety of which Winnicott gave the first and most successful demonstration. Here again, what is involved is a dysfunctioning of the frontiers of the ego which proves to be incapable of protecting the subject against the object's intrusions. Though separation anxiety was known of as early as *Inhibitions, Symptoms and Anxiety*, intrusion anxiety was only individualized much later. Winnicott described what he called *impingement anxiety*, where the subject feels as if he is being invaded by the other person's psyche; he thus has the feeling that his own psyche is being broken into and, ultimately, colonized or alienated. It seems likely that Winnicott's description was intended to be a criticism of Kleinian technique, which did not shrink from engaging in a sort of interpretative harassment depriving the subject of his own defensive activity and, in a roundabout way, leading the analyst to influence the patient to conform with his own desires. Non-Kleinian contemporary technique has insisted, on the contrary, on the necessity of respecting the subject's defences, even when they appear to be anachronistic and pathological, inasmuch as his possibility of changing his defensive strategy is very limited, and it is better to wait until he feels ready to do so. Respecting defences does not mean not interpreting at all. It means trying to evaluate the patient's capacity to take leave of his personal narcissistic organization which serves him as a shield in front of the object and allows him, to some extent, to strengthen his sense of internal cohesion, even though it has been much undermined by instinctual anarchy and the limitations of his relationship with the other.

Implosion anxiety

At one degree more, the danger of being intruded upon by the other is translated by implosion anxiety, which was described for the first time by Ronald Laing, if I am not mistaken. This symptom is difficult to interpret, for it is not easy to know if the implosion is the direct result of the way in which the subject is parasitized by the object, culminating in the explosion of his containing structure, or if the implosion is the manifestation of a defensive self-destruction aimed at stopping the colonization by the object. In this case, one can see the close relations that exist between implosion and explosion. Be that as it may, there are always important narcissistic anxieties in the background affecting the ego's sense of unity or personal identity when the implosion sets in as an intolerable consequence of being invaded by the object. It can be seen that here, narcissism must be given prominent consideration. Let me point out in passing that a current defence against such a danger is the adoption of a *false-self* organization to comply with the object's desires.

Fragmentation

It is logical to conclude with fragmentation. This symptom, often dramatic in character and perceived as a disintegration of the ego and fragmentation of its unity, can be expressed in very frightening ways. I want to insist, nonetheless, on subentrant forms of which the patient does not always speak, but whose existence is finally revealed after many years of treatment. Once again, non-neurotic structures occupy the foreground, which, as a rule, justify face-to-face psychotherapies in which the frequency of sessions will vary. The feeling of fragmentation ('Once I am outside, I feel I am in pieces') appears, then, at the end of the session, when the patient leaves the analyst. It is as though the reactivation of conflicts, fixations, and more or less disorganizing anxieties was tolerable as long as the analyst was present, providing the patient with support on which he could lean in order to tackle the most problematic zones of his psyche. As soon as this support is abandoned at the end of the session, it is as if the patient were unable to lean on a representation of the analyst-object after separating from him. He now finds himself alone, weak, destitute, more or less helpless, having to struggle against the demons awakened by the session. Some of my patients have refused to come to sessions in the morning, on the pretext that they had to go to work afterwards and that it took them a long time to recover their ordinary composure. All this indicates the extent to which the psychic equilibrium of these structures is based less on repressions than on splitting designed to keep away everything that can come and disturb mental functioning. The latter has to be maintained at a reduced, impoverished, and more or less operative level. Here there arises the question of protective amputations aimed at ensuring a mode of functioning that appears normal, at least to others. This last idea is open to discussion, for it is the patient who imagines that those around him notice nothing ('no scandals!'), whereas when the analyst disposes of another source of information, he realizes that the impression left by the patient's behaviour is quite the opposite of the patient's illusion that his states of mental disturbance are not visible. One thinks here of the alcoholic who claims to be walking straight and to reveal nothing of his state of drunkenness, by trusting himself, so to speak, to his inner feeling, whereas a mere glance is enough to reveal his zigzag progression and the deficiencies of his co-ordination and balance.

We have now considered in turn the most classic manifestations that emerge during the treatment (orthodox), then the observations that are noted more frequently in non-neurotic structures, where narcissism frequently plays a prevalent role. I am going to close this chapter by turning again to phenomena which I have already mentioned and begun to develop in other parts of this work. I am resigned to the fact that it is difficult to avoid repetitions.

Overflows: hallucinatory activity, acting out, somatizations

Hallucinatory activity

I will cite hallucination first of all because, of the three occurrences, it is the one that appears to be the most directly related with a form of psychic organization. In fact, as I have already pointed out, following César and Sára Botella, Freud returned, in 1937, in 'Constructions in Analysis' which may be considered as a postscript to 'Analysis Terminable and Interminable', to the problem of the need for construction, when the lifting of infantile amnesia is impossible and when one is witnessing the return of the traces of events prior to the fixation of memories and the acquisition of language. He draws on the example of cases where the material takes a turn which can be connected with hallucinatory activity. As I have dwelt at length on the importance of negative hallucination,[33] it is easy to recognize the role of hallucinatory activity in Freud's work, and its evolution in various stages. He deals successively with the hallucinations in paranoia, included in the psychoneuroses of defence. Then comes *The Interpretation of Dreams* and, 15 years after that, 'A Metapsychological Supplement to the Theory of Dreams' – where dreams and hallucination are declared to be identical, but for a few details. He then comes to the Wolf Man and the hallucination of the severed finger; then to 'A Disturbance of Memory on the Acropolis'. And finally, 'Constructions'. It is clear that even if Freud had the tendency to restrict the role played by hallucination after the discovery of analysis and the promotion of the concept of representation, the theory of hallucination never ceased to preoccupy him inasmuch as it was related, according to him, to an essential function of the psychical apparatus. Which led him to conclude that the primary processes tend towards hallucinatory expression. The Botellas have given numerous examples of hallucinatory functioning in the session, the existence of which I can confirm. A patient said to me, once he was lying on the couch: 'It smells of shit in here.' There is no need to add that he was presenting an obsessional structure. Another, on his way to the session, heard his mother, who lived a long way away, calling to him in the street. This fact appears to corroborate what I have already indicated concerning the property of the psychical apparatus to bring into existence, creating it from start to finish, *another reality* which presents itself as being just as real as the other and even claims to be a substitute for it. Such is the case of dreams. So hallucinatory activity is not to be corroborated or denied by the analyst, but it must, first and foremost, be accepted, heard, and, if possible, analysed. It was once customary to consider hallucination as 'an offshoot of the instinct' (or rather of the drive). The drive and wishful fantasy gave birth to hallucinatory forms of wishing. Today, we know that the phenomenon is much more complicated, resting probably on a negative hallucination before the latter is covered over by a positive hallucination. I can only refer the reader to my writings (*The Work of the Negative*) to show the importance of this concept which was present at the origins of psychoanalysis, during the period of hypnosis, and disappeared progressively with the invention of the psychoanalytic method.

Acting out

I have had the opportunity of showing on several occasions the extent to which the problem raised by acting out, taking the place of remembering, led

Freud into an impasse and pushed him to carry out an agonizing revision. In my opinion this was the main reason justifying the mutation which culminated in the last theory of the drives and the creation of the last topography. I contend, in fact, that the first topography is centred on representations (and affect) and that it draws its inspiration from the metapsychological model of dreams (Ch. VII). The disappearance of the reference to representation (conscious/preconscious/unconscious) in the definitions of the id, and its replacement by the reference to the instinctual impulses forming the id which tend towards discharge, place acting out almost automatically at the centre of these modifications. If as early as 1914, Freud proposed us the emblematic formula: 'The patient acts out instead of remembering', it was because, already at this time, some six to nine years before the last decisive theoretical changes, acting out was imposing itself increasingly as a reference for understanding the patient's functioning, the patient seeming to prefer this path of elimination than that of elaboration through remembering. As I have already pointed out, acting out, as a vicissitude of the drive, exceeds the framework of action, and the model which characterizes it can be present where no form of action is discernible, as Bion has eloquently shown. In fact, we must not forget the connection between remembering and acting out which covers that between the elaboration of frustration and its evacuation. Thus, the question of acting out (today we say enacting), which is so important in contemporary psychoanalysis, and that of repetition-compulsion as a form of constraint (in compulsion, there is *'pulsion'*, with its cortège of thrust and imperious obligation), cause the pendulum of theory to swing back once again to its axiomatic Freudian pole. For Freud, the drive is indeed the foundation of the psychical apparatus, and every important regression returns to it, as does every dedifferentiation of the psyche. We know that, in various quarters now, emphasis is placed on object relations, on intersubjectivity, or on the primacy of the other. This Freudian theory is thus strongly contested. It is reproached for its excessive and inappropriate biologism. It is not certain that the acquisitions of contemporary biology do not give unexpected backing to Freudian theory. In reality, where psychic processes are concerned, two paths, and perhaps even three, need to be contrasted. The first, and the most fundamental, is the shortest (in fact, it is a short circuit). The last is the longest owing to the detour imposed on the psyche so that it can fully measure the consequences of its choices or of the orientations it has been obliged to follow. Between the two, a middle way, not as short as the shortest, not as long as the longest, would be the path of what I call the *intermediate formations* pertaining to the primary processes. It is not just the length of the trajectory that has to be taken into consideration. One also needs to inquire into the nature of the acting out. There are forms of acting out whose aim is to satisfy erotic impulses. However risky they may be, they bear no comparison with forms of acting out mobilized by self-punitive or self-destructive behaviour. Here, each one will interpret them according to his beliefs. If, in certain circles, there continues to be ferocious opposition to the idea of a functioning related to the death drive, others find in these quasi-suicidal behaviours food for thought concerning this question which cannot be closed prematurely.

Somatizations

Psychoanalysis inaugurated its discoveries with a study of hysterical conversion. The problem of the importance of the relations between psyche and body for the knowledge of the unconscious was thus formulated from the outset. The rich harvest of Freud's investigations concerning hysteria accompanied the first steps of psychoanalytic thought, not without the support of a comparatist approach which, in Freud, never failed to situate the mechanisms of the various transference neuroses in relation to each other.[34] Thereafter, when the interest for conversion hysteria declined – one can already see signs of this in *Inhibition, Symptoms and Anxiety* (1926), where there is remarkably little discussion of it – there developed, at a date that is difficult to situate precisely, a curiosity for the so-called psychosomatic illnesses. The history of psychosomatic medicine from its beginnings to the present day is often obscure, marked by authors who have relegated their predecessors to the background, wave after wave. Though it had always been known that the psyche participated in the clinical picture of certain medical affections, this path of research was soon to become the rule. It saw a rapid expansion in North America especially, as a result of a growing extension of the knowledge of the psychological factors interfering in the course of an illness. Great names won renown in various respects, among whom the most well-known are Flanders Dunbar, then, Alexander, who ran the Chicago School and was a highly respected classical psychoanalyst for a long time. To simplify, the first investigators were primarily concerned to compare certain psycholog-ical and character constellations with certain clinical pictures in which, not infrequently, a figurative image, in other respects rather poor, was supposed to represent the psychical counterpart of a clinical picture of the internal medical pathology. Thus, ulcer patients were pictured as worriers; those with high blood pressure as 'over-tense', etc. After a while, these characterological profiles were called into question and the parallel that some ventured to establish between a psychical configuration and a physiological syndrome was criticized. Various currents of psychosomatic medicine shared the field of this discipline among themselves. In parallel to a more or less well-defined psychopathological current (Brisset, Sapir, Held), there soon emerged the Paris Psychosomatic School under the leadership of Pierre Marty (assisted by Michel Fain, Michel de M'Uzan, Christian David), which was the one that pushed the furthest an original conception, grounded in psychoanalysis, and defending ideas that were less simplistic and naïve than had been the case hitherto. Pierre Marty devoted his life to psychosomatics. The latter took such an important place in his thinking that he was led to say, at the end of his life, that psychoanalysis was no more than a branch of psychosomatics, whereas the contrary opinion prevailed. There can be no question of summing up in a few words the scope of Pierre Marty's work. I will simply cite the chapter headings, while referring the interested reader to the works which speak about them. We are indebted to him for the notions, among others, of:

- mentalization and dementalization
- operative thinking, later called operative life
- irregularity of mental functioning
- alteration of the preconscious (the preconscious receives and does not emit)
- essential depression
- progressive disorganization.[35]

It is difficult to enter into the subtle workings of all these mechanisms. It needs to be emphasized that, underlying them, there is a disorder of the function of phantasy which is seen here as deficient or, when its existence can be noted, of very weak functional value. It is as though the psychosomatic patient does not allow the deployment of investments in the direction of the unconscious or those coming from the unconscious. The associative poverty of the discourse is clear; when consulting patients are asked what they think of this or that part of their discourse, they classically reply, after a few words, by saying 'That's all.' The absence of psychical liberty is obvious. The domain occupied by the character neuroses as well as by the so-called behavioural neuroses is a remarkably extensive one. With the latter denomination, which Marty wants to distinguish from the former, it is behaviour that becomes the agency which soaks up anxiety and desire. As Marty himself says in a succinct formula: when one looks for desire in these patients, one finds money, cars (I would add today boats, and even planes), and women. Let us not forget computers. It is as though, for these subjects, fantasy activity was regarded as being 'dangerous', unreasonable to the point of leading the subject into madness (thus something to be mistrusted, to be got rid of and, in any case, to be controlled and restrained). Very often, pleasure is itself the object of a limitation when it is not immediately tangible. Marty's successors have described the *self-calming procedures* to which they accord a role corresponding to that of auto-erotism in 'mentalized' neuroses. It is in such cases that one can notice attitudes of exhaustion where the aim is to get rid of a state of tension rather than according a certain freedom to the psyche which can be a source of libidinal satisfaction.

These descriptions doubtless give the impression of being somewhat schematic when they are taken up by minds which are inclined to simplification using a reductive thought grid. But Pierre Marty's most remarkable discovery in my view is that of *essential depression*. The analyst sometimes witnesses the progressive destructuring of the psychosomatic unity of the patient, whose biological functions appear to deteriorate with a degree of rapidity and gravity which do not seem totally explicable by the severity of the symptoms presented and the observed biological dysfunctioning. Essential depression and the progressive disorganizations are reminiscent of my own descriptions of the *disobjectalizing function*, a concept, moreover, that has been adopted without difficulty by authors who are themselves psychosomaticians (C. Smadja,[36] M. Aisenstein).

I will conclude this chapter by raising two questions to which it would perhaps be premature to seek an answer. The first concerns the specificity of the descriptions of psychosomaticians. Are we to suppose that the original descriptions that they propose are exclusively limited to psychosomatic patients? I have shown elsewhere[37] that patients who do not present somatic symptoms and who may be regarded without hesitation as borderline could present many traits belonging to the descriptions of the psychosomaticians. It would seem that we are dealing here with a modality of the work of the negative which can be identified, transversally, in various mental states sharing more or less the same structure. The second question, which is equally difficult to settle, is that of the relations that exist between hysteria (with or without conversion) and psychosomatic manifestations. Although Marty's theory ventured to differentiate the two clinical entities, refusing interpretations of content when one was dealing with somatic patients (thus breaking with the path traced by the Chicago School and still followed by some Kleinians today), it seems to me that this opposition needs to be reconsidered. Not so much because hysteria and psychosomatic manifestations do not differ where their structural organization is concerned, but because of the observation of symptoms belonging to both series, hysterical and psychosomatic, in the same patient, either at different periods in the evolution of his illness or of his transference, or during one and the same period. Here we are faced with the mystery of certain evolutions in patients in analysis who, while they came originally for treatment of a neurosis, without warning and to the analyst's great surprise, develop, *during the treatment*, a real illness (cancer or systemic disease). An entire chapter of questions, which so far have received little consideration and are of great interest for future research – for instance, the domain of autoimmune diseases – could be opened here. There is no coincidence in the fact that I am citing those affections which raise the problem of the relations in psychoanalysis with effects that are attributable to the hypothetical death drive.

In any case, the interest aroused in France by Pierre Marty's thinking, and its developments, has made psychosomatics a discipline in its own right. It is enriched by its collaboration with psychoanalysts in the search for a definition of a field of original problems, demonstrating singular mechanisms, and different from those of the neuroses.

This is the moment for me to signal a confusion that can be attributed to Pierre Marty himself. After doing classical analytic training, his interest turned at an early stage (from the time of his registrarship at Saint-Anne's hospital) towards domains in which doctors themselves were seeking elucidation from those who had a good knowledge of mental mechanisms. Pierre Marty, who, at the time, was unaware of the writings of the English school, was struck by the difference between what was known of the functioning of the neuroses and what could be understood by means of psychosomatic investigation. It is perfectly legitimate to differentiate between what is observed in somatic patients and what is known of the neuroses. It is equally justified to compare non-neurotic structures with those that can be identified in psychosomatic affections. I consider, moreover, that psychosomatic structures are but a part of the domain which comes under the heading of non-neurotic structures. Here the most fruitful comparisons await us and deserve to be explored. Thus, when Marty speaks of poorly mentalized, or even dementalized structures, he does not seem to realize that they bear a strong resemblance to the descriptions made by those who have interested themselves in borderline cases. This is perhaps a good opportunity to recall certain facts that the psychosomaticians themselves found striking, such as the similarities between the mechanism of foreclosure described in psychosis and the more or less deficient mentalization of psychosomatosis. There is no doubt in my mind that a fruitful field of research will lead us to an increasingly close and precise comparison between psychotic functioning and psychosomatic functioning.

Thought disturbances

In the preceding chapters, one might have postulated the more or less mani-fest, more or less perceptible, more or less accentuated existence of thought disturbances. The latter have been given scarcely any treatment in Freudian psychoanalysis. Generally speaking, thought is a theme in Freud's work which had a brilliant start in the third part of the *Project* and then took on a different form in *The Interpretation of Dreams* (thoughts of the previous day and their repercussions in dreams). Thereafter, it appeared intermittently, in particular in the article 'Formulations on the Two Principles of Mental Functioning' (1911), and then continued its course with some difficulty in the case of the 'Wolf Man'. It reappeared above all in 'A Note upon the Mystic "Writing-Pad"' (1924) and, implicitly, with the articles of 1924 on neurosis and psychosis. It emerged again forcefully in the article on 'Negation' (1925), then in 'Fetishism' with splitting, a problem that would be re-examined from 1927 to 1938, until the end of Freud's work. Melanie Klein, forging ahead along the paths opened up by Freud – but which, in her eyes, were insufficiently signposted – continued the reflections on thought although it was never actually named as such. One had to wait for Bion[38] to see the development of a genuine theory of thinking, set out with imagination and rigour. Indirectly, in my view, Bion's thought should be linked up with Winnicott's considerations on space and transitional phenomena. Lastly, Lacan's work also plays a complementary role via language and speech.

It is interesting to compare Bion's alpha function, *which is unknown to the system and must remain so,* the role of which is to transform raw impressions of meaning into psychic material fit for elaboration by myths, dreams, and passion, and – seen from quite another perspective – the formation of the intermediate area which shelters transitional phenomena from which paradoxical thought processes can emerge, creating objects which both are and are not the internal or external objects that they represent. For my part, I have insisted on the usefulness of a model of the *double limit* (Green 1982) between inside and outside, as well as between conscious and unconscious through the intermediary of the preconscious. I have studied, through the work of the negative, the fruitful and fecund forms of negativity which may be contrasted with the sterilizing and impoverishing forms of the psyche. Giving serious thought to the negative seems to me to be absolutely essential for establishing a theoretical conception that is capable of accounting for thought processes.

Bion emphasized the role of the object's *containing function.* For my part, I have developed the idea of a *framing structure.*[39] I make the assumption that the child (whatever culture he is born in) is held by the mother against her body. When contact with the mother's body is broken, what remains of this experience is the trace of the bodily contact – as a rule, the mother's arms – which constitutes a framing structure sheltering the loss of the perception of the maternal object, *in the form of a negative hallucination of it.* It is against this negativized background that the future object presentations, sheltered by the framing structure, will be inscribed. This containing function will allow for the elaboration of the work of representations which undergo the transformations relative to the transition from the psychical representatives of the drive to the word presentations and the ideas and judgements drawn from the experience of reality. Thus outside and inside will provide the basis for a model of the double limit and a framing structure for the model.

It seems to me, today, that while psychoanalysis was able to develop without concerning itself overly with thought processes when dealing with well-structured transference neuro-psychoses, the appearance, in all their diversity, of non-neurotic structures has shown the necessity for a psychoanalytic conception of thinking in order to understand these manifestations. Clinically, there can be no doubt of this, and patients speak about it spontaneously. They themselves say that they are incapable of thinking. It is not easy for the interlocutor who hears these words to form a clear picture of what they are referring to. In fact, what these patients do not realize is that, as a precautionary measure and to avoid anxiety (which they do not succeed in doing), they are engaged in a process of whitewashing ideas and evacuating any thoughts that could favour or give rise to the creation of links. They manage to forget what they have just been thinking.

I would say that these patients stop themselves from developing their thoughts, as if they sensed that if they were to allow them to develop it would lead them precisely where they have no wish to go, rather like the television viewer who is zapping not only because he is bored, but because he imagines that the rest of the programme might make him feel uneasy, or even cause him displeasure. This activity, which can range from cutting off thoughts to evacuating them, has an undeniably debilitating effect. It will be seen that we are dealing here with a very different mechanism from repression or even from splitting. An even more radical measure is put into operation when the subject carries out a negative hallucination of the meaning linked to words, where the recollection of certain things that have been said is completely dissociated from the sense that was attributed to them, or that had been conferred on them by the analyst's interpretation. The domain of thought disorders is certain to develop, and it is not impossible that the advances of neurobiology (the breakthroughs achieved by G. Edelman and M. Solms raised hopes of this)[40] will inaugurate a new period in this domain where little spadework has as yet been done.

The vast panorama we have been studying, starting with representations and concluding our reflections on the question of thought disorders, has shown us a great variety of psychic formations in the composition of the material subjected to analysis and calling for interpretation. Let me say, to conclude, that analysability depends on the relations that can be identified in a given piece of material, from an *intrapsychic* modality (relations between a slip of the tongue, a phantasy, acting out, traced back to their semantic elements and psychic function) and, from a standpoint that is complementary to it, from the *intersubjective* perspective (in the axis of the transference). This is the thinking that guides my approach.

Notes

1 Freud, S. (1891). *On Aphasia*. London: International Universities Press, 1953.
2 Freud, S. (1924). The loss of reality in neurosis and psychosis. *S.E.* XIX, 185.
3 It is right to draw attention to the anteriority of an *early reality-ego* whose function is limited to localizing the external or internal origin of the excitations.
4 I have proposed the term affect representative (*représentant-affect*) to mark the correspondence with the ideational representative (*représentant–représentation*).
5 Green, A. 'L'affect', paper presented to the XXXth Congress of French-speaking Psychoanalysts. *Revue française de psychanalyse*, 34, 1970, pp. 885–1169; reprinted in *Le discours vivant: la conception psychanalytique de l'affect*. Paris: Presses Universitaires de France, 1973. And 'Sur la discrimination et l'indiscrimination entre affect et repésentation', a paper presented to the Xth International Congress of Psychoanalysis, Santiago, 1999, reprinted in *La pensée clinique*. Paris: Editions Odile Jacob, 2002.
6 Green, A. (1973). *Le discours vivant. La conception psychanalytique de l'affect*. Paris: Presses Universitaires de France. [English edition: *The Fabric of Affect in the*

Psychoanalytic Discourse, p. 303, trans. A. Sheridan. London: Routledge and The Institute of Psychoanalysis, 1999.]

7   Here we have an echo of R. Thom's concepts of *saillance* and *pregnance*.

8   In English in the original.

9   I have myself devoted a study to the passions: Passions et destins des passions. In: *Nouvelle Revue de Psychanalyse*, 1980, 21; reprinted in *La folie privée*. Paris: Gallimard, 1990. [English edition: 'Passions and their vicissitudes', trans. K. Aubertin. In: *On Private Madness*. London: Hogarth Press, 1986.]

10 Freud, S. (1933). *New Introductory Lectures on Psychoanalysis*, S.E. XXII, 90.

11 Translator's note: there is a play on words here in French between *mû* (from *mouvoir* = move, prompt, propel) and *ému* (from *émouvoir* = to affect, stir, rouse, etc).

12 Green, A. *La pensée clinique*, p. 207. Paris: Odile Jacob.

13 See note 1.

14 Ibid. pp. 219–220.

15 As far as the description of these states is concerned, I refer the reader to my Santiago report: *see La Pensée clinique*, pp. 221–237.

16 Ibid. p. 251.

17 Green, A. First published in *The International Journal of Psycho-Analysis*, 1975, 56.

18 Marty, P. (1976). *Les mouvements individuels de vie et de mort*. Paris: Payot; and, (1980) *L'ordre psychosomatique*. Paris: Payot.

19 Green, A. Après coup, l'archaïque. In: *La folie privée*. Paris: Gallimard, 1990. [Trans. note: this paper is not one of those included in *On Private Madness*. London: Hogarth, 1988.]

20 Freud, S. (1908b). Character and anal eroticism. *SE. IX*, 169; and, (1917) On transformations of instinct as exemplified in anal eroticism. *S.E. XVII*, 125.

21 Reich, W. (1933). *Character Analysis*. New York: Orgone Institute Press, 1945.

22 *S.E.* XII, 313.

23 *S.E.* IX, 170.

24 *S.E.* VII, 238–239.

25 Ibid. 175.

26 *S.E.* XXII, 91.

27 Freud, S. (1941[1938]). Findings, Ideas, Problems. *S.E.* XXIII, 299.

28 Freud, S. (1926d). *Inhibitions, Symptoms and Anxiety*. *S.E.* XX, 77.

29 Combe, C. (2002). *Soigner l'anoréxie*. Paris: Dunod.

30 Fonagy, P. (2001). *Attachment Theory and Psychoanalysis*. New York: Other Press.

31 Cournut, J. Deuils ratés, morts méconnues. *Bulletin de la SPP*, 1983, no. 2, pp. 9–26.

32 Green, A. (1980). La mère morte. In: *Narcissism de vie, narcissisme de mort* (pp. 222–253). Paris: Editions de Minuit, 1983. [English edition: The dead mother, trans. Katherine Aubertin. In: *On Private Madness*, London: Hogarth Press, 1986; reprinted in *Life Narcissism, Death Narcissism*. London: Free Association Books, 2001.]

33 See note 1.

34 See Green, A. (1964). Névrose obsessionnelle et hystérie, leur relation chez Freud et depuis: étude clinique, critique et structurale. In: *Revue française de psychanalyse*, 28 (5/6), pp. 679–716.

35 Marty, P. ibid.

36 Marty, P. ibid.

37 Green, A. Du sens en psychosomatique. In: *Interrogations psychosomatiques*, directed by A. Fine and J. Shaeffer. Paris: Presses Universitaires de France, 1988.

38 Bion, W.R. (1967). *Second Thoughts*. London: Heinemann.

39 Green, A. (1983). *Narcissisme de vie, narcissisme de mort*. Paris: Editions de Minuit. [English edition: *Life Narcissism. Death Narcissism*. trans. Andrew Weller. London: Free Association Books, 2000.]

40 See below.

SPACE(S) AND TIME

Space(s)

In 1970, Serge Viderman published *La construction de l'espace analytique*.[1] The title was an allusion to a notion which was not very common at the time. Moreover, the content of his book only offered a succinct treatment of what the title announced. In *L'enfant de Ça*,[2] written in collaboration with Jean-Luc Donnet in 1973, I proposed a theory of psychic spaces, purporting that each agency is related to its own space. Although, generally speaking, the concept of the object in psychoanalysis has been developed at length, not enough consideration has been given, perhaps, to the fact that the characteristics of an object have to be considered in relation to the space around it. At any rate, Freud did not have recourse to this kind of expression – which has only come into use on a large scale in contemporary analysis. Nowadays, there is no longer much need to explain what is being referred to. I have had occasion to point out that psychoanalytic theory has extensively elaborated the concept of space, whereas its reflection is a good deal less rich with regard to the question of time. Space and time are a priori forms of sensible knowledge, according to Kant, a statement the validity of which Freud called into question. Moreover, his object was not what pertains to consciousness but to the unconscious, which has scarcely any notion of time. But if one takes into consideration not consciousness or even the unconscious, but the psychical apparatus, one realizes that it is necessary to turn one's attention to space and temporality, which refer to conceptions that are specific to psychoanalysis.

At the outset, Freud was interested above all in the dream-space. This was a deliberate choice. It was precisely because he was trying to penetrate the mystery of neurosis, by analysing the symptoms furnished by psychoanalytic clinical practice, that he found that he was disturbed by interference between the conscious and the unconscious as he was trying to determine what belonged to each respectively. So he decided to shut himself away in his own sleep with the aim of eliminating all input from the external world and consciousness, leaving the field as free as possible for the internal world and the unconscious. Freud's initial procedures were all guided by the opposition between the world of representations and that of perceptions. The first can be either conscious or unconscious, whereas the second only belong to consciousness. An unconscious representation can be linked up with a conscious representation, and there is a useful means of comparing the nature of each of them. We know how Freud opposed the system of thing-presentations and the word-presentations corresponding to them in order to define conscious representation, whereas unconscious representation was only formed of thing-presentations. Both are part of the internal world, divided into two parts of unequal importance the first of which, relatively restricted, is consciousness, and the second, much more considerable part, is the unconscious. The external world is accessible to us through the perceptions furnished by the sense organs. This elementary description can be made even more intelligible by the model I have proposed of the *double limit* (1982).[3] In such a model, a vertical division separates the inside from the outside, whereas the inside is itself divided into conscious space and unconscious space. Such is the schematized formula by means of which the constituent parts of a theory of the psychic spaces of the first topography can be gathered together. Nonetheless, this basic cell must be completed.

As for the external world, Freud neglected to distinguish the contribution made by the primary objects. Although their external status as not-ego is incontestable, even if it is not the only one, they must be individualized as such within the multitude of objects in the external world. They will have their counterpart in the form of the representation of external objects in the psyche (at the conscious and unconscious levels). As far as the internal world is concerned, the picture that has been given so far needs completing. The conscious and unconscious levels are separated by a horizontal limit. But, in fact, it is less a limit than a buffer zone with considerable importance since it concerns nothing less than the preconscious. The nature of the preconscious is altogether problematic and interesting. Structurally, the preconscious is attached to the conscious (we speak of the system *Cs.-Pcs.*), though it can also be attached to the unconscious: it is the portion of the latter that is capable of becoming conscious. In any case, it is a zone of active exchanges permitting the circulation of investments and memory traces on either side of this frontier zone, and harbouring processes of transformation in which language plays an important role. We should note in passing that an important part of the ego belongs to the preconscious. The first topography, which implies differently structured psychic spaces, remains, as I have often pointed out, organized around the reference to consciousness (conscious/pre*conscious*/un*conscious*). Here there is an implicit conception of negativity, since, of these three agencies, the first is positive; the second is negative but capable of being positivized; and the third is negative without the possibility of being positivized. It remains that by making these agencies revolve around the axis constituted by consciousness, even if the unconscious differs in its system of functioning, one can observe a certain unity between them. This is clear where representations are concerned. We have already seen earlier that the representative modalities are not limited to the couple thing-presentation/word-presentation. The controversy is still open with regard to the question of knowing whether it is legitimate to speak of unconscious affects (see above). What is certain is that when Freud felt the need to go beyond this first topography and to propose another, he modified, at the same time, the relations between the agencies. He now introduced the drives *into* the psychical apparatus. Speaking of the id, he used an abundance of metaphors to give an idea of the world inhabiting it. We are familiar with the famous comparisons, albeit somewhat naïve, with the constantly seething cauldron (The witches' soup in Macbeth!) of instinctual impulses seeking discharge, in other words having scarcely any space for elaboration. And Freud adds that everything we know of the id can only be imagined by means of a comparison which negativizes everything that is known of the ego which is more accessible to investigation. Drawing up a list of the ego's functions is not very useful. What I want to emphasize above all is that, unlike the id, the ego offers the instinctual impulses a space for elaboration. Let us bear in mind that, according to Freud, the ego is only that part of the id which has differentiated itself as a result of its contact with the external world. And this allows for the postponing of discharge, the activity of binding, the work on representations which gives them access to rationality by means of the relation between cause and consequence, the control of motor activity, the possibility of postponement, and so on. At any rate, it can never be emphasized enough how, in formulating the second topography, Freud insisted on the importance of *the unconsciousness of a large part of the ego*. I have shown that this unconsciousness pertains more to the container than the contents.

The most complex structure in terms of space is undoubtedly the superego. First because of its double nature, rooted in the id and a product of a division of the ego. It is quite plain for anyone who is interested in the pathological effects of the superego that the latter sometimes proves to be so cruel that one cannot avoid thinking that its sources are indeed to be found in the id. But, on the other hand, the role of identification refers us to a problem arising from the division of the ego: one part is devoted to investing an object, whereas the other undergoes the alteration implied by identification. Freud makes three observations which should be borne in mind here: The first indicates that the child's superego is formed through identification, *not with the parents' ego but with their superego*. The second lends particular attention to the processes of internal elaboration which will culminate in the setting up of an *impersonal* agency (thus detached from primary parental objects), reflecting a system of *ethical values*. The third, which is not the least important, is that the superego plays the role of a *protective power of destiny*. When an individual feels abandoned by this protective power, the danger of suicide is to be feared. This ranges from suicidal impulses to attempts at suicide and then to the successful suicide attempt. Let us beware of speaking too hastily of blackmail. The complex and ambiguous structure of the superego can lead one to see it as a quasi-persecuting agency, always demanding fresh sacrifices at the level of instinctual satisfaction, but, paradoxically, as protective too, acting as a safeguard of life. One can see how difficult it is to imagine the system of exchanges which could define the space of the superego. It seems perfectly obvious that the superego surpasses the limits of a particular individual (this is already the case when identification with the parents' superego is involved); it continues into the cultural space guarding the values of a given social group and, beyond that, of a civilization. Thus individual superego and cultural value do not have watertight relations isolating them from each other; they stimulate each other mutually and potentialize the forces animating them. Cornelius Castoriadis has usefully extended Freud's initial observations on this point.[4] As for the ego, the question of the link between the representations and their energetic correlates is in the foreground here. Betraying cultural norms leads to despondency, mourning. But one can add that the processes of binding, much more than for the ego, bind aggressivity in order to metabolize its manifestations and convert them into socially acceptable forms of behaviour or even ones on which society places value, while at the same time establishing, within their ethical system, metaphorical links maintained by culture. Naturally, the question arises here of the relations between social reality and the way it wishes to appear through the manifestations to which it gives rise, which are supported by an ideology that is permanently nourished and considered as representing the shared beliefs of a given community.

One of the most remarkable elaborations of the transformations of the superego resides in the constitution of alterity. The Other does indeed seem to be at the root of every ethical system. We know that, in certain psychoanalytic theorisations (Lacan, Laplanche), this concept has a central importance even to the point of relegating to a secondary position Freudian concepts which do not take enough account of it.

It will be understood that a theory of spaces leads us to articulate various types of spatiality here, ranging from that in which the margin of manoeuvre – I would say the 'respiration' of the forces within it – is the most reduced, to the practically unlimited field of culture fixed by tradition which allows it to enrich itself and, above all, to be internalized so as to become part of the most fundamental elements of the psychic life of an individual and his relation to the generations before him and after him.

Time

The history of the treatment of temporality in psychoanalysis is a curious one, covering two periods. The first runs right the way through Freud's work. It is characterized by a continual growth in richness and complexity from the beginning until the end. The second period begins after Freud's death. In fact, it began before his death, as early as 1924, and had continued into the present. In contradistinction to the first period, where Freud was moving towards ever greater complexity, here one has the feeling that with the passing of time, the richness of Freudian thought has increasingly been eroded, and a simplifying consensus has been created to reduce temporality to a smaller common denominator marked by the hegemony of the genetic point of view. Although present in Freud's work, the latter has never been anything other than one of the constituents of an otherwise more complicated problem that causes the analyst difficulties when interpreting material which presents links with the patient's past and his history.[5] Before going into further details, we can note that the treatment of the history and of the past has been the subject of deceptions and has led analysts to fall back on such choices as the exclusive practice by the English school of making *here and now* interpretations, aimed at according exclusive importance to the actuality of what is happening during the session. I do not believe, for my part, that this loss of confidence in interpretations related to the past is an example to be followed. There are several reasons justifying this position, it seems to me. First, by alternating interpretations referring to the present and those referring to the past, albeit hypothetical and aleatory, the analysis is obliged to go back and forth between what is happening *here and now* and what is supposed to have happened *at another time and in another place*. Moreover, these *here and now* interpretations are frequently related to a conception of the cure in which a very distant past, often going back to the first two years, is experienced as present. It has to be understood as a resurgence of the first period of life (see M. Klein's 'memories in feeling') according to the Kleinians. In my opinion such a view is utopian. All material, whatever it is, comprises, as Freud had already shown for the screen-memories, elements belonging to different layers of the past which are intermingled and remodelled by a secondary elaboration when they surface in the material. Likewise, it does not seem legitimate to me to interpret material connected with relatively late periods of development (those of the Oedipus complex, or adolescence) as a defence in relation to what can be imagined in the way of earlier, sometimes primal fixations. We need to bear in mind here Freud's great disappointment in 1937 when he was obliged to accept that a complete lifting of infantile amnesia was utopian. Hence the interest he took in hallucinatory reminiscences, which he interpreted as translating manifestations of the return of the past belonging to a period when the registration of memories as such was not possible owing to the early character of the traumas and the absence of language making it possible to fix them in the form of memories at the time when they were experienced. As we shall see, Freud's point of view on temporality was formed by an accumulation of mechanisms of different types. However, with Melanie Klein, who was interested in the mechanisms of the very earliest period of childhood, the predominance of what she considered comprehensible from a 'genetic' standpoint was already affirmed. Her observations were not accepted by the adversaries of the Kleinian movement, and more especially by the American school which came to the assistance of Anna Freud. They proposed to construct what in their eyes was a 'truly' genetic conception, founded on observation and aiming to restrict the element of phantasmagorical speculation which, in their view, Melanie Klein took advantage of without supplying proof of what she was advancing.

For my part, I shall defend the point of view that Freud's hypotheses still have their utility, but that they must be understood as relating – as far as some of them are concerned – to different categories of patients and referring to various types of mental functioning. Once again, it is undoubtedly the increasing presence of non-neurotic structures on analysts' couches which has upset the homogeneity of yesteryear, replacing it with a multi-hued polymorphism.

General framework of the theory of temporality

Freud pointed out on more than one occasion that, in psychoanalysis, only the method is psychological. Analysis, *stricto sensu*, consisted in dissolving (this is the etymological sense of the term) psychologically a clinical structure composed of different symptoms, some psychological and others somatic, which combined their effects and were intermingled, giving birth to a distorted psychical activity. What Freud contended was that, from the beginning, the two series of factors, psychological and somatic, were intermingled, giving birth to psychical activity. This is why the concept of the drive, situated at the frontier of the somatic and the psychic was, in his eyes, particularly appropriate, implying as a consequence a 'demand made upon the mind for work in consequence of its connection with the body' (*S.E.* XIV, 122). Two problems are raised. The first is the way in which the psychic can be conceived as emerging from the somatic in development; and the second is the possibility in certain particularly regressive structures, of losing a portion of the attributes of the psyche won over from the bodily determinants to which they are linked. In other words, we once again see the importance of the idea of the plasticity and flexibility of the interactions between psychic and somatic. There is, as we know, only one reality, the brain; and when we speak of the psychic and the somatic, we are referring to two different levels of brain activity. The psychic is related to those parts of the brain which concern what we call the mind. Which does not mean that the psychic is not dependent on the mechanisms of the brain. The somatic depends functionally on the part (sub-cortical) of the brain which is related to the bodily organs at its periphery. Psychic expression concerns, in particular, the relations between the 'soul' and the body.

These remarks apply directly to the question of time. One aspect of time is obviously dependent on somatic influences (biological clocks, circadian rhythms, cerebral formations linked with time, developmental stages). I am not suggesting that developmental stages are exclusively determined by somatic factors, for they too are subject to psychological influences, as Spitz[6] was the first to show. It is undeniable that these patients are also under the control of somatic influences. In other words, the causality in question here, while being dependent on biological factors, can also be influenced by other factors described by Freudian theory (*Nachträglichkeit*, infantile amnesia, ignorance of time by the unconscious, etc.). Other factors, too, according to Freud, are supposed to have a biological origin (phylogenetic memory traces), although biology in no way confirms this hypothesis. But, notwithstanding this hypothetical origin, Freud still attributes them with psychological functions (categorization of psychic experiences). Ultimately, it is difficult to escape the impression that, when Freud describes repetition-compulsion, he does not have in mind a form of regression which relates psychic activity to the level of drive functioning, close to their biological moorings. Hence the temptation to translate the expression by repetition 'automatism'. We thus come to the conclusion that the Freudian conception of time implies an articulation of the levels of psychic functioning from the id to the superego.

As time passed, Freudian metapsychology (in the broad sense) lost its credit. It was short-circuited by other explanatory systems (object-relations theory); or, subjected to the spotlight of severe criticism, it was rejected in particular on account of its unverifiable speculations and replaced by theories of a more distinctly psychological nature. Criticism took a different course in France, but culminated in many cases in a rejection, albeit in the name of conflicting principles. The common idea was to recognize that Freud had made a discovery of cardinal importance, i.e. the unconscious, but that he had inserted it into a completely erroneous context. However, if we look at the matter more closely, there were not two authors who could agree on the right solution to rectify Freud's errors. Along with the criticism of his biological 'errancy', his solipsistic conception of development was considered inadmissible. It is not difficult, behind all these criticisms, to discover that all of them are related, in fact, to his theory of the drives. It was the object or, in other contexts, the subject (of inter-subjectivity) and the Other, that pushed the drive off the stage. Increasingly, the field of psychoanalysis became restricted to its method of treatment. This encouraged the abandonment and condemnation, in general, of methods of applied psychoanalysis owing to the criticisms of the representatives of disciplines which felt they were being colonised by psychoanalysis.

It is understandable that there has been an increasing unwillingness to adopt Freud's biological axioms uncritically. In fact, the opinions of psychoanalysts are divided into two camps. While some consider that Freud's biologism is but gratuitous speculation and have opted for a reinterpretation of his theory on more clearly affirmed psychological bases, others, on the contrary, think that Freud was *not enough* of a biologist, and, claiming to base the theory on more unquestionably scientific foundations, have wished to see it freed of all its pseudoscientific trappings in favour of an authentically scientific discipline of thought. This has resulted, on the one hand, in a psychological or psychologizing psychoanalysis, isolated from the natural sciences, and, on the other, in an allegiance to the neurosciences which as a rule have been hostile to psychoanalysis, considering it merely as a late representative of a spiritualist, not to say metaphysical, theory. From another point of view one can think that, even when they are inexact, Freud's theories have the merit of preserving the place of later discoveries which, in due course, have completed the body of psychoanalytic knowledge. This does not mean that we must accept blindly the acquisitions of biology inasmuch as many of them are foreign to the object of psychoanalysis. I will come back to this problem in the last part of this book. It would seem difficult to cease to make any further reference to biology, for we would then be in a more embarrassing position for resolving certain questions raised by psychosomatics,[7] biological discoveries in the field of depressions, and the effect of psychotropic drugs, especially in psychoses. Naturally, I am not saying that Freud's biological speculations can provide answers to these questions, but they can contribute to the search for adequate solutions.

Let us return to the problem of time. The rejection of Freud's hypotheses led progressively to the abandonment of the complex theoretical series of statements he had developed concerning time. Perhaps such a set of views was not easy to handle. By a sort of tacit consensus, the adoption of the genetic point of view became a point of concentration for all the problems associated with the organization of temporality. Even those who were not entirely in agreement with Hartmann followed the same direction. For it is impossible to say that Melanie Klein, Bion or Winnicott shared Hartmann's views. French analysts, under the influence of Lacan, and also many who were not Lacanians, resisted the American approach and engaged in a long-term battle with it. They insisted on the Freudian conception of *Nachträglichkeit* becoming aware in the process that many of their Anglo-Saxon colleagues did not even know what they were referring to. And it was then discovered that no English translation of the Freudian expression was satisfactory.

What is the current situation? Whatever differences there may be, it is clear that the developmental genetic standpoint has dominated the scene and eclipsed the other constituents of the Freudian conception. And yet, it cannot be said that the genetic point of view has succeeded in commanding unanimity. I propose to distinguish two principal trends. The first represents the prolongation of the classical psychoanalytic method, attempting to construct a coherent theory on the basis of the experience of the psychoanalytic cure. This position has not led to any general agreement. Melanie Klein's theory is not compatible either with Kohut's or with Lacan's, to confine ourselves to those. The second trend, which is also plural, is an attempt to construct a coherent theory of development on the basis of child and baby observation within a research setting. We are in the presence of a broad spectrum of constructions which range from Esther Bick to R. Emde and P. Fonagy – which sometimes have little in common and even criticize each other, when they are not fighting each other. We can find other approaches, for instances, those of M. Mahler, Roiphe and Galenson, D. Stern, etc. Beyond the differences – and even sometimes the oppositions – in these authors' 'discoveries', it is important to emphasize that sometimes they position themselves with reference to psychoanalytic theory, and sometimes they adopt an objectivist method which proclaims its scientificity and states that it is quite ready to reject many, if not most of the theorems of psychoanalysis, Freudian and post-Freudian. The problem of time, in this context, is dramatically reduced to questions of clocks, calendars and diaries, and to that which can be examined from the outside with the aid of interpretative grids ranging from the most biological to the most psychological in a so-called *continuum*. What about accessibility to the intrapsychic world then?

Another division appears to structure analytic thought. It contrasts and links the *intrapsychic and the intersubjective*. It is clear that the first of the two seeks to understand the functioning of the psyche from the inside with the help of the indications that we have of it owing to certain processes that emerge from it. Their paradigms can be found in dreams. By contrast, the intersubjective point of view is more linked to a relational perspective. Its paradigm is the exchange between two persons, child and adult, or between adults, as in the transference process of analytic treatment. The intrapsychic focuses on the roots of psychic activity, those that are the most deeply covered over, those that are the least accessible to direct exploration. The intersubjective explores the exchange that is observable from the outside by someone who is in a position to describe the processes taking place. Very few efforts venture to combine the two perspectives, as it would seem logical to do.[8]

Elements for a psychoanalytic conception of time

Before venturing to propose a psychoanalytic conception of time, it is necessary to review the different aspects of the overall picture. Freud discovered them step by step. His ideas show that initially his approach to the unconscious was three-pronged – that is to say, via the dream (*Traum*), the joke (*Witz*), and the drive (*Trieb*). This was the path he followed, exploring many fields along the way before arriving at his systematic conception of infantile development in the *Three Essays on the Theory of Sexuality* (1905d). I have thus felt it is legitimate to speak of a *tree of time* in Freud's thought.[9]

The development of the libido

This notion is the most popular and the easiest to retain and use, albeit often to the detriment of fidelity to the facts. Freud did not seek to give a complete view of individual development, but to present a picture which followed a progressive pattern from the mouth to the genital organs, and from the feeding situation to sexual relations. He endeavoured to explain how these different stages could be marked by fixations and give rise to regressions that would draw the psyche back to earlier stages linked to the erogenous zones and intensely invested objects. He was clearly referring here to the pleasure-seeking libido, governed by the pleasure/unpleasure principle. It is important to emphasize that, for Freud, the motor for development is the progressive replacement of one erogenous zone by another, succeeding it, until the Oedipal phase crowning infantile sexuality. The *diphasic status* of the libido separates infantile sexuality from puberty and post-puberty in its adult form.

Though it is undeniable that a developmental model of a linear type is obviously being described here, it still needs to be added that the evolution of psychic development is concentrated on the erogenous zones from an anatomical and functional point of view. These zones are made up of mucous tissues sensitive to excitation, which form areas of transition permitting communication between inside and outside. This explains the polarization of psychic experiences of which they are the source. But this linear movement is in fact relative. Freud stresses that each new phase of libidinal development co-exists with the one before it, comparing them to a series of lava flows one on top of the other. These fixations will provoke repressions forming a *discontinuous* memory of psychic events, leading to infantile amnesia. The continuity of memory cannot exist owing to the maintenance of defences, above all repression, which create gaps, or holes in the personal history.

Bidirectional models

Freud always believed that dreams had a memory function. But the principal characteristic of dreams is that, each night, we seem to be trying to undo the work which took place during the waking activity of the day before. In waking life, we give priority to progressive thinking. When we go to sleep, and dream, a mode of thinking inhabited by topographical regression sets in, trying to find some satisfaction for the waking fantasies that had to be repressed. This satisfaction is made possible by the lowering of censorship. Dream analysis shows the representation of events occurring during various periods of life. Dreams appear to be a *recurrent digression* (Green) occurring on the margins of ordinary time. The dream work demonstrates its indifference to the idea of time.

Repression

Herein lies the major cause of the incomplete picture we have of our psychic functioning, ruining the confidence that we are able to place in our conscious processes. Other defences can have a more radical (foreclosure or rejection), more paradoxical (splitting or disavowal), or more general (negation) character. I have proposed that they be grouped together under the heading of the *work of the negative*.

Nachträglichkeit

It is impossible to describe it in detail here. Trauma does not consist only or essentially in its original occurrence (the earliest scene), but in its retrospective recollection (the latest scene). The reason for this is that the later recollection occurs in a sexually mature body, whereas the body, at the time of the trauma, was only inhabited by a pre-pubertal sexuality (pre-sexual sexuality). Accordingly, the period of the primitive trauma could not have its full effect. It is thus often the recollection of the trauma that is more traumatic than the event which bears its name. This point leaves to one side the other traumas which can affect the ego, discovered much later by Ferenczi. Sexuality, in its essence, is premature; hence the inevitable disturbances linked to its existence. What is more, the analysis of the Wolf Man brought Freud back to the problem of *Nachträglichkeit* so that he could evaluate the influence of the observation of the primal scene on the patient's psychopathology. Freud thereby forced us to consider the role of the intrusion of parental sexuality, breaking into the child's mind and exciting his libido.

Timelessness of the unconscious

This idea, one of Freud's most audacious, still arouses criticism today. In fact, this concept is an essential cog in the psychoanalytic conception of time. It is linked with the primary processes, which are supposedly unaware of time just as they are of negation and doubt. We are always struck in psychoanalytic experience, by the persistence intact in adulthood, and even later, of childhood wishes. They reappear in the patient who does not seem to be aware that these manifestations belong to a very distant past. A striking example can be found in the sexual theories of children which continue to operate in the unconscious of adults.

Primal phantasies

Freud wanted to explain how the varieties of individual experience could be condensed into a few very limited and encountered phantasies (seduction, castration, primitive scene) in all patients. If they have their origin at the heart of the multiplicity and variability of the innumerable experiences that individuals undergo, how is it that we notice them appearing regularly in contexts where they seem to be organizing psychical activity? The question is a legitimate one. The answer that Freud proposed is widely refuted today because it seems to be in contradiction with the discoveries of biology. Freud postulated the existence of a set of primal phantasies – Lacan calls them *key signifiers* – representing phylogenetic memory traces whose role is to impose a certain order on the infinite varieties of individual experience by classifying them. The questions Freud raised deserve our consideration, but call for different explanations. However, according to him, these basic memory traces have to be re-experienced individually – here Freud takes his distance from Jung – in order to be efficient, which implies that individual experience cannot be short-circuited. These phantasies thus have a 'disposition for re-acquisition'.

Repetition as a substitute for remembering

Freud was long embarrassed by the transference. He considered it initially as a resistance, for it worked against remembering. He later discovered that some patients repeated by acting out instead of remembering. This means, para-doxically, that they seem to be incapable of remembering and can only use acting out, which then acquires this signification. It was this fact that led, in my view, to the second topography, which involved a considerable change. The role played by representation in the first topography was replaced in the second by instinctual impulses (representations were no longer mentioned in the Freud's description of the id). The reference to instinctual impulses bears witness to the increasing influence of the drives in the last phase of the theory. *In the second topography*, as I keep repeating, *the drives are included in the psychical apparatus.* In the first topography, only their representations were included in the psychical apparatus. The stage of 1914, 'Remembering, Repeating and Working-Through', was followed in 1920 by *Beyond the Pleasure Principle*, which proposes the theory of repetition-compulsion as a characteristic of *all* instinctual functioning, while adding to it certain special attributes which make it more deadly owing to the 'death drive'. The effect of the latter is clearly to undo any psychically significant or important temporal sequence in relation with the pleasure principle which could be in the service of the ego.

Forces of destiny

In parallel with its function of censorship, the superego plays the role of a protective power of destiny. This is not only because it is the guardian of tradition and ethics but also because, in conjunction with the ego ideal, it takes into consideration the consequences of planned actions and watches over the destiny of individuals. While the ego has the function of postponing the demands of the id, the superego is an orientator of time (Green). Its action is not satisfied with simply ensuring the primacy of rationality, but demands to be placed under a higher authority playing the role of 'parent of the human species'.

Events which cannot be remembered

In 'Constructions in Analysis' (1937d), Freud acknowledges the impossibility of recalling traumas experienced in the first ages of life (during the first two years) owing to the fact that they occur before language has been acquired, as I have already mentioned. Remembering thus assumes the unusual forms of hallucinatory states or uncontrollable repeated acting out.

Historical truth

Freud's concept of historical truth is often misunderstood. It is not a question of a truth that has been historically established, that is to say, validated by evidence. On the contrary, it is historical in the sense that the beliefs in question, which are powerfully invested as if they were true, are dependent on beliefs which already prevailed in the psyche of the individual at the time when they emerged, while claiming to have the status of eternal truth. These truths are, in fact, but resurrections, under a new cloak, of old convictions or ancient fables. They reappear in the present in a distorted fashion. Inasmuch as they are repetitions of the past that can no longer be remembered, they are truths which express themselves compulsively (as in religious beliefs). Insofar as the contents of these truths no longer represent the original conditions under which they emerged, they are illusions. This condition should not be limited to socio-historical manifestations. The compulsive quality of some psychic structures is in fact bound up with events which are relived in the form of uncontrollable compulsions. The fact that they are mixed, from the beginning, with influences from the environment should not make us overlook their repetitively compulsive dimension.

Such are the different aspects which bear witness to the complexity of Freud's conception of temporality. There is no need to underline the extent to which the reference to a genetic point of alone impoverishes this richness.

The determinants of time

It is time to regroup the different elements organizing the temporality of psychic structure. Different types must be distinguished.

Biological determinants

Some of them are evident. It is clear that maturation and development are, partially at least, under the influence of biological models, as are diurnal and nocturnal rhythms. Freud describes a typical historical sequence: early trauma which cannot be remembered, repression, return of the repressed taking, in certain cases, the form of a compulsion to repeat which re-actualizes the traces of the original trauma. It is also reasonable to assume that the immaturity of the brain is responsible for the impossibility of remembering early traumas and may explain their expressions in the form of hallucinatory states or acting out. In formulating the conditions which accompany these early traumas, Freud says that too much was demanded of the psyche during this period of immaturity.

Other determinants are entirely hypothetical. Such is the case of the very debatable ideas on phylogenesis, the transmission of acquired characteristics, and so on. As I have already said, though the answers given by Freud are unacceptable, the questions he raises are worthy of our consideration.

We are probably ready today to accept that a single model cannot describe the Oedipus complex, and that we need to recognize several models which cannot be entirely subsumed under the classical *Vaterkomplex*. I am not drawing here on the discoveries of observations based on developmental studies, but on what I have learnt from clinical experience. Instead of simply opposing pregenital and genital structures, it would be better to compare different models of organization on a clinical basis. The structures that are the most far removed from the Oedipal model will present the most compact experiences of time with a limitation of possibilities with regard to temporal resources. In other words, the rich network present in Freud's work is much more restricted here. The freedom necessary for creativity is lacking. Creativity goes hand in hand with freedom, and freedom with the capacity to move from one mode of thinking to another according to the circumstances. The importance of the compulsion to repeat is striking in borderline cases. It is clear in my mind that in describing the compulsion to repeat, Freud thought that the psychic activity observable in these cases was more dependent on instinctual functioning than on that of the unconscious. Do we have the right to infer biological factors in this case?

Psychic determinants

They form the specificity of the psychoanalytic conception of time. No other theory, outside psychoanalysis, defends comparable ideas. A general model can be sifted out from a large variety of modalities. Psychical activity, which is subject to the determinism of the unconscious, can rarely be envisaged directly, according to the scheme cause–consequence. Most of the time, the psychic follows a general model. If we consider X as an unknown experience (unknown as such because it is only apprehended retrospectively), it is unacceptable in part, either so as to preserve the organization of the ego, or for fear of the object's disapproval. It therefore has to be repressed. As such, it does not disappear; it remains in the unconscious and *is attracted by the pre-existent repressed* (Freud). Its contents combine with other earlier contents, present in the unconscious, and become an integral part of its organization. At a given moment, facilitated by certain circumstances (weakening of the censorship, increase of desire or wishes, disguises which deceive repression, symbolic reinforcement, life events, etc.), it resurfaces: this is the return of the repressed. *This is the real point of departure, and not the unknown original event, which can only be conceived retrospectively.*

I have described the process in terms of a linear temporal sequence for reasons of intelligibility. In fact, it is with the return of the repressed that we must begin. This can take a 'normal' form, that is to say a dream or a parapraxis or an act of forgetting; or it can reappear in the form of a symptom (benign, if it is a neurosis); or it can manifest itself in a transferential movement (even outside a regular transference process). The important thing is to understand that *it is only with this return that we can have an idea of what has been repressed or reduced to silence, obliging us to make assumptions a posteriori concerning the inaugural x which can only be grasped retrospectively and hypothetically.* This typical model functions by virtue of the structure of our psyche: the capacity to dream, the existence of unconscious primary processes, the function of *Nachträglichkeit*, and so on. The timelessness of the unconscious is a formidable reserve of dynamic purposive ideas and wishes charged with their unconscious meaning. It is more than probable that these constitute the basis of our pleasure in living. We need a set of psychic organizers and disorganizers to complete the picture.

Organizers

The paradigm for understanding the situation is the transference, where all these aspects are encountered. Instead of returning to the interminable discussions on the transference as a repetition of the past or as an experience that has never occurred before, I want to propose another conception. Both of the options I have just mentioned are true. The transference process cannot be entirely independent of the past; nor can it be a mere repetition of the past. What we can say, as Bion has already stated, is that we have to arrive at an *approximation* of the truth about the past, with the analysand's agreement. The psychoanalytic work must culminate in an agreement on a possible relation between the past and the experience of the analysis, overcoming the opposition between phantasy and reality between the analysand and the analyst. It is important to emphasize that it is now impossible to speak of a pure transference process, which is an ideal condition that is never encountered. We have before us different models of transference depending on the patient's psychopathology. This clouds our comprehension of what happens in the cure. The situation is aggravated by the diversity of techniques for analysing the transference. An always enigmatic question is that of the negative therapeutic reaction, with its cortège of endless repetitions, its impossibility of completing a work of mourning, its incurable feelings of solitude, of despair, of vengeance. It is in these cases that the past seems to be blocked, and the patient petrified in his protests. Here, the analyst sometimes has the feeling that the unconscious aim is to stop the course of time by repeating perpetually a stillborn relationship.

I should say a word about the cultural determinants of the organization of time. I am referring here to the superego, nourished by ancestral values. Without overlooking socio-anthropological aspects, what is important for a psychoanalyst is the manner in which a subject integrates what he has received from the values of his parental imagos, shared by the community to which he belongs. The superego and the ego ideal will have the effect of protecting the organization of time owing to the psyche's vulnerability to the assaults of the drives, the ego's dissatisfactions, and the disappointments of reality. An important criticism can be made of Freud's theories in the measure that they underestimate the influence of the Other. It is true that the theory of the drives neglects the importance of the object relation. It is impossible today to put forward a theory of the experience of time without recognizing *the time of the Other* (the object, the parental imago). Primitive experiences of time, which occur even before the sovereignty of the pleasure–unpleasure principle is established, are rooted in temporal sequences comprised of rhythms, tonalities, modalities, repetitions, etc. (A. Denis[10]) to which the object will give meaning and which will be linked to the alternatives of its presence and its absence. Furthermore, the time of the mother is different, in essence, from that of the child. The mother has to identify *regressively* with the child, and the child progressively with the mother. It is on the basis of the intermittent encounters between mother and child that the functions of the object will facilitate the entanglement of the feelings of love and hate, as well as those connected with construction and destruction, in the mode of oscillations between pleasant and unpleasant experiences. All these aspects contribute to the construction of the experience of time. Let us recall that Freud considered that the experience of time, which belongs to consciousness, is the result of discontinuous investments (see the 'Mystic Writing-Pad').

Disorganizers

Many of the points that I shall be mentioning here appear in the last part of Freud's work. The hypothesis that I am making of disorganizers is supposed to account, in part, for the failures of analytic treatment. Let us recall the main ones:

- early traumas which cannot be remembered, that is to say, elaborated, which cannot be integrated at the heart of the psyche
- absence-deficiency of the transitional area (Winnicott)

- repetition-compulsion
- failure of reparation (M. Klein)
- unbinding due to excessive projective identification and attacks on linking
- distortion of the ego which has become incapable of integrating the transformations of the drives and their evolution in more flexible structures which have the possibility of taking the paths of sublimation.

In all the situations I have described, it is plain that Freud underestimated the importance of object relations. Nor did he develop all the resources that may be expected of the ego, which is understood currently in terms of Self or Subject. All things considered, Freud's conception is still very useful for it shows the diversity of mechanisms which intervene in the regulation of time, within a psychoanalytic perspective of the psyche.

Polychrony: exploded time

An analysis of the different components of temporality shows the existence of a network of heterogeneous constituents. In the Freudian conception of time one can retrace different types of organization consisting of attributes of the psychic world: drives, unconscious ideas, memory, conscious experiences. The entire system cannot fail to evoke a *polychronic structure* of what are sometimes conflictual relations. The final picture will be one of *exploded time* (*temps éclaté*, Green 2001). Living organisms are governed by the arrow of time. Time is no longer reversible; life unfolds from birth to death. It is oriented from the past towards the future. Its paradigm is not entropy but organization (see below, E. Morin). Until Freud, we had been accustomed to thinking that the human psyche was always subject to the passage of time – human beings knew that they had to expect to die sooner or later. Death is certain; only the moment of its coming remains uncertain. While it is stressed that burying the dead is one of the distinctive signs of humanity, one can also say that one of the tasks of philosophy is to meditate on death.

What Freud contributed to our knowledge was absolutely revolutionary. At the beginning, we have an immediate experience of time. It is experience of the positive present caught between a past and a future. It is experience linked to the currents of consciousness. It is also connected with feelings of 'temporariness' and, more generally, with affects, ranging from ephemeral joy to interminable sufferings. However rich this experience is, though, it is not specific to psychoanalysis. One is also bound to say that psychoanalysis has contributed very little to its comprehension. What it has shown is that this familiar knowledge of time, experienced intuitively, is in fact but a small part of temporality, as any analysis shows convincingly. Moreover, psychoanalysis has tied this experience up with the successive phases of ontogenesis affecting the sensual body, subject to fixations and regressions.

181

Human consciousness of time is, to a certain extent, contradicted by other parameters of temporality. This is partly due to the structure of our biologically determined brain. This would seem to be the function of dreaming. Although reality obliges us to submit to the coercion of time from youth to old age, this hard necessity can be circumvented by a subsystem which is able to enact wish fulfilments at the heart of an internal world in which we immerse ourselves each night, and in which we believe quite as much as we do in the external world during waking life. Because this is the creation of our desires, we believe in it more than we do in what we call external reality which we are obliged to accept. Such is the basis of our beliefs in a timeless psychic reality. It would be wrong to suppose that this subsystem is indestructible. Nightmares and other disturbances of the function of dreaming indicate that cracks can occur, giving rise to raw forms of anxiety and sometimes leading to serious disorganizations.

But even if the function of dreaming, that is to say the system of thing-presentations, equally at work in phantasies, is not available, other solutions are possible owing to primary thought – processes which are unaware of time. I would emphasize the fact that primary processes are essentially comprised of representations – for the most part visual – accompanied by their affects. Surely the most revolutionary advance Freud made was that of showing the omnipotent capacity of the mind to resist the debasement of psychic processes subject to the passage of time. This ineluctable submission, which is another way of obeying the injunction to abandon wishes or phantasies, is based on the opposition of reality or the superego. This system requires the help of a special mechanism in order to avoid being submerged by anxiety – namely, repression. The price to be paid for its efficiency is that important parts of our memory are sacrificed; consequently, it is incomplete concerning certain important events of our past. Owing to this system which is capable of suppressing the effects of disappointment and of procuring the compensation of wish fulfilments through dreams and phantasies, as well as with the help of the omnipotence of thoughts, life can become tolerable and agreeable on certain conditions, and sometimes fascinating. But, in other unfortunate outcomes such as mourning, unhappiness, torments, nameless dread, time is an infinite torturing experience, to the point even of making us hope that death will intervene to deliver us from it.

My description so far only concerns the events of daily life, those that may be described as 'normal'. We must now turn our attention towards the processes that are met with in neurosis. I have already described the benign topographical regression that occurs in dreams. In neurosis, regression is not only topographical, but also temporal, with a return to the fixations of childhood. But here, we are still in the domain of representations and affect. Reversibility to normality, thanks to analytic treatment, can be reasonably hoped for if there are no disturbances in the ego's functioning. Finally, when the representational system is overwhelmed, and when regression brings the psychical apparatus back to the functioning consecutive to the early traumas, resulting also in disorganizations of the ego, repetition-compulsion is at work and there is a danger of a negative therapeutic reaction. There can be no denying that the forces of destruction play an important role in non-neurotic structures. In fortunate cases, love and pleasure finally overcome negative influences. A re-evaluation of the technique involving modifications of time (lengthening of sessions) may be called for in deep regressions (Winnicott).

Countertransference reactions can obscure the situation. Interpretations have a limited effect if the question of time is neglected. Constructions not only concern the past, but also the mental processes arising in the transference relationship. Finally, being conscious of one's own historical truth, that is to say, according to Freud, accepting that the truth can only be reached via its distortions, may be the last word of the analytic process.

This tripartite system comprised of normality, neurosis, and borderline or psychotic structure, has to be completed by a synchronic point of view. All of the mechanisms can come into play in any one of the aforementioned structures. What is important to remember is that all the processes described act together, often involving conflictual relations. Hence the idea of *exploded time*.

Timelessness and the denial of time

Among the specific characteristics of the psychoanalytic conception of time, there are two that deserve our attention owing to possible misunderstandings: timelessness and the compulsion to repeat. Both seem to challenge our most evident ideas about time. But each does so in its own way. To say that the unconscious is unaware of time, as Freud postulated, does not mean that we can escape the ravages of time. We get older each day, whatever our age. Our functions also age. When one thinks of sexuality, for instance, it is obvious that it undergoes changes, irrespective of individual susceptibilities. In the end, we are forced to acknowledge the decline of this activity which deteriorates like other psychic functions such as memory, attention, and so on. The same thing applies where sexual needs are concerned. It has been said that there is some advantage in no longer being tormented by the burden of sexuality when one advances in age. So what is the meaning of this enigmatic timelessness? I think that what Freud meant was that the memory traces of our libidinal desires and the capacity that we have of reinvesting them again is never lost and is always potentially active. It retains its vivacity and its possibility of being reinvested at the level of its traces, even when sexual potency is lost. Hence, insofar as the desires, wishes and phantasies that are part of our unconscious being are concerned, there is something in them that never wears out. We can think of it as a sort of reserve of life, hope, and of illusions, too, which at least make life tolerable when it has become less agreeable owing to the process of ageing. In the unconscious, wishes do not concern the things that we hope will happen; they take the form, in their representations, of *wishes that have already been realized*. All this necessitates a complex psychical organization which gives us the capacity of binding together wishes that have not yet been realized and wishes that have already been realized, according to a very specific meaning. They can thus be invested, preserved, stored up, while still remaining available when recourse to them is necessary to sustain what is alive in the individual, in his internal world, thus helping him to face the difficulties of life. Nostalgia.

A great change occurred in psychoanalysis when Winnicott developed the concept of illusion. Before him, Freud had fought hard to convince us of its harmful influence in psychic life, underlining in particular its negative aspects for the psyche, inviting us to analyse them, that is to say to dissolve it, in order to establish the undivided sovereignty of reason. But Winnicott has shown us how much illusion is important for the healthy development of the psyche. Accepting disillusionment implies that we have first been subject to illusion, a necessary stage in our development. When this is lacking in our development, a premature awakening to reality proves to be harmful to development.

The compulsion to repeat is of a different genre. Here, it is not only wishes that persist in our mind, or our infantile phantasies, which have never disappeared; it is the capacity for *actualizing* more or less complete configurations which are liberated and repeated endlessly, as if to give them a tangible reality. The actualization assumes the form of acting out in the psyche. All analysts have had the experience of the desperate sterility of the interminable repetitions in certain analysands in spite of intense analytic work.

Is this a form of timelessness? In principle, one could argue that it is. Except that, in fact, it is the opposite. Timelessness presupposes that the hope of realizing a wish or a phantasy is always ready for use if appropriate circumstances demand it: for example, when excessive frustrations arise. This can be observed at the level of unconscious formations, whose function is to maintain them. We should bear in mind that the timelessness of the unconscious concerns positive, desirable, hoped for events. On the contrary, the compulsion to repeat is not just an ignorance of time, or even a refusal to accept the limitations that reason or experience force us to accept. It is not a question of a rebellion against the limits of our omnipotence and the constraints linked with impossibility. *In fact it is a denial of time.* In the timelessness of the unconscious, the world continues to move forwards. We are the ones who remain eternally young and fixed to the illusions of our youth. In the compulsion to repeat, not only do we refuse to grow up, but we have the mad phantasy that we can *stop the march of time.* It is not only that we cling to the illusions of childhood; it is as though, in trying to stop time, we were committing a *murder of time.* The idea of murder here may anticipate our intuitions concerning the death drive. Even if we do not believe in Freud's concept, we should nonetheless accept that destructive forces are in operation, *first and foremost against the psyche of the subject* and also against the picture we form of others. A paradox can be formulated here. *Destruction destroys the representation of objects that we hate and also destroys the temporal processes connected with them.* Thus, by bringing about the destruction of temporal processes and by realizing death wishes addressed to the objects of our hate, the fixed, immobilized, petrified time that results prevents the idea of the death of these objects in the psyche. The object is hated, but its love and its presence remain vitally important. Thus the object's death has to be both sought after and warded off. The only way of satisfying these contradictory requirements is to freeze the experience of time and to deny the phantasies connected with them.

The difference between timelessness and the denial of time appears to coincide with the prevalence of Eros in the first case and that of the destructive drives in the second.

Binding and recognition

Is there a concept that would help us to transcend the differences between the experience of time, timelessness and the compulsion to repeat? I will propose, following Freud, the hypothesis of binding. With the experience of time (past, present, future) the oriented sequence implies submission to the arrow of time, from past to future, from birth to death. In the middle is our *present*, that is to say, our *presence* in the world. This sequence is absent in timelessness, though for the constitution of a simple wish, a sequence is required. Even if it is present in the unconscious, a certain number of elements must be gathered together, reunited and organized in a minimal way. This is true of the simplest operations of the psyche as well as for the subject's most primitive reactions. 'In the beginning', it may be assumed that no complete sequence is available. But even in the absence of a complete sequence, a minimal form of succession for forming a meaning is established, *in the absence of which no meaning is perceptible*. Later, a dialogue will link together two or several sequences. From this perspective, I contend that instead of opposing the theory of the drives and that of object relations, we should accept *an organizing structure combining the reciprocal effects of the drives and the objects in both directions*. Finally, in repetition-compulsion, we can see that the sequence is always in danger, as if it were stillborn. The conflict appears to be situated between the possibility of maintaining and developing links within a *sequence of sequences*, enriching the meaning, presenting it with all its nuances, details, correlations and contradictions and, at the other extreme, cutting short all concatenation of any kind (drives, thing-presentations, affects, word-presentations, representation of reality, etc.), the possibility of the sequence coming to an end on the spot. In a structure with a normal evolution, the task of the psyche seems to be to diversify the central propositions (including in them even its internal oppositions) with the aim of reflecting the complexity of the psyche when it has to account for an experience in relation to the external world and, above all, in the case of psychic experience itself. So when does the experience of time become really effective? I propose to consider the role of *processes of recognition.* With recognition, the experience of time not only knows what can be known but recognizes the existence of an object or a meaning and becomes capable of knowing itself.

To rediscover is to refind. Freud said that, in accordance with the reality principle, we do not find an object; we refind it. Thus, surely, with the existence of this second vision, an earlier vision is implied and a separation at the heart of time must have occurred.

To conclude, I will introduce here the idea of *causality*: constructing a causal relation presupposes the well-known sequence, 'if . . . then'. Psychoanalysis is in a particularly favourable position here because no other discipline has developed as much this field of the 'if'. It is a domain with infinite possibilities. By the same token, the *then* of psychoanalysis has opened up new avenues for psychic causality which have been left aside by science. They have been subject to many developments in the domain of art. Perhaps the specificity of psychoanalysis is to position itself between them, claiming an original status, which should be preserved at all costs.

Notes

1 Viderman, S. (1970). *La construction de l'espace analytique*. Paris: Denoël.
2 Donnet, J.-L. and Green, A. (1973). *L'enfant de Ça. Pour introduire la psychose blanche*. Paris: Editions de Minuit.
3 See note 1.
4 Castoriadis, C. (1999). *Figures du pensable*. Paris: Le Seuil.
5 I have discussed this problem in two of my works to which I would refer the reader: *Diachrony in Psychoanalysis* and *Time in Psychoanalysis*, trans. A. Weller. London: Free Association Books, 2002.
6 Spitz, R.A. (1958). *The First Year of Life. A Psychoanalytic Study of Normal and Deviant Development in Object Relations*. New York: International. Universities Press, 1965.
7 See note 1.
8 Green, A. L'intrapsychique et l'intersubjectif. In: *La pensée clinique*. Paris: O. Jacob, 2002. Initially published by Lanctot Editions, Montréal. [English edition: The Intrapsychic and the Intersubjective in Psychoanalysis, tr. A. Weller. *The Psychoanalytic Quarterly*, LXIX.]
9 Green, A. (2001). *Le temps éclaté*. Paris: Editions de Minuit. [English version: *Time in Psychoanalysis – Some Contradictory Aspects*, tr. A. Weller. London: Free Association Books, 2002.]
10 Denis, A. Temporality and modes of languages. In: *International Journal of Psychoanalysis*, 1995, 76, pp. 1109–1119; and Le présent. In: *Revue française de psychanalyse*, 1995, LIX, pp. 1083–1091.

CONFIGURATIONS OF THIRDNESS

Freud considered the Oedipus complex as the nuclear complex of the neuroses. He also described in detail structures that we prefer to call pregenital than pre-Oedipal, but it seems implicit in his thought that they only assumed their full meaning in relation to the crowning of infantile sexuality with the Oedipus complex. After his death, and as a result of various influences, the psychoanalytic community thought it had discovered something important by drawing attention to these pregenital forms which had not been studied sufficiently hitherto. Consequently, triangular Oedipal constellations were relegated to the background while increasing interest was taken in pathological states that were traced back to periods prior to the Oedipus complex. A great deal of reflection was then devoted to the importance of pregenital relations (they were also called pre-Oedipal) characterized by dual relations. The figure of the father was to fade increasingly until it became almost absent from the clinical picture. In the same way, castration anxiety saw its domain shrink in the face of anxieties linked to an exclusive mother–child relationship: anxieties of separation, intrusion, etc., of which I have already spoken earlier. The general idea was that if one managed to understand better the fixations related to the pregenital periods, one would be in a better position to cure patients who presented clinical pictures corresponding to them. Without overlooking the interest of deepening our knowledge of these pregenital phases and their associated pathologies, I think that it was an illusion to suppose that one was dealing, in these cases, with states in which the father could be declared out of play, so to speak, or of negligible importance. It was Lacan's merit to re-establish the paternal function, not only in neurotic cases with an Oedipal fixation but, in general, *in all pathology*, each form calling for its own particular theorization from which the place of the father could not be erased. Further, the swings of the theoretical pendulum led psychoanalysts, independently of Lacan's influence, to realize that the supposed moment of intervention of the paternal image should be situated much earlier. In fact, psychoanalytic 'discoveries' had been based to a large extent on the methods of observation of the mother–child relationship (M. Mahler). It should be noted that this position, which has a touch of positivist realism about it, was far from being shared by Freud since he had postulated the existence of 'an individual's first and most important identification, his identification with the father in his own personal prehistory.'[1]

But it is sufficient to look upon these first exchanges from a different angle to discover something other than that which had hitherto attracted attention. For my part, and no doubt as a result of Lacan's influence, the partial and slanted character of the mother–child relations and the descriptions to which they led, convinced me of the impasses of the dual relationship, especially in their application to the psychoanalytic cure, where the analyst and analysand are enclosed within a circular exchange which is difficult to get out of. Taking Lacan's reflections further, I was sensitive to the idea that triangular relations had been neglected and arbitrarily restricted to the Oedipus complex. More than a function, what we were dealing with was a paternal *metaphor*. It was then that the work of C. S. Peirce threw a decisive and fresh light on the situation for me, with his conception of triadic relations leading to the more general concept of thirdness. I attempted to apply this approach to ideas which I had already advanced without referring to a particular theory, as well as to cases which I had not as yet considered from this angle. Accordingly, I intend to study four domains:

- psychic processes
- the Oedipus complex
- the psychical apparatus
- language.

In all of them, the triadic nature of relations may be noted.

The analytic third

The necessary and adequate condition for establishing a relationship is that there be two terms. This simple declaration has many implications. It sets up the pair as a theoretical reference which is more fruitful than all those which use unity as a base. If we reflect even further on the implications of this fundamental duality as the condition for the production of a third part, we find the basis of symbolic activity.[2]

Developing this line of thinking, I recapitulated my description of *tertiary processes*.[3] In 1975, in another text dealing with the object in psychoanalysis, I observed: 'The analytic object is neither internal (to the analysand or to the analyst) nor external (to either of them) but is *between them*.' It is evident that this sentence was inspired by Winnicott. In fact, I made the hypothesis of a primitive triangular structure which exists even at the heart of the so-called dual exchanges between mother and child. This was to indicate the place of the father, even though at the very beginning of life he is not as yet a distinct person. He nonetheless exists in the form of his presence *in the mother's mind*.[4] This conception is directly related to symbolization. The classical definition of the symbol is of an 'object cut in two constituting a sign of recognition when the two pieces are assembled by those carrying them' (*Dictionnaire le Robert*).

There are in fact three objects: the two separated pieces and the object corresponding to their reunion. *In the session, the analytic object is like this third object, a product of the reunion of those constituted by the analysand and the analyst.*

Taking up these ideas, T. Ogden formed the concept of the *analytic third*,[5] which he uses for understanding phenomena occurring during the session.

Primary, secondary, tertiary processes

I will not be enlarging here on this subject which has already been dealt with before; and will simply underline the role of the tertiary processes, whose existence I have postulated as binding processes between the primary and secondary processes. Without a structure making it possible to pass from one field to the other, one cannot see how either of the two series (primary and secondary) can be linked up with the other; nor how analytic progress can be conceived of. Without wishing to postulate the existence of particular processes – though in fact the idea of alpha function all but necessarily implies it – Bion emphasized the role of *attacks on linking* in psychosis. Subsequently, I described a central phobic position[6] extending Bion's observations which I have developed in a personal way. I had described, then, without realizing it, a form of thirdness, without having access to the notion that would allow me to theorize it. In this case, it was a matter of making an adjunction to Freudian theory where Freud had limited himself to a binary opposition. It may be pointed out, moreover, that many theoretical systems are content to oppose the two systems, primary and secondary. It may be of interest to review them. Incidentally, when Edelman opposes primary consciousness and higher consciousness, *can the mechanisms of reentry, whose existence he postulates, not be considered as the equivalent of tertiary processes?* (See below.)

When one considers the general framework of the elements of Freudian theory, one notices that duality is the rule: drive dualism, contrasting pairs, primary and secondary repressions, primal and secondary phantasies, *avant coup* and *après coup* (i.e. the initial event and the fresh meaning attributed to it retrospectively at a later date), difference between the sexes, difference between generations, and so on. One could go on drawing up a list endlessly of the number of cardinal notions which form a pair and are inhabited by relations of synergy and antagonism within a subtle dialectic. There are two notable exceptions to this picture: the Oedipus complex and the two theories of the agencies of the psychical apparatus. Here, thirdness is manifest and unavoidable.

Perhaps one can conclude that, when a certain level of complexity has been attained, duality becomes insufficient for explaining relations and only a triadic relation enables us to understand the basis of the possible combinations. I have already touched upon the question of the relations between fixations to structures prior to the appearance of the Oedipus complex, and raised a few problematic points concerning their existence. Let us first step back a little before returning to the crux of the question.

The Oedipus complex

Every connoisseur of Freud's work has been struck by the fact that his first intuitions concerning the Oedipus complex date back to 1897. They can even be traced back to his trip to Paris, in 1895, when Freud had been impressed by the performance of *King Oedipus* at the Comédie-Française, with Mounet Sully in the leading role. If he goes back even further, the biographer will note that Freud had to translate for his 'Matura' (the equivalent of our A Levels) a few lines of *King Oedipus*. These anecdotal notations are only of interest in that they show the extent to which Freud was prepared, with reference to the culture of his time (the culture and not the customs), to be sensitive to what could emerge from quite another angle, i.e. the material of his patients, and to attribute the Oedipus complex with particular importance. I have already had the opportunity of commenting on the unusual length of time separating the first intuitions in 1897 and his complete (and short) theorization in 1923. However, every Freud reader will equally recognize that between 1897 and 1923, from *The Interpretation of Dreams* up until the descriptions of his *Case Histories*, he did not remain silent on the question. This is confirmed by the remarks made en route, each time that he presented a clinical case.

There was, then, a long period of latency, periodically interrupted by partial illuminations which only really pushed him to formulate the theory of the Oedipus complex once his ideas had matured sufficiently in him. It has always seemed to me that, before Freud felt ready to formulate a theory on the question, he needed arguments which went further than that which was revealed by the observations, albeit sufficiently eloquent, of the customs of his time and of pathology. He waited until he had found a source of reflection which he sought in ancient cultures and even much earlier. Greece played a decisive revelatory role. There is no space here to enlarge upon the importance of culture for Freud, but Greek culture certainly had pre-eminence, more than Jewish culture, and was probably on an equal footing with Germanic culture. The reference to Greece may have been due to the fact that, since it was not marked by Christianity (and anti-Semitism), Freud looked upon it sympathetically. But there was probably more to it than this. Greek religion was not dogmatic; people were free to believe or not to believe, which, for Freud, was surely of great importance in the development of his intellectual curiosity.[7] Be that as it may, Freud was interested, even beyond Greek civilization, in the study of so-called primitive societies, which led him to think that they might give us an idea, albeit an approximate one, of the earliest stages of humanity. We know – Freud says so himself – that this was in fact not so. This was in *Totem and Taboo* (1912–1913), where the Oedipus complex is omnipresent. Later, when he came to the study of group psychology and the analysis of the ego, he treated indirectly, through the figure of the leader, the relation to the father of the primitive horde. Soon, the *Urvater* and the *Vatercomplex* would be brought together in *Moses and Monotheism* (1939a).

In 1923, in *The Ego and the Id*, Freud gave the first, somewhat detailed version – and practically the only one – of his conception of the Oedipus complex. It is worthwhile citing the relevant passage:

> For one gets an impression that the simple Oedipus complex is by no means its commonest form, but rather represents a simplification or schematization which, to be sure, is often enough justified for practical purposes. Closer study usually discloses the more complete Oedipus complex, which is twofold, positive and negative, and is due to the bisexuality originally present in children: that is to say, a boy has not merely an ambivalent attitude towards his father and an affectionate object-choice towards his mother, but at the same time he also behaves like a girl and displays an affectionate feminine attitude to his father and a corresponding jealousy and hostility towards his mother.[8]

One cannot fail to be struck by this formulation which gives the impression of having been written, before its time, by a structuralist.

Later on, Freud was to enlarge this conception by putting forward the hypothesis that the Oedipus complex might encompass everything concerning the child's relation to his parents. This enlargement indicates that he was aware that the Oedipus complex could not be confined within the limits of a phase of infantile sexuality, however important it might be. Moreover, it is also necessary to think of the post-Oedipal situation – that is, everything concerning the genesis of the superego via identification and its effects in intra- and inter-systemic relations. In a study carried out some time ago now,[9] I showed that the Oedipus complex needs to be looked at today from a different angle. Though Lacan fought hard to show that the Oedipus complex was not limited to the Oedipus complex of infantile sexuality and that, drawing on the works of Lévi-Strauss in anthropology, it was necessary to consider it as a structure, I do not think that we can leave it at that. *I think that the historical and structural Oedipus complex must also be considered as a model for which we only have approximations.* Let me note in passing that the most extreme pathology never faces us with the extreme situations treated by tragedy, namely, the combination of parricide, incest and the incestuous procreation of children. At best – or at worst – only certain aspects of all these situations can be realized; but I do not know of an example in which the Oedipal tragedy is illustrated in reality. I refer the reader to my treatment[10] of this question for the details of my argument.

I would simply point out that this model is not so much represented by a closed triangle as by an *open triangle*. If there is indeed a complete relation between the parents and an aim-inhibited instinctual relationship between mother and child, there is no equivalent of it between the father and the child. And this leads me now to an observation of cardinal importance: *Of the three poles of this triangular structure, the mother is the only one to have a carnal relation with the two others, with the father and the child, even if they differ in their expression.* I think that part of the complications of feminine sexuality depends on this fact. Freud clarified things to a remarkable extent in Chapter VII of *Group Psychology and the Analysis of the Ego* (1921c) when he wrote:

> He [the child] then exhibits, therefore, two psychologically distinct ties: a straightforward sexual object-cathexis towards his mother and an identification with his father which takes him as his model. The two subsist side by side for a time without any mutual influence or interference. In consequence of the irresistible advance towards a unification of mental life, they come together at last; and the normal Oedipus complex originates from their confluence.[11]

In the model shown in Figure 11.1, it can be seen that the father comes between the mother and child, thereby modifying the direct investment uniting

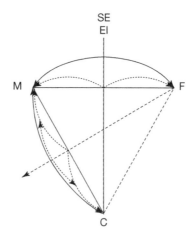

C = Child, M = Mother, F = Father, SE = Superego, EI = Ego Ideal

Figure 11.1 The Oedipus complex

them, and favouring separation. The child in turn responds to the break in the continuity of this tie with the mother by wanting to separate the parents united in the primitive scene. But these different interruptions of the trends between the mother and child and between the mother and father are paid for in the form of guilt and with the genesis of the superego and the ego ideal. The separation effected by the father now gives him a separate state of existence. He was not really absent before but only intervened indirectly via the mother (the father, in the mother's mind). From now on, he exists in his own right, as much as a separating, or prohibiting agent as a second object to be loved. The constitution of the Oedipus complex in the Oedipal phase also has the interest, by virtue of its positive and negative structure, of distributing the investments in the positive Oedipus through a positive tie with the mother (affect and tenderness) and a negative tie with the father (jealously hostile relationship). In the negative structure of the complex, the opposite obtains. In fact, the four constituents are in operation at the same time, giving rise to more or less pronounced repressions. Only vestiges survive. But let us note the impasse which often accompanies the predominant choice on the side of the negative Oedipus.

The construction of this model gives rise to various observations. Affects are included in it that can be associated with Eros, and, in certain extreme cases, with the drives of destruction. The last theory of the drives is thus confirmed by it. Moreover, the model contains a clear reference to bisexuality. Contrary to an opinion that he had heard advanced, Freud stressed that it is not only sexuality with persons of the same sex that is repressed (homosexuality), but the two components, heterosexual and homosexual. Furthermore, the model shows the relations between desire and identification. Though desire is always subject to the action of repression, in variable proportions ranging from sensuality to tenderness, it seems to me that what is most interesting is the fate of the affects of jealous rivalry. One of the most remarkable achievements of the Oedipus complex is undoubtedly that hostility is successfully transformed into identification. The paradox of the Oedipal injunction has already been noted on many occasions: 'Be like your father, take him as a model, but don't allow yourself to do everything he does and obey his prohibition against possessing your mother.' In other words, it is less a matter of accepting a total and complete prohibition than of accepting the prohibition of an incestuous choice, maintaining the object-choice of the sex of the object of desire, and effecting a displacement on to another person. Finally, one cannot emphasize enough the importance of the outcome of the Oedipus complex in the genesis of a superego that is at once prohibitive and protective, as we have already seen.

Today, and this began as early as 1960,[12] the death of the Oedipus complex has been announced on the pretext that in our contemporary societies the place of the father is no longer maintained in its traditional role. For their part, certain psychoanalysts, always sensitive to the lessons to be learnt from the most manifest clinical expressions have, as I have already said, militated in favour of recognizing the early mother–infant relations from which the father is assumed to be excluded. Winnicott was not afraid of admitting, on occasions, that he could observe no trace of the Oedipus complex in many of his patients. The fact is undeniable, with arguments to support it both from Lacan and Winnicott. They invite us, however, to ask ourselves if the theory should only reflect the most apparent reality or if the latter should not be understood as expressing the singularities of the theory. Jean Laplanche adopts a comparable approach when he contends that what can be observed in all societies is the generation gap and that, whatever the context, adults always have to bring up children, owing to their biological prematurity, bringing them to the status of adults. In other words, Laplanche centres all his effort on the analysis of the vicissitudes of the affects of the Other on the subject. As far as I am concerned, I cannot detach myself from the fundamental basis of the Oedipus complex – namely, the double difference of the sexes and the generations presiding when the subject is born. With reference to this basis, whatever the individual's sexual choices are, he still cannot overlook the fact that he is the result of a sexual relation between two parents of an earlier generation, themselves separated by the difference of the sexes and that, throughout his whole life, he will have to elaborate this origin. However far his personal choices take him in an attempt to avoid reproducing the situation – and infantile sexuality in all its aspects is involved here – it is still true that that is where he comes from.

Today, all sorts of social pressures, with guilt-inducing effects, exist to make sure that the rights of more or less persecuted minorities are recognized. Though one can scarcely deny the persecution, the recognition of rights remains problematic, as Pierre Legendre has well understood. Even when it concerns sexual choices considered by previous norms as deviant, such as homosexuality, transvestism, or even transsexualism, all these situations which were once regarded as marginal, and even, in certain societies, heavily sanctioned, are now supposed to become the object of pride. The most recent of the measures under discussion is the adoption of children by homosexuals. The remark will doubtless appear more shocking than the fact itself. We know that adoption is often a ruse employed by paedophiles to quietly satisfy their sexual leanings. Such discussions very often sidestep the real issue and are the object of mediatic complaisance, nobody wanting to be outdone in the 'why-not-ism'. Studies carried out on such children have been very superficial and, at any rate, are not convincing. It is well known that the child has a very considerable capacity to absorb unusual situations. But what he is capable of introjecting, without being too surprised from the point of view of his consciousness – he has already introjected many other things! – does not fail, however, to continue its path below the surface without any symptom emerging on the surface till much later (latency), and gives one to suppose that unconscious conflicts exist in him. Especially as no one wants to disturb the provisional equilibrium that he has acquired by exciting his psyche from the outside on the pretext of making investigations. In point of fact, we have to accept our current state of ignorance concerning the novelty of the situations encountered, and above all to recognize that the effects on a child of being brought up by a homosexual couple will rarely manifest themselves before adolescence. A certain amount of experience has already been accumulated. This concerns children of a heterosexual couple who have separated after the homosexuality of one of the two parents has been revealed in broad daylight. As both parents retain the right of visit – or provide a shared guardianship – it is possible to observe the way in which the child responds when he stays with the new homosexual couple. Certainly, nothing permits us to say that a pathology is operative, but one has to take into account the child's love for the parent, even if he has turned out to be homosexual. There is also a need to recognize the necessity of sustained and nuanced psychological monitoring. Let us say in any case that it is with a macroscopic paedo-psychiatric clinical approach that we will succeed in furthering our knowledge.

As for paedophilia, it is a domain that seems to be shrouded in great confusion. For it is true that all the forms exist, from the isolated instance of paedophiliac acting out which is not backed up by the organization of a sexual choice oriented in this direction, to incestuous or criminal paedophilia which indulges in very destructive acts towards children who have been seduced. It seems to me on the one hand that a differential evaluation is necessary in each case and, on the other that the so-called therapies of deconditioning are not sufficient for solving the problem.

In any case, one fact is striking. In the relationships involving acts of paedophilia reported in the media, many causal mechanisms are invoked. In particular the past of certain paedophiles who themselves have been the object of seductions and violence in their childhood, frequently by their ascendants. Yet, mention is hardly ever made of the theorizations originating in Freud, which means that *the notion of infantile sexuality, discovered in 1905, remains today – notwithstanding the existence a certain superficial knowledge – almost a century after, unheeded*. It seems to raise too many problems when one no longer considers it solely from the point of view of the victim. Nor do the theoretical developments offered to the media make any mention of the *infantile sexuality reactivated in the paedophile by the attraction exerted on him by his victims. Nor is there any question – horresco referens – of invoking the existence of infantile sexuality in the children who become victims of paedophiles*. This gives us a good idea of the considerable resistance with which culture opposes psychoanalysis, even when it becomes common practice to invoke the role of the 'drives', a term which is often loosely misused, and which is restricted to the domain of the most reproved deviations of sexuality. The argument of monstrosity suffices to qualify the matter, which, of course, only concerns those who can under no circumstances be deemed to belong to civilized human community. How are we to explain, though, the network of complicity resulting in the disappearance of legal files, in affairs being stifled and dragged out, and in the paralysis of the arm of justice as well as that of medicine? It is as though it was being claimed that paedophilia is a necessary activity for the distraction of the population, rather like hunting or fishing.

All these observations merely show the degree to which it is rash to claim that sexuality no longer plays such an important role as it did in Freud's time. Not only has its role not diminished, but also one can perhaps add that, since Freud, the agents at the origin of sexual traumas have become far more cynical.

The agencies

I will not expand on this question which has already been given sufficient treatment in earlier chapters. Nevertheless, whether it is the model of the first topography or that of the second which is in question, we find a situation with three terms. I have pointed out the differences between the first topography, which is centred around consciousness, is more homogeneous, and has no place within it for the drives, and the second which rectifies this situation. It should nonetheless be noted that the three agencies of the first topography can be reduced to two large subsystems, since Freud concludes by regrouping the conscious–preconscious system which he contrasts with the unconscious. A few observations are called for before continuing.

Few authors are ready to relativize, as Freud did, the importance of the first topography once he had created the second. For the large majority of them, both topographies are in fact used according to the circumstances, each demonstrating its pertinence in relation to a defined problem. There are some authors who content themselves with the first topography, expressing many reservations about the second and wishing to do without it. There is no particular reason for such an attitude. Lacan, for example, clearly remained very faithful to the logic of the first topography. When he decided to take up the question of the applicability of his ideas to the second topography in the Seminars after 1968, the result was not very convincing. In effect, invoking grammaticality to account for what Freud was speaking about concerning the id represented a challenge. Few of his pupils, moreover, followed him on this matter. Lacan's attitude was very understandable in the light of the highly critical position he always held concerning any biologizing point of view within psychoanalytic theory. In this respect, Laplanche's position is not very different from Lacan's.

I have stated my reasons for adhering to the turning-point of 1920 and explained why Freud's proposition of his second topography should be followed. I would like to come back to the place that he accorded, in 1923, to what he had spoken of in the first topography. There is a chapter in *An Outline of Psycho-Analysis*, entitled 'Psychical Qualities', which, it seems to me, gets right to the bottom of this question. If, indeed, as he asserts, the theory of the drives forces us to accept the prevalence of an energetic point of view and to recognize *the forces which are active within the psychical apparatus*, the wish to construct a theory that brings together physiology and psychology is accentuated. For, if the unconscious is essentially made up of representations – leaving the question of affects to one side for the moment – the relation to psychology seems to me to be larger than the physiological foundation of the drives. It is a question, in short, of recognizing that the activity of representation, initially highly influenced by its link with the somatic through the mediation of the drives, becomes as it were more psychological with the pair thing-presentations/word-presentations. In the critique he undertakes of his own work in the *Outline*, Freud gets to the heart of the problem by focusing the discussion on consciousness. Throughout his life, he never ceased to repeat that the equation psychic = conscious was false. Concerning psycho-physical parallelism, he draws attention to the fact that many psychic or somatic processes have no conscious psychical equivalents. He adds: 'It of course becomes plausible to lay the stress in psychology on these somatic processes, to see in *them* the true essence of what is psychical and to look for some other assessment of the conscious processes.'[13] Freud recalls that psychoanalysis 'explains the supposedly somatic concomitant phenomena as being what is truly psychical and thus in the first instance disregards the quality of consciousness'.[14] I note the expression 'supposedly somatic'. It seems to me that this reserve indicates that what is labelled as somatic is not always what is meant by the term. Once again, we come across the idea of an elementary or primitive psyche rooted in the somatic, but that is already of a psychical order in a form that we are unable to conceive of. It is understandable, then, that the reference to consciousness only alludes, within such a perspective, to a psychical quality. This will also be the case, then, for the unconscious.

As far as I am concerned, I can certainly envisage the existence of unconscious somatic processes – in the biological sense – at one extremity of the chain. One could postulate the existence, in the proximity of the latter, of processes that can be encountered in certain affections of a psychosomatic order, involving 'poorly mentalized' psychical forms and in which the interactions between what is somatic and what is psychical occur in both directions: either a somatic aggravation is translated by psychical impoverishment or an increase in psychical conflict is translated by a worsening of the illness. It is sometimes the case that the latter has the last word, as in the *syndrome of essential disorganization* described by Pierre Marty. Another category is that of the disturbed economic, dynamic and topographical exchanges with reality. This is psychosis, which Freud defined as entailing the repression of reality and the deployment of destructive drives. I have underlined on several occasions the role that I ascribe to negative hallucination, which may, or may not, be accompanied by positive hallucination.

A very rich subject opens before us here, and requires us to take into consideration hallucinatory activity in psychosis and hallucinatory activity in general, especially in neurotico-normal states, in the topographical regression of dreams.[15] Let me repeat what I said earlier, namely, that if it were necessary to select just one of the characteristics that can be identified in the last conception of the psychical apparatus for its value in clinical applications, it would be the *ego's unconsciousness of its own resistances and defences.* For it seems to me that this is what the system is aiming at in order to account for the difficulties encountered in clinical practice. One now understands what is really at stake for the ego. It is not enough to say that it is captivated by the subject's imaginary identifications (Lacan); one still needs to disclose what is at stake in such an organization. What is at stake here are the relations of misrecognition and recognition of the unconscious governed by the agonistic and antagonistic processes that I have chosen as a subtitle for this book.

At another level, pathological organizations are characterized, as Freud indicates, by the conflict with the drives. Either the latter triumph over the superego in perversion, engendering disturbances of certain functions of the ego in splitting, or, on the contrary, the neurosis takes on the aspect of the negative of perversion. We also need to speak of the conflicts of agencies between the ego and the superego, which can be observed essentially in the narcissistic neuroses, mania and melancholia. It can be seen that, in such a grid, my theory of gradients finds a new application. And one can say that the clinical issues cannot be confined within a conception of the psyche which gives them uniform functions on all levels. Psychoanalytic practice shows that the modes of apprehending the psyche are not the same in the treatments of psychosomatic patients, psychotics, perverts, neurotics or depressive subjects. Moreover, all the psychic functions need to be re-evaluated, such as the value of language, the value of representations and affects, the empire abandoned by the compulsion to repeat, and so on.

Likewise, questions also need to be raised concerning the functions of the dream or their failures. As I have already said, it is perhaps necessary to return to the Aristotelian formula, which speaks of the *dreamer's psychical life.* I have maintained that, if the dream is included within a series which also comprises anxiety dreams, nightmares, nocturnal terrors, sleepwalking, stage IV dreams, blank dreams, etc., this rich range would eventually make it possible to establish certain links between neurotico-normal states, in which the function of dreaming is preserved and has its role to play in the internal equilibrium of the psyche and the legibility of desire, and the other manifestations which are encountered more frequently in non-neurotic structures. Sleepwalking, in my opinion, deserves to be considered separately and has not been sufficiently studied by psychoanalysts. For, though certain studies have indeed been devoted to it when it is a central symptom, the role it plays in clinical situations involving non-neurotic structures where it is encountered is not always examined in detail.

Language

The question of language in psychoanalysis raises particular problems which justify a separate chapter. Though, at first sight, the question does not appear to belong to a chapter concerning the configurations of thirdness, it seems to me that its inclusion here is perfectly legitimate. One only has to consider the three personal pronouns. The existence of a third person (masculine or feminine, singular or plural) refers to the absent third party. But the problems of the relations of language, speech and discourse are worthy of a chapter to themselves. I therefore refer the reader to Chapter 12.

Thirdness

We now come to the study of thirdness proper. I only became aware of the importance of this concept relatively late in my psychoanalytic career (1989).[16] Peirce made it possible to conceptualize the relations of linguistics to semiology, helping us to get out of the enclosed position in which Lacan had sequestered us, enabling us to extend our reflections, beyond language as a system of word-presentations, to semiology which equally includes thing-presentations. The work of Peirce is considerable. It is of such complexity that I am obliged to recognize that I do not grasp all the aspects of it. I shall confine myself, accordingly, to considerations that are essential for me, and will only describe them with the purpose of introducing the reader to his philosophy and to the advantages that the psychoanalyst can derive from it. It first needs to be noted that Peirce proposed his ideas before the principal theses underlying Freudian theory were even established. Let us limit ourselves to a few preliminary, but important remarks. Peirce's lucidity in adopting certain axioms should be acknowledged. He writes: 'It is the instincts and sentiments that constitute the substance of the soul. Cognition is but the surface, its point of contact with what is external to it.'[17] Peirce distinguishes the modes of relating to Firstness which bears witness to the position of the subject; he refers to the citation that I have just made. He then considers the *dyadic* relation, the paired relation destined to circularity. This is reminiscent, then, of the criticisms contesting the interest of the so-called dual relation. He comes finally to the *triadic* relation, which is the one I am concerned with. Peirce envisages the situation of the concrete subject by bringing together, in the same acceptation, the materiality of the sign and its function of representation. He calls *representamen* everything that is concerned by the analysis of the intelligence of the sign, including in this analysis the representation of the one who analyses the representation. The third reference becomes inescapable here: it is at the beginning of the discourse. The latter includes both the object, the point of departure for the discourse, and the discourse about this object which leads back to the subject of the discourse.

From such a point of view, the subject, the object to which *the subject* is attached and *the object produced by this relation constitute an irreducible triad*. Though it is said that the *representamen* is what language signifies, one cannot dissociate from this signification the impulsion that it gives to whoever is in a position to recognize it. Hence the definition of *representamen*:

> A *Sign* or *Representamen* is a First which stands in such a genuine triadic relation to a Second called its Object as to be capable of determining a Third called its *Interpretant* to assume the same triadic relation to its object in which it stands itself to the same object.[18]

Note that the interpretant is not the person who interprets but a constitutive element of the sign. It designates the necessary connection between the interpretant and some possible other, in the position of interpreter. There is interpretation, not in the sign, but by the sign, for a third term. Peirce is sensitive to the central dimension of conflict: 'The second simplest characteristic common to everything that presents itself to the mind is the element of struggle.'[19] It is clear how the application of Peirce's ideas is interesting for psychoanalysis insofar as the referential position of the *representamen* refers us to all the forms of representation, and not only to word-presentations. Intuitively, I would say that such a conception sheds much light on the dream work, and not only on the analysand's discourse. Peirce's work did not escape Lacan, who cites it without dwelling on it, even though, in my view, he owes him a lot. However, influenced perhaps by the spirit of the times, he preferred to turn towards Saussurean linguistics with a view to defending his theory of the unconscious structured like a language. I have shown the interest and the limits of such a thesis.

At some point along the way, I proposed – without always pursuing my reflections to their conclusion, and before coming across Peirce – a *theory of a generalized triangular structure with a variable third*, and stated that, although it was still necessary to try and think in terms of a modality in which the third term would refer to a triangular structure, this did not mean that in psychoanalysis we always have to come back to the Oedipal structure. It is perfectly possible to envisage triangular relations in which the third term would not represent the paternal function. On the other hand, it seems to me that it is important not to let oneself be imprisoned by the dual relation. With a view to proposing a general figure, I will recall the example which I made use of before: We are in the presence of a ternary structure comprising the subject, the object and the other of the object, this other not being the subject. Thus, for example, the child's relationship to the mother would refer to one of the mother's other objects, a sibling, or an object of the mother's desire other than the father, sustaining this or that passion. The *other of the object* could also concern another object of the mother's own childhood: her own mother, her own father, or one of her brothers or sisters, a wet-nurse or housekeeper. It is not difficult to grasp, then, the multiple possible applications of thirdness.

Notes

1 Freud, S. (1923). *The Ego and the Id*. *S.E.* XIX, 31.
2 Green, A., from the Inaugural Lecture of the Freud Memorial Chair at University College London, 15 October 1979. Also in *On Private Madness*, p. 19. London: Hogarth Press, 1986.
3 Green, A. Note sur les processus tertiaires. In: *Propédeutique, La métapsychologie revisitée* (Annexe D). Paris: Champ Vallon, 1995 (1st publication, 1972).
4 Green, A. The Analyst, Symbolization and Absence in the Analytic Setting. In: *On Private Madness*. London: Hogarth Press, 1986. Originally published in French in 1975.
5 Ogden, T. (1994). *Subject of Analysis*. New York: Jason Aronson Inc.
6 Green, A. La position phobique centrale. In: *La pensée clinique*. Paris: Editions Odile Jacob, 2002. (Originally published in *Revue française de psychanalyse*, 3, 2000.)
7 Green, A. (1992). Oedipe, Freud et nous. In: *La Déliaison*. Paris: Les Belles Lettres.
8 Freud, S. (1923). *The Ego and the Id*. *S.E.* XIX, 33.
9 See Green. A. (1992). Oedipe, Freud et nous. In: *La Déliaison*. Paris: Les Belles Lettres.
10 See Green, A. *La Déliaison*. Paris: Editions Hachette, 'Littérature', pp. 131–143.
11 Freud, S. (1921). *Group Psychology and the Analysis of the Ego*. *S.E.* XVIII, 105.
12 See J. Lacan: Subversion du sujet et dialectique du désir dans l'inconscient freudian. In: *Ecrits*. Paris: Editions du Seuil, 1966. [English version: The subversion of the subject and the dialectic of desire in the Freudian unconscious, tr. Alan Sheridan. *Ecrits: A Selection*. London: Routledge 1977.]
13 Freud, S. (1940a [1938]). *An Outline of Psycho-Analysis*. *S.E.* XXIII, 157.
14 Ibid. p. 158.
15 G. Lavallée has made an extremely interesting study on this subject: Le potentiel hallucinatoire, son organisation de base, son accueil et sa transformation dans un processus analytique. In: *Revue française de psychosomatique*, 19–2001.
16 Green, A. De la tiercéité. In: *La pensée clinique*. Paris: Editions Odile Jacob, 2002. First published in *Les monographies de la Revue française de psychanalyse*, 1989.
17 Peirce, C.S. *Le raisonnement et la logique des choses* (Conferences à Cambridge, 1898), Cerf, Passages, 1995. [English edition: *Reasoning and the Logic of Things*. Harvard University Press, Cambridge, MA, 1992.]
18 Peirce, C.S. *Ecrits sur le signe*, p. 116. Paris: Editions du Seuil, 1978. (English edition: *Philosophical Writings of Peirce*, Selected and Edited by Justus Buchler, pp. 99–100. New York, Dover Publications, 1955.)
19 Ibid. p. 95. (English text: p. 89.)

12

LANGUAGE – SPEECH – DISCOURSE IN PSYCHOANALYSIS[1]

From the moment that the only injunction given to the analysand, in the form of the fundamental rule, enjoins him to *say everything* that comes to his mind and to *do nothing*, psychoanalysis cannot neglect the study of language and speech, as it is refracted by the analytic situation between two partners. In fact, apart from certain arrangements reduced to their minimum, the lever of analysis rests on two props: silence and interpretation, or alternatively internal speech and enunciated speech. The analyst who undertakes to inform himself about linguistics is entering a maze where he will have to sift out that which seems to him to be fruitful *from his point of view*, from that which he can afford to ignore as it only concerns him very remotely, without however contesting the value it may have for others.

What conclusions will he draw from it? First, that language is a *form*. More precisely: 'The activity of language is meaningful in the measure that an enunciator produces forms so that they are recognized by a co-enunciator as being produced in order to be recognized as interpretable' (A. Culioli). Comprised in this definition are the references:

- to a couple enunciator/co-enunciator
- united by conventions concerning forms (acceptability)
- produced and recognized
- interpretable.

When one examines these forms more closely, one notices the mutual influence of a system of monomorphic sounds (that is, exclusively constituted by sonic forms of which all language is constituted) and polymorphic conceptual references (referring to thought elaborated from heterogeneous elements: imagination, reason, movement, etc.). These two intersecting spheres of sound and meaning constitute the indivisible nucleus of language which reaches us via the language spoken by a community using speech as the singular expression of a speaking subject. Two levels are to be noted: the first is that of the composition of the sounds belonging to language (thought-sound), itself subdivided into grammar, syntax and vocabulary; the second is that of the operations which have a bearing on the meaning; it coincides with the first. One soon comes to the conclusion, as Darmsteter has already observed,[2] that languages are living organisms (which Darmester ventures to say are subjected to Darwinian transformism). This reference obliges us, then, to relate the functions that are specific to living organisms and those that are specific to man; and, within the latter, to link up the life of words and the life of thought. The languages spoken by human beings are subject to influences connected with life. Spoken by humans, they depend on their characteristics, which belong only to man. The relations between language and thought have to be taken into consideration. Three levels must be considered: life, language and thought, which are themselves operative at the level of the community and of the individual (language and speech). It can be seen immediately that, of these three levels, language is the one that is defined and circumscribed the best. For, the reference to the life of words presupposes knowledge which provides a better explanation of the activity of language and speech than of the form of life which animates them. Similarly, relating language to thought requires that there is agreement about what thought is; however, if we consult the philosophers, we are far from arriving at a univocal conclusion.

Concerning the life of words, a special place should be accorded to sexuality, as the works of P. Guiraud have shown.[3] Since language brings into relationship, at the minimum, a pair enunciator/co-enunciator, we cannot minimize that which characterizes the most intense of relations, namely, sexual eroticism. It is against this background that the dynamic of language manifests itself.

The activity of which Culioli speaks implies recognition. And, beyond that, at an even more general level, language is traversed by contradictory mechanisms, some aiming to preserve forms, others to change them – thereby destroying the earlier forms. There is thus a surprising convergence between certain linguists and the Freud of the last drive theory.

The question of speech and language would doubtless not have had such an important place in psychoanalysis had Lacan not centred his conception of the unconscious on language. But, before coming to this, we need to examine his point of departure. The relations between Freudian thought and language are not always clear, which allows some of my contemporaries to affirm with firm conviction that, in Freud's work, the question is rarely one of language, whereas others contend that it is the only question.[4] To bring the debate back to essentials, let us recall a remark made by Freud in *An Outline of Psychoanalysis* to the effect that 'the presence of that connection [i.e. with speech] makes it safe to infer the preconscious nature of a process.'[5] In fact, Freud had already made it clear in the *Papers on Metapsychology* that the unconscious is only constituted of thing-presentations, 'the first and true object-cathexes'. Without forcing the facts, one can say that the principal aim of Freud's work was to underline the difference between thought governed by language, as illustrated by what he referred to as secondary processes, and the thought of unconscious processes (first topography), or related to the agency he called the id (second topography). This in no way detracts from Lacan's innovative thinking, with the sole reservation that he presented it as a return to Freud, which is inexact. Lacan had as an excuse the fact that, at the time when he began theorizing, Freud's work had been brought into disrepute. But if one had shown interest in Freud as an author worthy of seeing his thought and concepts analysed with the same rigorous approach that is applied to philosophers, the results of the enquiry could under no circumstances lead to Lacan's conclusions. This is what emerges in any case from the analysis made by Riceour.[6] Why did Lacan not have the courage to say from the outset that in examining Freud's work, he was led to prefer a new thesis which differed from Freud's – namely, 'The unconscious is structured like a language'? It would have been more risky, but many useless controversies might have been avoided. In fact, Lacan wanted to cover himself with Freud's backing in order to get across a message which he feared would not be accepted without this high patronage. However, at the end of his life, when he was assured of his success, he revealed his hand. 'The unconscious did not originate with Freud,' he asserted, 'but with Lacan.' This at least was clear, while coinciding with the admission of the failure of his teaching. It is true that, with the passing of time, Freud's fate was scarcely more enviable.

And yet anyone who sets aside concerns about Freud's patronage, who turns his attention towards tropes and considers the detail of the logical conditions of changes of meaning (synecdoche, i.e. reciprocal absorption between what is determining and what is determined; extension of meaning, i.e. metonymy and metaphor, catachresis),[7] cannot fail to see their similarity with Freud's descriptions of the transformations which operate in the unconscious. But it is only – at the very most – a parallel suggesting the relations that exist between the transformations of language and those that occur in the unconscious. The question that arises, then, is one of knowing if, when the analyst listens to his analysand's speech, it is the operations of language which attract his attention and mobilize his specific mode of thinking or, if it is his work, centred on the transformations effected (hypothetically) at an unconscious level, which engage his listening and require a mode of thinking that is quite different from the linguist's. There is no question as to what the answer is.

Lacan could not let go of his reference to the signifier, however much he profoundly transformed the meaning and the work which it occasions in the psyche. In fact, Lacan did not take account of Freud's evolution when he modified his theoretical system and went beyond the theoretical foundations of his first topography by proposing the last theory of the drives (1920) and the last conception of the psychical apparatus (1923). Whatever one may think of the derivations that followed Freud's last conceptions – with Hartmann, Melanie Klein, W.R. Bion and D.W. Winnicott – Lacan's conceptions, a consequence of the vigorous manner in which he had shaken up the psychoanalytic theories of his time, seem to me further removed from the Freudian corpus than those of the other authors I have just mentioned. Moreover, they did not feel the need themselves to affirm their allegiance to Freud or to pride themselves on being faithful to him.

In short, the real question – there is no other – is this: *Does Lacan's work provide a better answer than that of his contemporaries to the questions raised by psychoanalytic experience in the second half of the twentieth century? Without beating about the bush, the answer, in my opinion, is no.* For, as the founder of psychoanalysis had sensed at the end of his life, psychoanalysis would have to deal increasingly with modes of thinking that are alien to ordinary common sense.[8] He had thus already foreseen that the mode of thinking proper to the neuroses would be insufficient. And even, which was perilous, that the intellectual means for approaching the specificity of this mode of thinking found in non-neurotic structures would be cruelly lacking.

In other words, without renouncing anything of the analytic technique founded on the fundamental rule, that is, speech in its entirety animated by free association, Freud's last theorizations suggested that the gap between this speech and the psychical processes inferred beyond consciousness would increase more in non-neurotic structures than in those now qualified as neurotico-normal. Should one conclude that Lacanian theory continues to be true for the analysis of neuroses. I fear that, even in this case, just when one thinks that it might find confirmation, it proves inexact.

Psychoanalysis is based on the use of speech. However, this use marks it with certain particularities. Since 1973, I have described this as *speech delivered lying down to a hidden addressee.* What I mean is that the requirements of the setting give this speech, which has to obey the fundamental rule, a field that alters its ordinary conditions. For free association is correlative of topographical regression, which may be compared with the verbal communication of the mental state of reverie, if not of dreaming. *And yet in Lacan's work this specific feature of the psychoanalytic verbal exchange is never taken into consideration.* A linguist as eminent as Culioli himself admitted that if he had had to take an interest in dreams, he would only have been able to approach them from the angle of the dream narrative. Analytic speech has achieved a true conversion of everything it expresses in language (thing-presentations, affects, one's own bodily states, compulsive manifestations, attempts at acting out, and even desire itself). Now it is difficult to claim that one is close to the truth of the discourse when one considers that this conversion into a homogenizing verbalization succeeds in dissolving in language the particularities of all the registers outside-language of the psyche. This is why I contend that psychoanalytic discourse is *the result of the transformation of the psychical apparatus into a language apparatus* (Green 1984).

Everything depends how the implications of this are used. Will there be an attempt, by means of thought, to rediscover the colours of the transformed register or will speech be treated in a homogenizing manner (thus mutilating the psyche of its diversity, neglecting the coefficient of conflictual tension which inhabits speech. Speech is liable to overflow, in the most highly charged moments, beyond the sphere of language, through hallucinatory activity, somatization and acting out)?

Even if we remain within the field of linguistics, and notwithstanding the very widespread craze which led to its theory receiving the backing of numerous intellectuals, one cannot fail to notice certain of Lacan's omissions and to raise certain criticisms. I will not expand on the positions of Deleuze and Guattari who, on the pretext of criticizing the hegemony of the signifier, preferred in its stead a theory of fluxes disavowing the Freudian construction. It is nonetheless revealing that they left behind the examination of schizophrenia in order to develop their theses. Without going into their arguments at all, P. Aulagnier also based herself on the material of psychosis in order to demonstrate the inadequacies of the concept of the signifier and to defend a theory closer to Freud's thought.[9]

Would it suffice to amend Lacanian theory on this point to make it acceptable? This is what Rosolato and Anzieu have done, each in his own way: Rosolato with his conception of the *demarcation signifiers* arising from the five senses[10] outside language, and Anzieu, who, in agreement with Rosolato, preferred the domination of *formal signifiers*[11] regarding them as more adequate for supporting his conception of the skin-ego. Laplanche has proposed the idea of *enigmatic signifiers* which go beyond the sphere of language.[12] This is why he later called them *enigmatic messages*, alluding to the signs coming from the mother's preconscious (of which she is unconscious) addressed to the child, charged with sexuality, and resulting in a real seduction. But why do these authors continue to refer to the signifier, even when modifying its meaning and function, if it is not because, in spite of everything, they only renounce in part the primacy of the linguistic signifier, as if they considered that it should nonetheless serve as a fundamental paradigm and model? In other words, it is as if only language could express meaning, and as if all the other systems of signs referred to it. Th. Sebeok (1974) pointed out, however, that if this were the case, one would not understand why the latter have survived.[13] However, while remaining on the side of the linguists, they overlook all their affirmations which are contrary to the Lacanian interpretation. A few remarks will suffice here. Jakobson – who nonetheless counted Lacan amongst those closest to him – defined the six functions of language, designating the first among them as the *emotional function*.[14] This fact certainly did not escape Lacan, but as he had taken up a clear position against affect, he never spoke about it, counting probably on the lack of curiosity of those who had embraced his theses. Natalia Avtonomova, a Russian linguist, has criticized, in Lacan's work, the hypertrophy of the functions of language as a method, and the impoverishment of language as an object.[15] She rejects, in turn, the formula of the unconscious structured like a language. However, generally speaking, linguists have gone their own way, ignoring Lacan's work. Chomsky, a partisan of a conception of the unconscious which owes nothing to psychoanalysis, remaining attached to biology, disregarded it. I will leave Derrida's critique until later.

However, notwithstanding the success of Lacanian theory and its place in the field of contemporary psychoanalytic theories alongside those inspired by other leading authors whom I will not be mentioning here, a possible misunderstanding needs to be noted. Lacan founded his theory at the time when Saussure was being rediscovered, at the beginning of the 1950s. The source of his inspiration was the *Course of General Linguistics* in the edition of 1916, put together from the notes of Ch. Bally and A. Sechehaye. Now, more recently, the studies by R. Godel,[16] R. Engler,[17] S. Bouquet,[18] F. Rastier,[19] C. Normand,[20] have made an important reappraisal of what has to be called the ideology of the reporters of the *Course*. Saussure distinguished the linguistics of language from the linguistics of speech. However, Bally and Sechehaye greatly minimized, if not completely suffocated, everything related to the linguistics of speech. Certainly, Lacan did not lose sight of speech. It is mentioned in the title he gave to his Rome Report in 1953. I think, though, that he would have developed his point of view differently had he been aware of the reflections of Saussure which do not appear in the *Course*.[21] It is striking to note that the term *signifier* is rarely used in the *Course*. Saussure preferred instead 'vocal figure'. He himself points out the ambiguity between *word* in the sense of *global sign* (*signifier* + *signified*) and *word* in the sense of *signifier* (cited by S. Bouquet). What Lacan says of the signifier, i.e., that it is 'what represents a subject for another signifier', adds still further to this ambiguity. Nowadays, some linguists divide linguistics into a *logico-grammatical* field and a *rhetorico-hermeneutic* field (S. Bouquet and F. Rastier). There has been a wish to pull Saussure towards the first while minimizing the significance of the second, in which his place is no less important. Today, the concept of speech according to Saussure has been replaced by that of discourse, which fits in better with my conception which underlines the heterogeneity of the signifier and is compatible with the idea of an articulated whole.

Among the uses of the word 'discourse', the one that interests psychoanalysts the most is related to a 'qualification of the associative link in language'. Now it is this link which undergoes significant transformations in free association. I have described – discovering with surprise that I am in agreement here with Darmsteter who had underlined the role of radiance and linkage – the phenomena of *irradiation* (*retroactive reverberation–anticipatory annunciation*) in analytic listening, and specified, in a more detailed manner than is usually the case, the processes that it implies. Likewise, it seems to me that Lacan underestimated the role that Saussure attributed to *value*, which was quite distinct from that attributed to the signified. Furthermore, Saussure had raised the question of what is outside language: 'the significations of ideas, the grammatical categories outside the field of signs [. . .] may exist externally to the linguistic domain; it is a very shaky question to examine, at any rate by anyone other than a linguist.'[22] This is what C. S. Peirce would do. In fact it is impossible to dissociate language, as it is conceived of by psychoanalysis, from the general system of representation. Saussure speaks of a thought-sound, just as Freud speaks implicitly of a thought-body in connection with the concept of the drive. The key issue is the triple reference of the body, the sign and the idea. According to Saussure, the linguistic domain of *thought* becomes that of the '*IDEA IN THE SIGN*' or of the vocal figure which becomes *SIGN IN THE IDEA*. For Saussure, whoever says sign says signification, and whoever says signification says sign (with its two indissociable constituents). For him as for Freud, *it is the point of view that creates the object and not the contrary*. And it is here that the psychoanalyst refers to body language. Let me mention in passing the distinction proposed by H. Atlan between brain-psyche and psyche-language.

Saussure's successor in the Chair of Linguistics in Geneva, in 1913, Ch. Bally, criticized his mentor's intellectualist conception and proved to be in agreement, without knowing it, on very many points with psychoanalysis. He was not listened to. But it may be that, at the beginning of the twenty-first century, linguistics, or at least a certain tendency within it, is changing course so that a more complex vision of Saussure can emerge – the path reopened by Ch. Bally making it possible to construct the triangle Saussure–Peirce–Freud. Herein lies, it seems to me, the hope of an interpretative linguistics which has before it an immense field of work. It could be, though, that a certain obscurity or misunderstanding will continue to hang over the question of language, which will have to be lifted.

Henri Meschonnic vigorously rejects the solution which consists in departing from language in favour of communication. But he soon goes on to denounce the poverty of our way of thinking about language. There is an almost unavoidable temptation to link together *language and concept* and to confine language within this relation. In Meschonnic's view, we should follow Spinoza in his defence of a theorization of *the affect-concept*. Meschonnic wants to re-establish the poetry of language through the reference to rhythm. And if what matters is above all to read poetically (and no doubt to *hear* affectively), it is because what is important is to open oneself to *the encounter between concept and affect*. Freud makes a central opposition between representation and affect; Saussure between the vocal figure and the idea (the signifier and the signified). Meschonnic's thesis proposes the linking together of affect and concept. There is a hint here of a distant reference to a dualism between body and mind which is persistently said to be outmoded. We will have the opportunity of returning to this, for, of course, I do not believe in an essential dualism: body and mind are taken together, as it were, in the same envelope, in an inevitable monism. There remains a structural dualism in which the difference of thought imposes itself on our body against its will. The position adopted by Meschonnic may elucidate the question of language in psychoanalysis decisively.

It appears to me that everything began with the Vienna circle and the turning taken by phonology. From this moment, linguisitc research turned towards the creation of concepts from phonological units of language whose opposing relations were significant, *without however having any meanings*. Roman Jakobson marked the domain of phonology and poetics within the framework of structuralist thought. There were close links between him and Claude Lévi-Strauss as well as Jacques Lacan. We have already noted the censorship that Lacan imposed on Jakobson's thinking by not taking into account this function of language which he was the first to describe – namely, the 'expressive or emotive function'. Structural linguistics banished emotion from its preoccupations, yielding to the fever of investigating purely conceptual structures. *In short, the concept repressed the affect*, in spite of the studies of Ch. Bally, neglecting the nuances introduced by Saussure who preferred the term vocal figure to that of signifier. The vocal figure gives an important place to the *voice*. Yet linguists have minimized the role of the voice, often so as to throw themselves into speculation on the concept alone (relation between the terms). They have treated the voice 'abstractly', whereas it is the mode of transmitting affect.

Not enough attention has been given to the fact that Jakobson wrote the preface to the book by Ivan Fonagy, a pioneer of the relations between psychoanalysis and language, and whose work was concerned with the *instinctual bases of phonation* and the affective values in phonology.[23] Consequently, one can see that it is at the level of the smallest units of language, in their relations with the voice, that the link between concept and affect is the strongest, without it ceasing to intervene at higher levels of complexity. Psychoanalysis, which only approaches this problem from the standpoint of what the patient is saying in the session, cannot afford to neglect this dimension, for no one will deny that the voice is an important diagnostic instrument in the cure. Lacan missed this by overvaluing the concept separating representation from its affective quantity, where the affect is cut off from its correlate, just as he also separated the signifier from the signified.[24] It was a fatal error for, at the level of the signifier, affect occupies a place from which it cannot be dislodged. This is what Saussure called the thought-sound. *The thought-sound presupposes the link affect-concept.* Psychoanalysis was to encounter this problematic issue in the division that Freud made between representation and affect. It must be added that the concept of the psychical representative of the drive embraces a unity which would later have separate outcomes. Freud understood the affective value of the phoneme in *Beyond the Pleasure Principle*, analysing the *Fort-Da* – which, in the mouth of his grandson became '*o-o-o-o*' – *da* – linking melancholia with disappearance: '*o-o-o-o*', and the expression of joy at its reappearance: the short *da* [there]. And this is why, although it does not lack depth, Lacan's analysis of it still misses the essential issue. This has been elaborated by other psychoanalysts who have not shrunk before the complexity of the phenomenon and who have not hesitated to face up to a lack of 'purity'. Lacan's position seems forced. For, to conserve the link affect-concept is to recognize the necessity of representing the body in thought and vice-versa. Affect is here the condensed form of a complex ensemble comprising emotion, sensation, sensoriality, in short, the whole sensible dimension of experience. One only has to read the *Ecrits* to notice that it is never missing.[25] The solution had to come from poetics, with Meschonnic, confirming that it is indeed on this side that the light shines. I have already pointed out that in the jungle of linguistic theories, it is with poetics that the analyst feels most at home, whereas the patient's discourse is the most prosaic possible (Green 1984).

Herein lies the mystery of the psychoanalytic exchange.

Notes

1   This chapter makes reference to various earlier studies including: Le langage dans la psychanalyse. In: *Langages*, Paris: Les Belles Lettres, 1984; Le langage au sein de la théorie générale de la représentation. In: *Pulsions, représentations, langage*, Lonat: Delachaux and Niestlé; *La cure parlante et le langage* (in press, Bayard Presse); Linguistique de la parole et psychisme non conscient. In: *Cahiers de L'Herne*: Ferdinand de Saussure, 2002. (In press.)

2   Darmsteter, A. *La vie des mots*. Paris: Le Champ libre, 1979 (first published, 1887).

3   Guiraud, P. (1978). *Sémiologie de la sexualité*. Paris: Payot; *Dictionnaire érotique*. Paris: Payot, 1978.

4   I refer the reader to my work: 'La cure parlante et le langage', a lecture cycle organised by the French Association of Psychiatrists (in press). See also: 'Le langage dans la psychanalyse'. In: *Langages*. Paris: Les Belles Lettres, 1984.

5   Freud, S. (1940 [1938]). *An Outline of Psycho-Analysis*. S.E. XXIII, 162.

6   Ricoeur, P. (1992). *De l'interprétation. Essai sur Freud*. Paris: Le Seuil.

7   See note 2.

8   Freud, S. (1940). Some Elementary Problems in Psycho-Analysis, *S.E.* XXIII, 282.

9   Green, A. Réponses à des questions inconcevables. In: *Topique*, 37, pp. 11–30, 1986.

10   Rosolato, G. (1969). *Essais sur le symbolique*. Paris: Gallimard.

11   Anzieu, D. (1994). *Le penser*. Paris: Dunod. In my view, this work does not have the place it deserves in psychoanalysis.

12   Laplanche, J. (1990). *Nouveaux fondements de la psychanalyse (avec Index général des problématiques)*. Paris: Presses Universitaires de France, 2nd edition.

13   Sebeok, T. (1974). Comment un signal devient signe. In: *L'unité de l'homme*. Paris: Le Seuil.

14   Jakobson, R. (1963). Linguistique et poétique. In: *Essais de linguistique générale*. Paris: Editions de Minuit.

15   Avtonomova, N. (1991). Lacan avec Kant: l'idée du symbolisme. In: *Lacan avec les philosophes*. Paris: Albin Michel.

16   Godel, R. (1957). *Les sources manuscrites du CLG de F. de Saussure*. Geneva: Droz.

17 Engler, R. *Bibliographie saussurienne*. In: *Cahiers F. de Saussure, passim*.

18 Bouquet, S. (1997). *Introduction à la lecture de Saussure*. Paris: Payot.

19 Rastier, F. (2001). *Arts et sciences du texte, formes sémiotiques*. Paris: Presses Universitaires de France.

20 Normand, C. (2000). *Saussure*. Paris: Les Belles Lettres.

21 Saussure de, F. *Ecrits de linguistique générale*. Paris: Gallimard, 2002.

22 Saussure de, F. De l'essence double du langage: In: *Ecrits de linguistique générale*, edited by S. Bouquet and R. Engler. Paris: Gallimard, 2002.

23 Fonagy, I. (1983). *La vive voix*. Paris: Payot.

24 Green, A. (1973). *Le discours vivant. La conception psychanalytique de l'affect*. Paris: Presses Universitaires de France. [English version, trans. Alan Sheridan. *The Fabric of Affect in the Psychoanalytic Discourse*. London: Routledge, 1999.]

25 One example among many: 'Ce couple de l'*hic et nunc*, dont le coassement jumeau n'est pas seulement ironique à faire les cornes à notre latin perdu, mais à fleurer un humanisme de meilleur aloi en ressuscitant les corneilles auxqelles nous revoilà bayant, sans plus n'avoir pour tirer nos auspices de la nique de leur oblique volettement et du volet narquois de leur clin d'oeil, que les démangeaisons de notre contre-transfert' (*Ecrits* I, p. 463. Paris: Editions du Seuil, 1966). [Translator's note: this passage appears in a text entitled, 'La situation de la psychanalyse en 1956', which it seems has not hitherto been translated, so I propose something along the following lines: 'The twin croak of this duo *hic et nunc* is not only ironic in dog-earing a page of our lost Latin, but in having a whiff of a humanism of better quality by reviving the crows of our distracted yawning, leaving us with no other means of drawing our omens from their mocking, sidelong fluttering and derisive winks, than the itchings of our countertransference.']

13

THE WORK OF THE NEGATIVE[1]

From the adjective to the noun

The negative is not an individualized notion as such in psychoanalytic writings. In Freud's work, it figures as an adjective. Negative hallucination, a concept to which I attribute a central importance, was mentioned on several occasions by Freud during the hypno-cathartic period. The idea was common in Bernheim's circles. Freud gave several examples of it at the beginning of his work; then the notion was eclipsed in the theory, only reappearing incidentally in a note in 'A Metapsychological Supplement to the Theory of Dreams' (1917d). Two particular mentions of it must be recalled here: the first defining *neurosis as the negative of perversion*; the second characterizing a regrettable evolution in the treatment, namely, *the negative therapeutic reaction*. It can be said that Freud's work is situated between two limits. But there is still nothing there to justify the noun, 'the' negative, for this form of thinking is quite far removed from Freud's. The idea re-emerged during Lacan's Hegelian period, though he paid little attention to it.

When one consults the systematic index of the major concepts of Lacan's *Ecrits* drawn up by Jacques-Alain Miller, one sees that it is given scarcely any place among the Hegelian categories (B, 2C). An attentive reading of the author of the index, as well as the list of Freud's terms in German, confirms this. Thus there is no anteriority for the introduction of the negative as a concept in psychoanalysis, any more in Lacan than in Freud. Moreover, in Hegel's work, it had a relatively limited significance in this direct form. One thus comes to the conclusion that it is perhaps in some of the contents of psychoanalytic theory that the negative has to be discovered, even though the term is not mentioned, and that an analysis of it will bring us many surprises. There exist many 'traces' of the negative in Freud – a negative that is, so to speak, unconscious of itself beginning with the concept of the *un*-conscious. But many other forms bear the trace of it too: mourning and object loss, identifications in relation to desire, and, last but not least, the immense continent of the death drive.[2]

212

The negative at work in Freud and thereafter

When one follows the thread of Freud's work, the idea not just of the negative but also of the *work of the negative* appears in the concept of defence. The theory of repression illustrates very clearly the work of the negative. Even before repression (*Verdrängung*), in his major work, *The Interpretation of Dreams* (1900), Freud had advanced the idea of the dream-work. He took the expression up again in 1915 when he described the work of mourning. These are the two cases where Freud explicitly uses this idea. After him, psychoanalysts enlarged its field of application (*work of delusion*, Racamier and Nacht; *work of melancholia*, B. Rosenberg). In truth, if the psychical apparatus is conceived of as the locus of processes of transformation at the heart of the agencies, and between them, the very idea of work is consubstantial with it. Throughout his work, Freud wavered between the description of repression as a paradigmatic defence, characterizing the defensive process in general, and another sense in which repression, however symbolically connoted it may be, is never more than one of the modes of defence, identifiable in particular in normality and neurosis. The application of one of my ideas can be found here, where one and the same concept is allocated to two places: (1) the representative of the series which has validity for the series as a whole, and (2) a term of the series. It can be seen, moreover, that this quasi-categorial use can be identified in some contemporary authors (J.-C. Rolland).[3] However, the differences between repression and other defences explains Freud's need to individualize the description of it. Let us recall the defence which he calls *Verwerfung*, which Lacan proposed to translate as *foreclosure* because he saw it as a mechanism of expulsion from the symbolic signifying chain. Since then, while the validity of the distinction is accepted (it is a question of something that is not *suppressed* but *abolished* inside, Freud himself says in the case of President Schreber, 1911), other translations have been preferred, such as *rejection*. A long period of time passed, then, before Freud came, after introducing the concept of the death drive, to dealing with the problem of negation (*Verneinung*) in 1925. This article alone would justify the concept of the work of the negative. Whereas hitherto, Freud had only been concerned with problems in relation with the unconscious (repression or foreclosure), now he was interested in negation proper, that is to say, in a phenomenon linked to language, and thus to consciousness. What is quite remarkable, however, in this short work, is the way in which Freud links up the forms of the negative between themselves; he asserts, for instance, that negation is the intellectual substitute for repression. He thus proceeds to consider the functions of judgement (intellectual activity), opposing two forms of the negative recognized outside the field of psychoanalysis (A. Culioli). On the one hand he divides the judgement of attribution into good and bad, the latter being the support of a wish to incorporate the good; the negative consists, then, in refusing to take the bad into oneself, with the intention of rejecting it outside of oneself. The judgement of existence, *posterior, in Freud, to the judgement of attribution,* must decide if something that exists in the unconscious also exists in reality. The task of this other form of the negative is thus less one of judging what is to be incorporated and what is to be *ex*-corporated, than of determining whether the thing that is in the mind is also in reality or not. Freud ended the article by referring to the 'language' of the most primitive instinctual impulses, that is, oral impulses (incorporation–excorporation), in which he saw the original materialization of what would subsequently become affirmation or negation. Let us recall in passing Freud's remark in *The New Introductory Lectures on Psycho-Analysis* (1933) according to which almost everything we know about the id is negative in character, compared with the ego. In short, we find ourselves faced with this paradoxical situation in which the noisiest and most assertive of the agencies of the psychical apparatus, the id, can only be conceived of by negativizing what we know of the ego, with which we are much more familiar. By reversing Freud's remark, it could be said, in another sense, that the ego is the id 'in the negative' (or 'negativized'). It is very revealing to note that Freud's article on negation has only been the subject of particular attention in France owing to Lacan and the Commentary by Jean Hippolyte[4] whom he invited to his seminar. Nowhere else – in the world dominated by Anglo-Saxon influence – has it given rise to any comparable reflection.[5]

And yet, Lacan was not the only one to develop the destiny of the negative in psychoanalysis. It was by means of a very different approach, essentially clinical rather than philosophical, that English psychoanalysis developed notions which are associated with it. With Melanie Klein it was the description of *denial*, understood differently from that which is described in the article on negation, and sometimes translated into French by *dénégation*. It can also be linked up with the concept of projective identification which is concerned with a comparable problematic. But above all, two authors after her were to accord an important place to the negative, namely, W. R. Bion and D. W. Winnicott. In *Learning from Experience*,[6] Bion introduced, a third category, Knowledge, alongside Love and Hate. That is to say, he attributed intellectual processes with a psychic function equivalent to that of love and hate, wherein it is easy to find traces of Eros and the drives of destruction. Bion's theoretical imagination led him, then, to divide Knowledge into positive Knowledge and negative Knowledge (K and –K). As a result, the negative entered contemporary psychoanalysis by another door. Bion's description, based on the analysis of psychosis and psychotic structures, is quite remarkable. Bion describes a process in two phases: in the first, projective identification expels from the psyche the elements which cannot be assimilated and elaborated following experiences of frustration. This psychic relief only lasts for a short while. The evacuated elements attempt to return to their original dwelling place; the psyche is then obliged to effect a new evacuation in which the psyche *as a whole* (and not just the undesirable elements) is subject to expulsion, leaving the psyche bloodless, inhabited solely by 'denuded' object relations (Bion). It is worth recalling here the fundamental dilemma of the psyche according to Bion: either frustration is evacuated by means of excessive projective identification, and, consequently, the psyche is impoverished or, there is an attempt to elaborate frustration (which implies being able to tolerate frustration initially). For his part, Winnicott – at a rather late stage, it has to be said – also came to recognize the place of the negative of which he had a premonitory intuition at the end of his work. It was in the last version of his article 'Transitional Objects and Transitional Phenomena', the first chapter in *Playing and Reality* (1969), that he described the part played in a female patient by 'the negative side of relationships'. For these patients who have been subjected to particularly disorganizing experiences involving traumatic separations, *only what is negative is real*. After a phase during which the object's absence has been unduly prolonged, it becomes equivalent to a loss and, *whether the object is there or not no longer makes any difference for reality is thenceforward identified with this negation of the object*. Winnicott concluded that, when the experience of separation goes beyond the child's capacity for tolerance, a disinvestment of the object may be seen to occur, with the result that the latter finally disappears from the psyche.[7]

But it is not only in pathology that the weight of the negative can be observed. When Winnicott describes the characteristics of transitional objects by saying: 'the object both is and is not the breast', not only is he defining a particular category of objects endowed with a very important function for the psyche, but he also manages to overcome the traditional opposition between being and not being, which brings us back to a new variety of the judgement of existence mentioned by Freud. This process, however, which is closely tied up with symbolization, can deteriorate (the transitional object symbolizes the uniting of two separated things, the baby and the mother, instead of initiating their separation). In those cases where only the negative is real, Winnicott says that patients who have been subjected to these traumatic experiences come to doubt the reality of the thing that they symbolize.

Let us return to Freud and continue our examination of the forms of the work of the negative that he discovered. The last of them, which had a very promising future but was subjected to an important semantic alteration by other authors, was *splitting or disavowal* (*Verleugnung*). Freud became aware of the singularity of this mechanism with the study of fetishism. He then described the form of defence in which the child's ego, faced with a traumatic situation caused by perception, is subjected to splitting (*Ichspaltung*) and thus has to tolerate the coexistence within it of two judgements. Neither prevails over the other, and each of them attributes an equal value to the other. One can easily imagine the consequences which can result when the pleasure principle and reality principle are endowed with the same value, the first being unable to renounce its claims, while nonetheless leaving a place for the second which seems ready to consent to the situation. It is rather like the fetishist who, following a perceptual experience, refuses to draw any lessons from it, preferring to maintain, in his judgement, the idea which suits him. It is of fundamental importance to point out the difference between repression, which affects *instinctual impulses or representations*, and *splitting*, or *disavowal*, which is primordially the *disavowal of a perception*. This is illustrated by the intellectual recognition that the mother (and later women) *does not have* a penis, and by the necessity of choosing a substitute on the periphery of the sexual organs (suspender belt or any other female accessory), which *has to take its place* and becomes indispensable for obtaining pleasure. Yet another case in which the ego is unconscious of its own defences! By making reality intervene via perception, Freud was opening up a new field of investigation for psychopathology. It is probably no coincidence that Freud wrote this article *after* having tackled the problem of the loss of reality in neurosis and psychosis. At the start, disavowal and splitting were put forward as an explanation for fetishism. However, though they can legitimately result from perceptions, they pose problems for the analyst as modes of psychic functioning calling for an analysis which relates – owing to the links of fetishism with reality – to the problem of judgement. Two remarks come to mind. The first, which I have already mentioned, concerns the fact that Freud came back to the question of splitting in *An Outline on Psychoanalysis*, giving it a very wide significance and implicitly making the link between perversion and psychosis. Chapter VIII of the *Outline* must be considered as an important development of the work of 1927. It is clear that had Freud lived longer, he would have attributed a much more important place to splitting. Freud freed himself increasingly from the neurotic paradigm involving above all intrapsychic conflicts in order to interest himself in relations with reality. It is thoroughly remarkable, moreover, that Freud returned again to this question in his uncompleted article, discovered after his death, 'Splitting of the Ego in the Process of Defence' (1940e), where he appears to hesitate between two positions: the first, which consisted of thinking that there was nothing new in what he was going to write (as if he thought that he had never spoken about anything else); and the second which induced him to think that what he was broaching was completely new and of unsuspected importance. This place taken by the conflict between the beliefs of the internal world and what we learn from the reality of the external world allows us to take up again and extend the conclusions of the article on Negation concerning the judgement of existence. What is involved here is a protest against a traumatic non-existence: the mother's lack of a penis.

César and Sára Botella (2001) have found a felicitous formulation resuming the situation of the judgement of existence: 'Only inside, also outside'. But every coin has its reverse side. Freud approached the question of reality in a rigorous manner and by linking it up with psychical reality. After his death, and in certain psychoanalytic movements with a tendency towards simplification and reduction, the reference to reality was, as it were, demeaned, reducing the theory to the level of Monsieur Homais.[8] And there was a period when analytic technique set itself the ambition of bringing the patient back to reality (in particular in psychoses), as if proposing that the patient see things through his analyst's eyes was going to transform his vision. This presupposed that one could quite simply disregard his psyche and ask him to jump over his shadow. It seems that we are coming back to this again, in other contexts (intersubjectivity).

We know that the concept of *splitting* was widely used by M. Klein and her school. However, all these authors, Bion included, used this concept in a different way from Freud. For Freud, it was essential to maintain the existence of two functions, one linked to the recognition of reality, the other adhering to the misrecognition of it. In the work of Kleinian authors, the use of *splitting* and its generalized form, *minute splitting*, is closely linked with projective identification, and retains nothing of the function of recognition postulated by Freud. In fact the basic hypothesis has changed. By projective identification, the Kleinians are above all alluding to a mechanism of evacuation from the psyche involving the projection of certain parts which seek to make their return through an identification with the projected parts. I have proposed certain developments of the function of splitting, by way of extending Freud's thesis, and have described a syndrome of *subjective disengagement by the ego*, where the patient adopts a general position of withdrawal. He responds with indifference to interpretations concerning his transference and his mental functioning, adhering to them occasionally in an ephemeral way, but without their leading to a judgement on the part of his ego; that is to say, without the patient undertaking to recognize fully the manifestations of his unconscious (i.e. that they belong to this system), and without his becoming conscious of the conflicts within him and the consequences that such disengagement implies. It seems to me that this is an important issue in certain treatments, whose fate is different from that of the negative therapeutic reaction, and where the narcissistic wall behind which the subject shelters seems to resist a thorough analysis. These cases may be compared with the anti-analysand once described by J. McDougall (1978). It is in these circumstances that the question of the status of the object provides material for discussion. It is all very well for the theoreticians of object relations to mention the insufficiencies of Freudian theory, but they have little sensitivity for their own insufficiencies. This is the moment to recall, once again, how any excessive unbalance in theories stressing the link with the object results ipso facto in contrary theories which shift the accent on to narcissism. Subject unbinding, which I have characterized as a process of disengagement sustained by a more or less omnipotent fantasy of self-sufficiency on the part of the ego, has the aim of escaping the object's control, of asserting the ego's freedom through its quasi all-powerful capacity to undo its ties with the object and, if necessary, with itself. I shall come back to this question when considering the manifestations of what I call negative narcissism.

At any rate, it is the series of different concepts that Freud examined, that is, repression, negation, splitting and disavowal, which I have gathered together and called the *work of the negative*. What is the basis for this selection among the defences and how can bringing them together under one heading be justified? Let us note that these different processes have in common a decision, thus a form of judgement. This judgement has the task of deciding, and, in all cases, of having to give an answer in the form of yes or no; which is not the case for other mechanisms of defence such as reversal against the self, turning something into its opposite, isolation, cancelling out, reaction formation and sublimation. I thus attribute this series with a cardinal role which can be linked, as Freud had already done in his article on Negation, to the drives of destruction. At bottom, there is a fundamental choice to be made, in the first person, between, 'I accept' or 'I refuse', which has far-reaching repercussions for the psyche.

Let us beware, however, of thinking that accepting is always good and refusing always bad. We would not survive, in our current state of civilization, if we did not recognize that everything begins with the idea of the drives being excessive or prone to excess, immoderation, *hybris*. This indeed is what Morin asks us to consider by designating the human species as *Homo sapiens demens*. The alternations of yes and no involve a subtle dialectic, ranging from the most alienating forms of alienation to the most sublime forms of sublimation.

Negative hallucination

A special place has to be reserved for negative hallucination. After progressively falling into disuse in the course of the history of psychoanalysis, the fortunes of negative hallucination have been variable. Just as I insisted earlier on the differences between repression and disavowal and their respective links with representation and perception, it must be emphasized that negative hallucination is related to perception. Clinically, it is characterized by the contrary of positive hallucination. The most schematic definition of the latter characterizes it as an objectless perception. *Conversely, negative hallucination is the non-perception of an object or of a perceptible psychical phenomenon.* It is thus a phenomenon involving the erasure of what should be perceived. In the past I defined it as representation of the absence of representation, but such a definition is perhaps subject to ambiguity inasmuch as it tends to preserve a confusion between representation and perception. Moreover, it is better to avoid including the term 'absence' in such a definition, owing to the fact that it is associated with a context which is also susceptible of inducing error. Absence, loss, and non-existence due to non-perception are categories that it is better to keep separate.

Before going any further, let me clarify the relations between positive and negative hallucination. In 1915, Freud's conception of hallucination underwent an important mutation. As I have already pointed out, whereas the whole of the first period of his work was based on the opposition between the memory system, of which representation is the product (re-presentation), and the perceptual system, which assures our relation to the present, in 1915 he found he had to revise the terms of this relationship. After comparing the dream–image and hallucination with a fine toothcomb, he concluded that there were no criteria which made it possible to establish their difference. One can measure the importance of what was at stake: hallucinatory wish fulfilment, dreams as wish fulfilments (later modified into *attempts* at wish fulfilment, hallucinations (of hysterics and psychotics), concluding with the equivalence dream-hallucination. From then on, Freud found himself obliged to defend *reality testing* which alone made it possible to differentiate the 'innocent' and temporary psychosis of the dream and its pathological (acute or chronic) form. In 'A Metapsychological Supplement to the Theory of Dreams' (1917d), he was led, with regard to hallucination, to insert a note which apparently only has an incidental function but in fact is the germ of a theoretical revolution: 'I may add by way of supplement that any attempt to explain hallucination would have to start out from negative rather than positive hallucination.'[9]

Let us observe in passing how typical is the expression of patients who seem to be affected by a sudden emptiness of thought and express their disturbance by saying, 'My mind's gone blank.' This is not the same thing as saying 'I can't remember any more what I was thinking about', or 'I've forgotten'. The *mental blank* seems to me to translate the subjective state of the patient, or of the person seeking help, in a manner which should attract our attention. With this sole notation, Freud gives us a glimpse of a whole psychic constellation at the origin of hallucinatory production. The latter results from a dual action based on an interface:

- On its external side: an undesirable, unbearable or intolerable perception leads to a negative hallucination which translates the wish to reject it to the point of denying the existence of the perceived objects.
- On its internal side: an unconscious representation of a wish (abolished) presses towards consciousness but finds itself hindered from doing so by the barrier of the system *Pcpt.-Cs*. The latter gives way to the pressure and the space occupied by the denied perception is left vacant.[10] It seems to me that this picture gives us a more complete view of the psychopathology. It is worth pointing out that negative hallucination, which can be encountered punctually in all circumstances, even the most normal, can also occupy a predominant place in psychosis, either in isolation (this is the repression of reality postulated by Freud) or as a preliminary stage to the onset of hallucinatory psychosis. Although Freud does not say so explicitly, negative hallucination plays an essential role in the concept – difficult to conceptualize – of the repression of reality.

What is of considerable interest in the Freudian position is that it does not limit, as is usually the case, the field of perception to that of sensoriality, i.e. to relations with the external world. In fact, Freud adds to it the field of *internal perceptions*. Perception can affect internal excitations arising from organs, perceived through awareness of the state of the body. It is worth recalling here the classical delusion of negations (known as the Cotard syndrome), where the patient is led to assert that he no longer has any organs and that he is thus immortal; and, more recently, alexithymia, as described by Sifneos, which is not without incidence in the psychosomatoses.

But it is undoubtedly in another field of activity that the concept helps us to understand strange clinical phenomena during the treatment. One of the original aspects of the Freudian conception of language is that it attributes it with the function of perceiving our thought processes. Putting this remark of Freud to good account, I have described phenomena of *negative hallucinations of thought* in patients who – depending on the case – do not acknowledge, even after the analyst has given precise circumstantial details, having said such and such a thing, or having accepted the interpretation which was given of it and which was recognized as the truth at the moment when this material was interpreted. I thought it was legitimate to assert that it was not a case of repression; for, as a rule, when the memory is put in context, the repression is lifted and the patient remembers what had been forgotten. In the present case, it is as though there is a real dissociation between the sonority of words and their conscious meaning on the one hand, and their unconscious meaning as it has been presented by the interpretation, on the other. It is this meaning that is neither perceptible nor recognized. In psychoanalytic treatments of borderline cases, this is where we find we are faced with one of the most tenacious forms of resistance.

As for psychosis, Freud's work provides us with abundant material for reflection, with the prodigiously rich analysis of the hallucination of the severed finger of the little Sergueï Pankejeff, in the account of his infantile neurosis given by Freud. These enrichments of the theory are not simply additions which leave intact the other parts of the field with which they are concerned. Here is one of the conclusions I presented in 1993:

> The work of the negative will no longer involve psychical activity as it can be imagined independently of the positive aspects of consciousness; it will concern itself with the relation to the object caught in the cross-fire of the destructive drives on the one hand, and the life or love drives on the other. The work of the negative thus comes down to one question: how, faced with the destruction which threatens everything, can a way be found for desire to live and love? And reciprocally, how should we interpret the results of the work of the negative which inhabits this fundamental conflict, i.e., the dilemma which we are caught in between the anvil of absolute satisfaction, to which omnipotence and masochism bear witness, and the hammer of renunciation for which sublimation is a possible outcome? Beyond this conflict looms detachment, a step towards the disinvestment

which is supposed to free one from all dependence on anyone or anything, so as to be able to encounter oneself at the price of murdering the other person.[11]

The problematic of negative hallucination is extremely diverse and I must, once again, ask the reader to kindly refer to the relevant chapter in my book, *The Work of the Negative*, of which it forms an essential axis. In effect, it is necessary to pursue our reflections on the relations between perception and representation and to analyse what I have tried to translate by means of an image – namely, that of an internal representation, more or less abolished, encountering an external perception which reactivates it from reality. When this situation refers to a trauma, I have made the comparison with two trains, representation and perception which, starting from opposite directions, are rushing at full speed along the same rails, destined ineluctably to have a catastrophic and mutually destructive collision. Claude Balier, in his studies on the psychopathology of violent forms of behaviour, has found this to be meaningful and useful in throwing light on what was happening with his patients.

All these considerations should lead to a re-evaluation of the Freudian theory of perception which has been humorously baptised as the Theory of the Immaculate Perception. It seems, in fact, that it is an infinitely more subtle, double-sided mechanism allowing a new perceptual registration to coexist with another activity formed by a representational flux which remains unconscious most of the time. In certain pathological structures, however, the latter can reach the subject's consciousness, which is split between perceptual activity and representational activity.

In 1967, in my study on primary narcissism, I postulated the existence of *primary decussation*, where the innermost and the outermost psyche of the subject crossed when exchanging places. The description of such a movement is necessary for understanding projection. Later on, I wrote in *The Work of the Negative*: 'Perceiving is not knowing, but re-cognising; re-cognising means following once again the path of a movement defined by its substitutive value for touching which is described as desirable or undesirable, or, failing that, acceptable or unacceptable.'[12]

One of the most fruitful applications of the concept of negative hallucination which does not concern psychopathology but is an integral part of normality, is to think of the situation of *holding* described by Winnicott as a framing structure, the memory of which will remain when the perception of the mother is no longer available owing to her absence. In 1967, I proposed the formula: 'The mother is caught in the empty framework of negative hallucination and becomes a containing structure for the subject himself. The subject constructs himself where the nomination of the object has been consecrated in place of its investment.'[13]

Negative narcissism

I am now going to set out briefly my conception of the death drive.[14] I shall not be undertaking an examination of this concept as it was defined by Freud. I have already examined it critically and have proposed to give it an acceptable content which tallies with clinical experience and contemporary theory.[15] My interpretation of the death drive is based on the assumption of a negative narcissism considered as an aspiration for the level zero, an expression of what I have called the *disobjectalizing function* which does not simply apply to objects or their substitutes, but to the objectalizing process itself. Here we encounter once again the major role of destruction through disinvestment. The objectalizing function is not, in effect, limited to the transformations of the object, but elevates psychic functions to the status of object, on the condition that they are always the vehicle of a *meaningful investment*. It is thus the investment itself which can be objectalized. When the disobjectalizing function is put to the service of negative narcissism, disinvestment undoes that which investment had succeeded in constructing. Negative narcissism is clearly a sort of extreme measure which, having disinvested objects, directs itself, if needs be, towards the ego itself, disinvesting it. In fact, psychic processes are prey to a permanent oscillation between the effect of the objectalizing function and its antagonistic contrary, the disobjectalizing function. Thus, a scale can be imagined which would begin with the most complete accomplishments of investment, capable of distributing itself along a spectrum ranging from love of the object to sublimation; then, following a regression, it would arrive at a stage where object investments give way to narcissistic investments which are withdrawn from the object (as is the case in positive narcissism); and lastly, at a final stage whose extensions are infinite, it would end up disinvesting its own ego. This is the effect of a negative narcissistic structure in which it is the ego itself that is impoverished, disintegrating to the point of losing its consistency, homogeneity, identity and organization.

This view is coherent, but it is perhaps excessively schematic. When one thinks of the clinical pictures which illustrate the last eventuality, certain affections come to mind for which theory gives but a very imperfect explanation – notably, forms of destruction in which unbinding is the fundamental and primordial mechanism. It exists in almost pure, disentangled forms, whereas I think that in borderline cases, for instance, the effects of unbinding and binding are combined. But in this clinical field, we encounter catastrophic or unthinkable anxieties, fears of annihilation or breakdown, feelings of devitalization or of psychic death. I have already alluded to anorexia, somatic disorganization, essential depression, all of which seem to obey this mechanism. Here, too, though, there is a need to nuance what we are saying. The clinical occurrences I have just described are often the consequence of a more complex state in which disinvestment – sometimes affecting the most vital functions, such as appetite – represents the counterpart and ultimate defence against the unleashing of instinctual chaos.

I have already mentioned the book by Colette Combe which confirms my views and enriches them considerably.

The ego's sense of self-disappearance

Before closing this chapter, I want to make a few propositions concerning a clinical picture encountered in certain cases which share common characteristics.[16] This elaboration has seemed to me sufficiently interesting to be worth reporting, even in rough outline. The patients I am going to speak about here present, more or less at the centre of their clinical picture, a symptom that is sometimes experienced as a mechanism which they are subject to, and which they do not understand, and sometimes as an aspiration for a desire which, paradoxically, takes the form of *self-disappearance*.

These patients have all experienced traumas characterized by abandonment, by a separation from the mother – either a physical separation or, alternatively, of the kind which I have described in my work on *the dead mother*. In cases where there has not been a real separation, it would seem that the child experiences his mother as inaccessible, which, with a word that condenses many situations, I will call the mother who is *elsewhere*. Now, this mother, who is 'elsewhere', progressively becomes for the child the object of an ambivalent, perpetually demanding fixation, infiltrated by *hainamoration* (Lacan), without the feeling of passionate love, which lies behind the recriminations, being given any recognition. As a consequence of this situation, an incapacity to tolerate frustration is often observed. In these circumstances, an internal reorganization occurs, in which the subject who has experienced distress, negligence and an absence of interest (this, at least, is what he complains of consciously) considers his mother as a child whom he has to take care of. The mother's presence–absence is such that, if the subject tries to think about the maternal object itself, he feels he is faced with a void or a hole. In a complementary manner, the child is simply used to quench with his blood the thirst of a maternal vampirism from which he says he suffers; but the analyst ends up interpreting the ardent need to be used as nourishment for the object. Moreover, there is a seesaw relationship here: 'Either she has to vampirize me or I have to invade her!' All this is relived in the transference, which is destined to periodic disillusionments as the analyst is unable for long to provide either relief or distance in relation to the conflict. The subject sometimes imagines that the analyst is applauding his pain and his distress and sometimes that he is indifferent and unaffected by his suffering. The perpetually sought-after consolation is never salutary. Speech is a locus of a strange transformation. It appears to pass right over the patient's psyche; it speaks of the conflict without being inhabited by it. The figure of the Other is always adverse; it is an Other which is no longer loving. It is 'emptied of love' (*désamouré*) (as if it was required elsewhere without one knowing either where, how or why). As for sexuality, it frequently assumes traumatic or perverse forms, discharging itself frenetically, giving the impression that it consists less of pleasure than of furious aggression. During sexual acting out, when there is no possibility of living these situations as a revenge against the trauma, reversals can be surmised between the victimized object and the cynical aggressor through unconscious and silent identification. The transference is often relocated, actualized, mis-recognized. In speaking of relocation, I do not simply mean a lateral transference whose link with the central transference is easily recognizable. Often, the forms of behaviour involved suggest a need for control and mastery. One frequently observes the development of very extreme sublimations which have the aim of pleasing the ego-ideal and play a more or less efficient role as a protective shield and as a means of insulation. The processes of recognition occur outside the setting, and rarely in the session; the patient bringing to the session what he has become conscious of outside the session. Generally speaking, one witnesses a hatred of the other sex. I am referring especially here to cases of women who have the greatest of difficulty in effecting and accepting the change of object. The father never acquires the same importance as the mother; in any case, not before a long time has been spent in the analysis. It is when he finally becomes an object of desire that the Oedipus complex is recognized for the first time; and the bond between the parents (primitive scene) becomes thinkable, at least implicitly. A certain degree of mourning for the primary object then occurs, with the appearance of feelings of love and tenderness for the mother as well as for the father. It is as if the analysand had finally accepted that the child is not everything for the mother. One understands, retrospectively, the extent to which a blockage of identification has prevented mourning. It is striking, however, that it is at this moment that the picture is transformed and that marks of love coming from the mother finally (!) appear – in an evanescent manner initially – which had never been acknowledged before. All other objects that have played the role of parental substitutes have been more or less dehumanized – with exceptions that almost have a status of extraterritoriality; that is to say, one's own children with whom one is united by the same flesh. One sees patients giving them exclusive signs of love – except during sudden surges of passion which do not last. In short, therapy has above all helped them to accomplish a deferred mourning. These cases bear witness to a sort of maternal omnipotence of a very particular nature since it consists, over a long period of time, of the feeling of never having been understood. It is omnipotence, then, from which one cannot benefit any more than one can imagine competing with the Oedipal mother. And yet, this omnipotence is coupled with a considerable degree of fragility if the subject dares to follow his own path by reversing his sense of being abandoned by the mother into one of abandoning the mother.

Let me conclude with two remarks, one on sexuality, the other on the ego. It appears that sexuality is unacceptable here because it began, in a form that cannot be remembered, with events where the subject was forced, events that are imagined or that were actually experienced. The question of desire does not arise, for it is, so to speak, absorbed by an irresistible curiosity for a generative experience of jouissance in which a considerable amount of rage, aggressivity and anger are mingled. One could almost say that its object, inasmuch as it was invested by desire, even seems to have disappeared or to have left the scene as a result of an unconscious decision to disappear. There is a pull towards non-being. The whole idea of Oedipal rivalry is absent; transgressive guilt is probably bound up with its sanction, experienced as a collapse, the consequence of the experience of abandonment in which desire itself is effaced. The rupture of this primitive tie has a retroactive effect on other instinctual ties. As for the ego, it seems to sustain itself through its opposition, which can take the form of a primary anality in association with a tendency to idealization, a tendency to disparage instinctual life ('bodies are meat', one patient said to me) and to engage in constrictive sublimatory interests which never satisfy the ego ideal. In extreme cases, the process of self-disappearance is set in movement, representing the ultimate attempt to escape from a constrictive and traumatic situation. It remains difficult to interpret. I have postulated that it is as if the ego were allowing itself to be pulled irresistibly into the wake of the object, which is itself carried along by a movement of distancing to the extent that it is only punctually present, before disappearing completely.

Notes

1 The title of this chapter is the same as that one of my books. See A. Green, *Le travail du négatif*. Paris: Editions de Minuit, 1993. [English edition, trans. Andrew Weller. *The Work of the Negative*, London: Free Association Books, 1999.] Clearly it is only possible here to give a very partial view of it.

2 Concerning all these points, see Chapter 3 of *The Work of the Negative*.

3 J.-C. Rolland uses repression almost exclusively.

4 Spoken commentary on Freud's 'Verneinung' by Jean Hippolyte, in the *Ecrits*. Paris: Editions du Seuil, 1966.

5 Introduction and response to Jean Hippolyte's Commentary, *Ecrits*, pp. 369–380 and 381–400.

6 Bion, W.R. (1962). *Learning from Experience*, p. 47ff. London: William Heinemann, Medical Books; reprinted London: Karnac Books, 1984.

7 Green, A. The intuition of the negative in playing and Reality. In: *The Dead Mother, The Work of André Green*. London and New York: Routledge, 1999.

8 Trans. note: a character in Flaubert's *Madame Bovary*.

9 Freud, S. (1917d [1915]). *S.E.* XIV, 232.

10 Green, A. *The Work of the Negative*, p. 171. London: Free Association Books, 1999.

11 Ibid. 185.

12 Ibid. 210.

13 Green, A. Primary narcissism: structure or state. In: *Life Narcissism, Death Narcissism*. London: Free Association Books, 2001. Cited in *The Work of the Negative*, p. 210.

14 See Green, A. *The Work of the Negative*, Ch. 4.
15 Green, A. L'invention de la pulsion de mort. *La pensée clinique*. Paris : Odile Jacob.
16 The ideas that follow arose from the exposition of three clinical cases presented at my Seminar on 'The Principles and Practices of Psychotherapies Carried Out by Psychoanalysts'. I would like to take the opportunity of thanking Marie-France Castarède, Guy Lavallée and Josiane Chambrier whose patients – to whom they listened – have stimulated my own reflections.

14

RECOGNITION OF THE UNCONSCIOUS

Field of misrecognition

As the subtitle of this work is *Misrecognition and Recognition of the Unconscious*, the reader might think that its content gives very unequal treatment to the first and the second. In fact, there is recognition because there has been misrecognition. As for the latter, it seems it is inevitable. In analysing its forms throughout the preceding chapters, and in as complete a manner as possible, I have said implicitly what has to be recognized if the subject is to be able to live the conflicts between the conscious mind and the unconscious mind in a way that is tolerable. Am I claiming that consciousness is recognition? There is no reason to think so. Where there is recognition there is *prise de conscience*, insight, that is to say, an inward-looking vision (I have proposed the term *introvision*). Nonetheless, we are bound to ask ourselves if consciousness is indispensable for recognition. But let us return for a moment to misrecognition. What can be noted about it is the existence of a double grid. Misrecognition is blindingly evident when we enter the heaviest sectors of pathology. One can even argue that, the more the individual is marked by pathology, the greater the misrecognition will be. Psychoanalysis was born and developed, at least during the time of Freud, out of the analysis of the neuroses, forms of pathology neighbouring on normality; I have shown that from the time of the second topography, this was no longer quite true. I have even contended that the modifications which marked the last part of Freud's work foreshadowed, in a way, the future, that is to say our present. I am quite sure, in fact, that Freud knew intuitively that, in the future, psychoanalysis would have to deal increasingly with non-neurotic structures.[1] From the beginning, Freud was obliged to recognize that normality was also inhabited by the unconscious, at least by certain of its particularly rich formations. Thus experiences such as dreams, phantasies, slips of the tongue, bungled actions, acts of forgetting, etc. are common to both 'ill people' and 'normal people'. This is even true of the experience of transference which is not restricted to the analytic cure and can appear in a variety of circumstances that lend themselves to it. It is not only what I shall call the normality of the ordinary man which shows vestiges of the unconscious; exceptional personalities reveal many aspects of it through their sublimation and their creativity. In fact, the analysis of cultural processes is equally enriching for noting the presence of the unconscious (systems of values, institutions, cultural creations, social organizations, etc.). I have just cited successively 'ill people' and 'normal people', whether they are ordinary or exceptional. One category is missing, namely, psychoanalysts. That they have to suffer the misrecognition of their unconscious is the very least that can be said, since psychoanalytic training rests on this postulate, without which it would not require the analysis of the future psychoanalyst (second fundamental rule, according to Ferenczi). But that is not all. The fairly detailed examination that I have made of the different doctrines which have occupied the field of psychoanalysis since Freud shows us that they present conceptions of the unconscious that are very different from each other, and even further removed from the work of the founder of psychoanalysis. It is worth noting a current tendency in certain psychoanalytic movements which presents the idea of a *continuity* between consciousness and unconsciousness. In short, such a conception which, in Freud, could only apply to the system *Cs.-Pcs.* here embraces the unconscious as well. What is contested, then, is the idea of a radical discontinuity between *Cs.-Pcs.* and *Ucs.* And if one adds that with the second topography in which the id replaces the unconscious, the question is no longer even one of discontinuity even but of a real break – which is perhaps the deepest reason for its rejection – then one realizes that adopting this position implies a fundamental disagreement with Freud's ideas. The answer will be: 'Why not? Does not science consist in demonstrating the errors in the knowledge of earlier epochs?' True enough. But what is at stake here is the consistency and coherence of the psychoanalytic conception of the psyche. As far as my present purpose is concerned, the question raised is that of the relation between misrecognition and recognition.

Factors of recognition

In analysis, recognition depends on a certain number of factors. I have already called attention to the more or less serious role played by pathology. Are we dealing with a fixation of sexuality, coexisting with ego integrity? Or, on the contrary, does the disturbance concern the structure of the ego, subjected to more or less extensive splitting? Or again, do the symptoms not result from a regression of the superego which not only brings into play a sense of guilt, but is the seat of widespread self-destruction?

Apart from pathology and its effects on the psychical apparatus, recognition depends on other factors. The first among them is the supposedly facilitating effect of the setting. When it is not applicable owing to the fact that the patient cannot tolerate its stringent conditions, insight is not facilitated and recognition, often punctual, can be cancelled out after having been accepted; or it frequently becomes stagnant, or even sterilized. It is evident that what is at stake here is nothing other than the *analysis of the transference. But, as we have seen there is transference and transference.* Recognition is optimal when a certain type of pathological structure is in harmony with the creation of the setting and gives access, without too many difficulties to the relations between the psychoneurosis, infantile neurosis and transference neurosis. All this comes down to two factors: first, the capacity to sustain, against all the odds, a regular psychoanalytic process; and second, a receptive sensibility, which is open to interpretation, with a felicitous mix of moderate resistances and insight. Here the question could be raised of the complex relations between interpretation and construction. The difference between them is generally recognized as resting on what is always the circumstantial and partial nature of interpretation. This progresses step by step, and, it could be said, bit by bit. On the other hand, constructions, which always have synthetic implications, provide the analyst with the opportunity of recovering a portion of the analysand's past from the narrative as a whole, which, among the fragments submitted for interpretation, gives it a meaning that it did not possess before the beginning of the narration.

A very remarkable trait of the process of insight (*prise de conscience*) resides in its *nachträglich* character. Thus *Nachträglichkeit* (*l'après-coup*), which we have seen at work, constantly taking up the elements involved in the reappearance of an earlier constellation which is enriched *a posteriori* with an additional meaning through the adjunction of fresh elements, finds itself in a different context here. Insight happens in relation to a process *that has already occurred.* The patient says exceptionally: 'I understand what that means', but is more likely to say, 'I *now* understand the meaning that I have to give to what happened before', the before in question perhaps concerning a very distant memory in the past; or again, 'I understand *now* why I did this or that and what the meaning was of the choice I made concerning such and such a decision while rationalizing my reasons for doing so.' Surprisingly, no element of the verbal material has an exclusive claim to be interpreted.

I have pointed out elsewhere that in the patient's discourse, no element isolated by linguistics has a particular privilege. Depending on the case, interpretation can concern a phoneme, the object of a slip, or another form of slip concerning a more extended unit of the discourse. It can also concern a homophony, a somewhat singular turn of phrase, or a sequence of phrases of variable length. In other circumstances, affect will be called into question for serving as a mask for its contrary (the classical case of hate dissimulating love or of love whose ambivalence makes one suspect the existence of hate: a bungled action, a repetition that is more or less compulsive, etc.).[2]

It would be wrong to think that the analytic process follows the progression of interpretations in such a way that the latter are always gaining more ground, constantly diminishing the share of what remains unanalysed. Quite to the contrary, even in the most comfortable of analyses, the conflict between the resistance and the interpretative elucidation resembles an undecided battle. Each piece of ground won over from the adversary can be the object of a more or less partial, a more or less temporary reconquest by neurosis. As Freud says, when he remarks that the overcoming of resistances is the most arduous task of psychoanalysis, the final decision remains uncertain, for 'it seems as if victory is in fact as a rule on the side of the big battalions'.[3]

Interpretation is really the noblest part of analytic work, requiring of the analyst the most acute sensibility, tact, perspicacity, benevolent neutrality, and that indefinable tone which makes it possible, at each instant and in an unforeseeable manner, to 'see' what has been heard, in a light which reveals what had been hidden within the folds of the discourse. But it has to be used pertinently. Here two contrasting caricatural attitudes exist which I shall just mention in passing. The first is the well-known attitude of silence which can be taken so far that it is reminiscent of the tomb. This, moreover, is often true of analysts who do not hide their mistrust of interpretation, or even their conviction that it is useless. Let me add that this attitude tends to encourage the idea that *by always keeping quiet, one never makes a mistake; but nor does one give the patient the possibility of recognizing anything.* And the question is to know whether what is most important is that the analyst appears as a Zen master, an image that is favourable for the patient's recovery, or, better still, a corpse of a Zen master which manifests itself at the bottom of the tomb; or, if such a silence is not responsible for a deleterious analytic atmosphere, letting the analysand fall back into his original *Hilflosigkeit*, withering away, session after session, on the couch. It is not uncommon in these cases for a decompensation to occur which sometimes even results either in the pure and simple interruption of the analysis or in periods of hospitalization of varying duration. These attitudes of abstaining from interpretation are frequently found in Lacanian psychoanalysts. Just as caricatural is the opposite extreme in which the analysand finds he is exposed to a barrage of interpretative artillery fire, subjecting each of his sentences to simultaneous translation, often in the terms of Kleinian praxis and theory. I have already pointed out that I consider this to be a factor of asphyxiation in the analysis and, a return, of which the analyst himself is unconscious, to suggestion. In fact, while being as receptive as possible to what comes to him from his unconscious as he listens to the patient's discourse, the analyst must also listen carefully to the way in which he thinks the patient is integrating the analyst's interpretations. H. Faimberg has rightly insisted on the role of the analyst's listening to interpretations.[4] It is not enough to cast the interpretation like a bottle into the sea. One still needs to know if there is any chance of its message being received by an addressee in the vicinity.

These two extreme positions of complete interpretative silence and a permanent barrage of interpretative activity only represent two extreme currents. The whole of contemporary psychoanalysis seems to be racking its brains to find ways of obtaining a modification in the patient which corresponds to the idea that the analyst has of his cure. Thus one hears the most diverse things that are scarcely compatible with each other: the analyst must seem 'real' to the patient, in other words, that's enough of interpreting the unconscious! We have to accept the necessity of unusual variations such as the more or less occasional adjuvant role of other therapists, even for the most common indications of analysis. The machine for inventing departures from the setting has been set in motion; it will not stop for some time.

The effects of interpretation deserve a more detailed discussion. Emphasis is usually placed on the sense of distance that has become possible, the increased control of impulses, displacements and sublimation. We should also recognize the importance of *self-reflexivity* as a mediating structure between the forms of the conflict and the capacity to tolerate them.

Return to the notion of cure

Though recognition plays an important role in the process of recovery, it is important to note how this notion has evolved since Freud's death. The year 1937 was decisive in this respect. At the beginningn of 'Analysis Terminable and Interminable', he wrote:

> Experience has taught us that psycho-analytic therapy – the freeing of someone from his neurotic symptoms, inhibitions and abnormalities of character – is a time-consuming business.[5]

Hitherto, this result was supposed to be achieved by the complete lifting of infantile amnesia. But in 'Constructions in Analysis', written just a few months later, Freud realized that such a result was impossible to achieve.[6] Moreover, it was now that he understood the role of hallucinatory states in the session. Considered in the light of the results of analysis as they are known to us today, some 65 years after, Freud's goal of the complete lifting of infantile amnesia seems rather unrealistic. Whatever technique is employed, for none can boast of obtaining significantly better results than the others, it is rare to witness such a personal mutation, or, as Freud puts it, such complete freedom. Accordingly, quite different views than the ones he held have since been defended. Winnicott, for instance, vigorously defended the idea that it is better for a patient to remain lively, even at the price of retaining some of his symptoms, than for his psyche to be totally cleared of the symptoms encumbering it and transformed in such a way that he loses all his vitality. Basically, the truest thing that Freud said about the results of analysis, condensed in a succinct manner, is that what is essential is to be able to love and to work – words that are devoid of any theoretical pretension and sufficiently close to life's observations. I will also cite Bion who, in one of his most audacious observations, pointed out that it was much easier to look like an analyst than to be one. His requirements, no less exacting than Freud's, led him to say that many who had the label of being psychoanalysts were hardly so in his eyes; and, furthermore, that he considered Bach, Beethoven, Plato, Monet, etc., as great psychoanalysts. I am sure that there are many who will be ready to contradict such a statement. But I think that, for Bion, any person who, through his creativity and his works, advances our knowledge of the mind, whether they be poets, philosophers, musicians or painters, could be considered as a rightful member of the psychoanalytic community. Perhaps what he meant was that the production of a work of culture, recognized as such, was the proof of a recognition of the unconscious, without necessarily being accompanied by insight. This amounts to saying that a successful analysis cannot short-circuit access to sublimation and frequentation with the great works of culture. It can be seen that the positions of Winnicott, like those of Bion, demonstrate a high degree of freedom and refuse to allow the destiny of analysis to bow to any kind of conformism vis-à-vis social norms; nor do they defend demagogically positions that can be likened with those of certain terrorists (not reneging on one's desire).

Today, it seems to me, the question of recognition is posed in completely new terms. Freud's position, which may be suspected of being normative, has been replaced by the need to answer a fundamental question: 'What does the individual do with his conflicts?' In posing this problem, one is implicitly referring to the vicissitudes of these conflicts which depend on the potential charge that they contain in the relations of Eros and destructivity.

Forms of unconscious recognition

The idea I am going to put forward now is likely to raise a good deal of controversy. I want to speak of the existence of forms of unconscious recognition. The paradox is immediately evident: if recognition is recognition of the unconscious, how could there be an unconscious recognition? There is a touch of contradiction *in adjecto* here. And yet, what I want to say is that, when the psyche achieves a certain result through the activation and development of creativity under the impulsion of Eros, it is this result which takes precedence over the recognition of the unconscious and gives it expression. The latter is not completely lost since psychoanalysts will be able to turn towards the products of this creativity in order to recognize in them the place and the mark of the unconscious. This, it seems to me, is the domain of art. And, in my opinion, it is what justifies the position of someone like Bion. This brings me to a point that

I have deliberately left out of this book, first to avoid lengthening it any further, and second because it would have to be examined from all sides for its interest to be appreciated. I am referring to what is known as *applied psychoanalysis*, an unfortunate term if ever there was one.[7] Others have been proposed: psychoanalysis outside the setting; psychoanalysis beyond the walls, but they do not seem much more satisfying to me. I think that the clearest denomination is that of *the psychoanalytic approach to works of art and cultural productions*. Personally, I consider that psychoanalysis took an unfavourable turning after critiques – often in the form of a volley of reproaches – had been addressed to psychoanalysts who had ventured upon this kind of activity by specialists from certain disciplines who were defending themselves progressively against the intrusions, which they judged to be illegitimate and unfounded, of psychoanalysts into their own domain. What is certain is that a psychoanalyst cannot propose a psychoanalytic interpretation of a work of art or of a cultural interpretation without having prior knowledge of the question. Nor without their being a risk of his own subjective structure surreptitiously intruding into his work. Let us note a paradox in passing. Freud's work on Leonardo has been recognized as containing some unquestionable errors, and other very probable ones (the famous *nibio*, for instance, where the kite flies away and returns decked with a vulture's feathers; Leonardo's earliest childhood in the exclusive company of his mother who brought the full weight of maternal seduction to bear on him, etc.). And yet, notwithstanding the constant denunciations, Freud's work is still taught in courses on aesthetics in university faculties throughout the world; and Shapiro himself, one of the most merciless to track down Freud's errors, considers that this work bears the mark of such originality that, unlike many others, it cannot be shelved.[8]

Sublimation is not an 'instinctual vicissitude' like the others.[9] Attention should be drawn to what can only be referred to as a sublimatory passion in certain creative individuals as well as in certain investigators of truth. If sublimation presupposes a diversion of sexual aims, it leaves the field free for a passion that has nothing to envy in relation to being in love. Freud was animated by a love for the truth which cannot be said to be present in all psychoanalysts, today even more than yesterday.

Discontents in our civilization

The fate of psychoanalysis can never be completely dissociated from the ideals of the culture in which it flourishes; the tradition and epoch within which one is speaking has to be taken into account. Without launching into generalizations that are always schematic, and without claiming to be able to talk about domains which call for specific areas of competence that I do not possess, when one compares the situation of the 1930s with that of today, the discontents in civilization of which Freud spoke have worsened considerably in spite of certain facts which remain to be interpreted, such as the liberation of moral codes and the lifting of many repressions which weighed very heavily in the past. Following the Second World War, the discovery of the horror of the concentration camps of totalitarian regimes, the disasters provoked by the atomic bomb, the conquest of space, the computer revolution, the processes of mediatization and global-ization, it would seem, merely to speak of the western societies in which we are living, that psychoanalysis – though not hindered in its practice – finds itself today in a perilous situation. There is a possibility that it will not survive unless it responds to the preoccupations of our time.[10] Many authors have already noted that our world does not encourage people to seek knowledge of themselves, to tackle internal conflicts, to analyse the unconscious. At best, facts of this order leave people indifferent; at worst, they are denied, other explanations, more mechanical are preferred. The notion of 'progress in spirituality' (Freud) is no longer a topical concern. More or less everywhere, the model that has become the common ideal is one that is oriented towards action, towards increasing power and wealth. Some may think this pessimism is excessive, but it is none-theless the conclusion I feel bound to come to. But perhaps I am only following the inclinations of age, which always push one to think that 'things were better before'. I think, though, that since 1930, we have witnessed increasingly what I would call a '*disillusionment with the spirit*'. Those civilizations that had placed the spirit at the forefront of their value systems and witnessed the construction of admirable cultures of great spiritual significance did not escape the advent of horror. The considerable knowledge accumulated has been constantly used to conquer material possessions, whereas spiritual and cultural values are of interest to fewer and fewer people compared with the numbers engaged in other, more physical activities (sports and music). The more societies evolve, giving individuals the power to improve their material situation and to fight against the evils which made them suffer and unhappy, the more, proportionally, violence is unleashed, insensible to the pain inflicted on others whereas one had hoped for the contrary. It is not pessimistic indulgence that is inducing me to write these lines which could make me pass for a bird of ill omen. Just like Freud who, after having drawn attention to the ravages of the destructive drive, appealed to the response of Eros, I can only formulate hopes that analysts will in the future find the means of achieving a reconciliation with the spirit. No good news to announce, then; no solution to propose; just a simple wish.

I am now coming to the end of my reflection. Right at the beginning of this work, before writing the first line, I registered my intention to follow the suggestion of my friend who expected an 'outline' from me. Now that I am coming to the end of the work, I realize that it scarcely resembles an outline! But I attribute this to the length of the book, which cannot legitimately be described as an outline. Yet, if one takes into consideration that, having gathered them together, I am transcribing here the essential ideas that have informed my writings from 1954 to 2002, i.e. a period of almost 50 years, the length of this volume does indeed represent the outline of this mass of writing – half of which would have been sufficient according to certain of my friends. But could I have done otherwise? I have written over the course of the years, depending on the inspiration of the moment and the problem to be resolved, what I thought needed to be said.

Notes

1   Freud, S. (1938). Some Elementary Lessons in Psychoanalysis. *S.E.* XXIII.
2   Green, A. Le langage dans la psychanalyse. In: *Langages: 2ème rencontres psychanalytiques d'Aix-en-Provence.* Paris: Les Belles Lettres, 1984, pp. 19–250.
3   Freud, S. (1937). Analysis terminable and interminable. *S.E.* XXIII, 240.
4   Faimberg, H. Listening to listening. In: *International Journal of Psycho-Analysis*, 1996, 77, no. 4, pp. 667–677.
5   Freud, S. (1937). 'Analysis terminable and interminable'. *S.E.* XXIII, 216.
6   Freud, S. (1937). 'Constructions in Analysis'. *S.E.* XXIII, 255.
7   See Green, A. (1992). *La déliaison.* Paris: Les Belles Lettres.
8   Shapiro, M. (1982). Leonard et Freud. In: *Style, Artiste, Société.* Paris: Gallimard.
9   See the chapter on sublimation in *The Work of the Negative*, ibid.
10 I mean as an institution. It goes without saying that there will always be people who will go and see an analyst with a view to elucidating what they do not understand by themselves. Psychoanalysts survived in the popular democracies of Eastern Europe during the time of Stalin.

PART THREE

Situating psychoanalysis at the dawn of the third millennium

This addendum is an attempt
to circumscribe the cultural environment of psychoanalysis.
It shows the relations of proximity, often more unfriendly than friendly,
which the related disciplines maintain with psychoanalytic thought.
In my opinion, they show how,
contrary to what is claimed,
psychoanalysis, more than a hundred years after,
has lost nothing of its subversive power.

— 15 —

PHILOSOPHICAL REFERENCES

Is it really necessary to include a chapter of philosophy in a psychoanalytic work? Between those who think that philosophy alone can really throw light on what psychoanalysis advances and those who do not hide their mistrust of any dialogue with it, I will adopt a nuanced position.

It is not unusual to identify certain philosophical references which may have played a part in Freud's judgement, beyond the immediate influences of his time. His correspondence during his youth with Silberstein[1] relates how he met Brentano, how the latter tried in vain to turn him away from medicine by inviting him to embrace a philosophical career. Anzieu has drawn up a balance sheet of what Freud owed him.[2] But, quite independently of that, one is struck by certain convergences with authors of the past in whom one finds the germ, as it were, of Freudian concepts. More recently, one is also surprised by the evolution of some of his ideas and the use to which they have been put in contexts far removed from psychoanalysis. Nor can one help thinking that Freud provided many philosophers with grist for their mill.

I am concerned here, then, with incidents which are only of a certain interest because, as a rule, they are passed over in silence. Thus, there is frequently a tendency to see Plato as one of the sources of Freudian inspiration, whereas Aristotle, it seems to me, is more influential; and Spinoza, often cited, tends to overshadow Kant. Hegel, whom Freud found obscure, played a role in Lacan's development thanks to Kojève. Nietzsche posed Freud with a difficult problem to resolve, and the latter admitted that he had avoided reading him. There remains the role of the philosophy of Schopenhauer who was also recognized by the inventor of psychoanalysis.

After Freud, modernity was obliged to come to terms with him. Today, it is psychoanalysis which has to come to terms with postmodernity. Foucault circumvents it, then goes beyond it. Deleuze set the amphitheatres alight by suggesting it should be buried in the name of the Anti-Oedipus (with the complicity of Guattari, whom one had to take at his word when he proclaimed himself a psychoanalyst). Derrida deconstructs it and leaves it behind. Habermas, sociologizes it. Lyotard 'forgets' it in his examination of postmodernity.

In the end, it is the epistemologists – who are not philosophers – of contemporary reflection who give his thought its best extension in the advances they have made in the field of hypercomplex thought. Philosophy served as an introduction to the definition of a new horizon of knowledge towards which it is no exaggeration to say that Freud opened up certain paths even before the need for a new way of thinking had become apparent.

Before Freud

Aristotle

Aristotle's *On the Soul*³ never ceases to astonish the psychoanalyst. I will make a selective reading of it for the purposes of this exposition. From the very first pages, going beyond the traditional problematic which has been studied throughout the entire history of philosophy, the Stagirite affirms: 'It seems indeed to be the case that with most affections the soul undergoes or produces none of them without the body' (I, 1). And if psychoanalysis can be pleased about such an affirmation – for it sees in it the germ of the notion of the drive – what follows only reinforces this recognition, for Aristotle discerned that 'movement is eminently characteristic of the soul' (I, 2), lifting himself, with this proposition, above his predecessors. Three features emerge from his analysis: movement, sensation and incorporeality. This thesis, discussed at length, comes up against the ever-present mystery of the union of the soul and the body. As he is developing his line of reasoning, Aristotle encounters the notion of the subject (I, 4) in relation to discursive thinking. 'Is it then somehow possible that this [the soul] be a unit?' (I, 4). One gets a glimpse here of the theory of the psychical apparatus advanced by Freud several centuries later. In such an apparatus, the tripartition is the reverse side of the unitary reference to the psyche in that the latter is distinct from the neurological or the cerebral. In fact, in his demonstration, Aristotle struggles against the difficulty of conceiving intellect as the most perfect form of the soul, but one which cannot be totally separated from the other attributes revealed by his examination. Among these, the category of the appetites (I, 5) raises the most difficult problems. The propositions are then reversed. It is not the body which gives the soul its unity but rather the soul that gives the body unity. The particular paths taken by the thinker are of more interest than his conclusions, so I will not dwell on these here (relations of substance with matter and form). On the other hand, let us note that Aristotle concludes that the body is subject and matter (II, 1). Having tried to go beyond the problem of multiplicity and unity, he is bound to arrive at the idea of a principle of different faculties: the nutritive, perceptive and intellective faculties and movement (II, 2). It was from this confrontation that the theory would emerge which, in my opinion was to be decisive for Freud. For the major interest of Aristotle is that he never forgets – nor underestimates – the imagination, desire, pleasure (and pain), even if he situates them outside the intellect. The soul, he says, is not a body but 'belongs to a body' (II, 2–3). Does it participate in it without being it, just as Freud sees the psychical anchored in the somatic but already belonging to the psychic in a form unknown to us? As one reads on, one comes across astonishing observations such as, 'if they [living things] have the perceptive faculty they have also that of desire' (II, 3). No less surprising is the remark that reproduction, at the heart of the nutritive soul, is the most natural of the functions for participating in the eternal and in desire. Aristotle could not abandon the idea of a triple causality. On the subject of the primitive soul he envisages the relations of the body to nutrition and reproduction. He then turns to the vast field of the sensitive soul. What concerns me here is the tangible and the faculty of touch. Which organ is proper to it? The flesh? Let us dwell a moment on the idea developed by Aristotle that sense is a sort of average between contrary sensibles (II, 11–12). Can this not be applied to the Freudian position which only ever treated of relations (average) of pleasure–unpleasure, leaving aside, though without overlooking their importance, the extremes of jouissance and pain. 'For that which perceives would be some thing extended, but what it is to be perceptive will certainly not be extended nor the sense; rather, they will be a formula and capacity of what perceives' (II, 12). 'Psyche is extended; knows nothing about it,' writes Freud in his posthumous notes.[4] Aristotle then turns to common sense (or the sixth sense), whose principle of judgement enables us to discern clearly.

Aristotle finally embarks on the most interesting part of his treatise by discussing the functions of knowledge. He separates two fields: local movement on one side, thought and intelligence on the other. Just before he had considered the boundary as that which makes it possible to judge two things at the same time from both sides of it (III, 2). Freud complicated this postulate in the definition he gave of the drive and in the division between id and ego. Nonetheless, he added to it the superego which reunites the two (it has its roots in the id and results from a division of the ego which gives judgement its ethical dimension). Aristotle is careful never to forget to situate this or that function of knowledge in an intermediate position between two others. He recognizes the dependence of the imagination, considered as 'superior' in relation to its more elementary forms. It is 'movement produced by perception in activity' (III, 8).

The great mutation is operated by the intellect, 'that whereby the soul thinks and supposes' (III, 4). The sensitive faculty and the intellectual faculty are quite distinct. Intellect is considered here as separate from the body (IV, 4). Having made this distinction, the need for a reunification makes itself felt, for how is one to judge the formal essence of flesh! The intellect thinks and can can be thought. The answer postulates the identity between the thought-subject and the thinking object (III, 4). The intellect is capable of becoming all things and is capable of producing them all (ibid). He is led to distinguish between different types of intellect.

Having thus approached the question of knowing how sensation 'judges', he considers the case in which the object is pleasant or painful. 'Avoidance and desire are, in their actualized state, the same thing, nor are their faculties different either from each other or from the perceptive faculty, but their way of being the same thing is different' (III, 7). *Lust und unlust prinzip!*

Imagination is what takes the place of sensation in the soul. 'The soul never thinks without an image' (III, 7). One understands, then, that in the imagination, the soul makes up for the lack of sensation by exciting the senses which put it in touch with itself. Although it does not occur to Aristotle to refer to them, one is led to think of dreams. With the imagination, Aristotle introduces us to the domain of interiority. Imagination only deserves its denomination by the way in which it is constituted, which only occurs through the mediation of an excitation coming from something other than it, in reality. It is thus this self-reality, so to speak, created by it, which Freud was to call the psychic reality of the internal world.

The intellect is comprised of forms (III, 8). At this point, a new distribution of the faculties grouped by parts proves necessary:

• the nutritive part;
• the perceptive part.

With no change. There then follows:

• the imaginative part;
• the desiring part.

One can see that the imagination holds, in short, the middle ground between desire, which gives birth to it, and the intellect, which sets about understanding it. But here, then, is the conclusion that philosophers over the centuries seem not to have read: 'If then one makes the soul tripartite, one will find desire in all three parts' (III, 9).

Desire is thus the principle of unity; depending on the case considered, it is distributed in the different parts making up the diversity, thereby influencing the nutritive soul and the sensitive soul. The admirable 'impartiality of the intellect' (Freud). This being the case, it is movement that is reinterpreted, since it always concerns the loss or the search for an object.

However, once again, all these divisions reoccur. Hence a new insight proposes two principles of movement, namely, desire and intellect. It is clear that the philosopher cannot bring himself to allow desire to occupy the whole terrain of the psyche. Consequently, Aristotle distinguishes between practical intellect and theoretical intellect, just as Freud does in the third part of his *Project*.[5] The object of desire becomes the principle of practical intellect (III, 10). Division triumphs. But suddenly there is a return of unity: 'the object of desire is the point of departure for action' (ibid.). The conclusion finally imposes itself: 'We have shown, then, that it is the sort of capacity of the soul that is called desire that produces movement' (III, 10). Aristotle is Freudian. He must have read *The Interpretation of Dreams*! Let's continue:

> There arise, however, desires opposed to one another. The opposition of reason and the appetites invariably leads to this, and its occurrence to those creatures enjoying resistance, while the appetite supports its case with the immediate facts. Inability to see into the future underwrites the appearance that what is immediately pleasant both is so and is absolutely good. In form, then, that which produces movement is a single thing, the faculty of desire as such. But first of all is the object of desire, which, by being thought or imagined, produces movement while not itself in motion.
>
> (III, 10)

There is no need for a desiring machine.

Aristotle's thinking is constantly brought back to the dimension of movement, just as Freud's is to the drive. 'The organ whereby desire produces movement is something bodily, whose investigation belongs with that of the common functions of body and soul' (III, 10). Is this the reason why Freud situates the drive at the frontiers of the psychic and the corporeal?

Another point in common between the philosopher and the psychoanalyst is that of not dissociating the human from the animal, not exaggerating their difference, but taking it into account. Man is a higher animal. Whence the observation that irrational desire triumphs over rational desire, sometimes at the heart of living nature. Do we know for sure that only animals endowed with motility possess a nervous organization? The drive is but the reverse side of action, the result of its interiorization. But in Aristotle one finds the idea of the lava flows of the different layers of the drives, an idea Freud was to put forward later: 'whatever has pushed something else produces in that thing an act of pushing, the movement occurring through a middle item' (III, 12). To conclude, speech is left to the tangible including in its manifestations hearing, 'whose function is that of perceiving certain signs, and language, that of communicating with others by means of signs'. I fear that, as Beaufret once said to me, this freedom of thought that existed prior to the beginnings of Christian thought, can no longer be found in philosophy or at least will not be found again for a long time.

Kant[6]

A priori, no philosophical work is further removed from psychoanalysis than Kant's, notwithstanding the use Bion made of it which involved reinterpreting psychoanalysis profoundly. What is more, today, it is from Kantism that the adversaries of psychoanalysis draw their arguments, defending a formalism in the colours of contemporary cognitivism. There exists, however, within the Kantian corpus, one work in relation to which the psychoanalyst can feel he has made a fortunate encounter, and this is *Anthropology from the Pragmatic Point of View*.[7] It is in no way a secondary work, for its French translator, M. Foucault, tells us that it had been taught for some 30 years until Kant withdrew from the Chair of Koenigsberg. Thus it was not published until 1797. It is worth recalling Kant's observations on the difficulties involved in establishing the foundations of an anthropological science. For if man feels he is being observed and examined, he is 'embarrassed (disturbed)' and 'hides himself. He does not want to be known as he is'. Kant does not say why. Another possibility for man is to examine himself: 'If the motives are at stake, he does not observe himself; if he observes himself, the motives are out of action'. For such is the pragmatic objective, which claims to provide knowledge of man as a *citizen of the world*.

As early as the First Book, a chapter entitled 'On the Ideas We Have without Being Aware of Them' attracts our attention, but Kant attaches this subject to *physiological* anthropology, even though he liked to give sexual love as an example of it.[8] Kant observes that I only know myself as *I appear* to myself; in other words erroneously. And yet, having studied all the criticisms that appearance is subject to, he nonetheless comes to its defence. However strong man's tendency to deceive is, the virtues, even acted, are in the end awakened. It is difficult to imagine that this can assume the value of truth. Throughout his writing, in contradistinction to Aristotle, a voluntarism which privileges activity and the will, and which he cannot get rid of, serves as a guarantee for his spiritualism (cf. the *intellectual pleasure* in communicating his thoughts[9]). One can already sense psychology en route. Everything which escapes the will, such as dreams and fantasies, is suspected of illness; and it is after having banished them as such that it is noted that they can also occur in healthy individuals. I will not dwell either on the weakness of his description of the attributes of the psyche or on his reflections on mental illnesses. Though the latter are merely the reflection of the knowledge of the time and cannot be the object of criticism, on the other hand, the explanations that Kant gives of them are singularly lacking in depth. Tribute should be paid to him, though, for having accepted to reflect on mental pathology; for after him, there was a marked tendency to avoid venturing into these mysterious and obscure regions.

In comparison with Aristotle, this reading would seem fastidious were it not for the interesting evocations – still seen from the perspective of noting convergences with Freud's thought – awaiting us in the Second Book. They pertain to pleasure and pain. The first is an 'advancement of vitality'; the second a 'hindrance of life'.[10] In §62, we come across the *pleasure principle*,[11] the source of which is attributed to Epicurus. The principle of constancy is implicitly evoked in the *even state of temper*. This announces, after reflections that are often obscure, the Third Book, which discusses, among others, the faculty of desire: 'Desire (*appetitio*),' writes Kant, 'is the self-definition of the power of the subject to imagine something in the future as an effect of such imagination. Desiring without emphasis on the production of the object is wish' (p. 155). Many of the descriptions that follow of the affective life are commonplace and moralizing. Fortunately, in the chapter on the passions, our interest is rekindled. In §80, Kant writes: 'The subjective possibility of having a certain desire arise, which precedes the representation of its object, is *propensity* (*propensio*). The inner *compulsion* of the faculty of desire to take this object into possession, before one is acquainted with it, is *instinct* (like the mating instinct, or the parental instinct of an animal to protect its offspring, and so forth).' But morality quickly gets the upper hand again. Passion is an illness; the passions are the blight of reason: they are, without exception, bad. Kant does not say if they are avoidable. Kant makes a revealing choice here: the form of well-being which seems to agree best with humanity is a good meal in the company of friends. One is astonished here at the omission of love; the lines that follow have little in common with Plato's *Symposium*.

The work closes with considerations of little interest, if the truth is to be told, on character, temperament, physiognomy, with scarcely any originality and too frequently accompanied by moral recommendations. Flashes of lucidity make up for long pieces of conventional eloquence: 'foolishness rather than evil is the most striking characteristic of our species'.[12] If Kant is so prolix in making moral recommendations, it is because he is profoundly pessimistic about the human condition, a point he has in common with Freud. I will let him speak for himself by citing one of the variants of the text:

> The spirit (*animus*) of man, as the totality of all ideas which can be accommodated within it, has a range (*sphaera*) which comprises the three premises of the faculty of cognition, the feeling of pleasure and displeasure, and the faculty of desire. Each of these premises is split into two divisions, the field of *sensuousness* and the field of the *intellect* (the field of sensuous and intellectual cognition, pleasure or displeasure, desire and rejection).[13]

Sensibility can be considered as a weakness, but also as a strength. We are not far away from Freud here. In terms of his moral preoccupations, is he more on the side of Kant or Aristotle? He would very much have liked, no doubt, to have been able to reason with the freedom of the first, and he thus borrowed more than one theoretical concept from him; but, like Kant, he was in search of an ideal balance, a little mistrustful of the passions which were in danger of disturbing his need for lucidity.

Schopenhauer

Freud referred on several occasions in his work to the connection between the philosophical conception of Schopenhauer and his own theory. It is not a question, then, of an occulted source. Nonetheless, the meeting points are so astonishingly close that they deserve to be pointed out in detail. 'For all amorousness is rooted in the sexual impulse alone, is in fact absolutely only a more closely determined, specialized, and indeed, in the strictest sense, individualized sexual impulse, however, ethereally it may deport itself.'[14] Like Freud, Schopenhauer extends considerably the domain of the sexual (it is the final aim of every human aspiration), which brings us closer to the first theory of the drives in which Freud opposes the species and the individual in the different forms taken by the will to live. Certainly, this consciousness, far in advance of its time, is accompanied by often astounding naiveties when the author indulges in generalizations which show that the fundamental intuition gives way to visionary temptations. Nevertheless, Schopenhauer is free enough to recognize ambivalence, or the coexistence of love and hate. By joining a metaphysics of death to that of love, he leads us to Freud's last theory of the drives, even though the idea of a death drive was foreign to him. However, both authors are united by the same stoicism towards death; with the consolation, in Schopenhauer, of the idea of immortality, sustained by the will to live. Perhaps, ultimately, the pivot around which the two theories turn is the idea of representation.

In short, the more knowledge approaches the idea of an instinctual basis of the psyche, the more the Stoic ethic imposes itself in *counterpoint*.[15]

After Freud

M. Foucault

In a work of 1954,[16] the content of which betrays the date of birth, M. Foucault, who was probably en route towards his *Madness and Civilization* (1961), focuses on the relations between mental illness and personality. Freud's shadow, which alternately fascinates Foucault and pushes him irresistibly to reject him, hangs over this reflection. Having presented an overview of the principal affections listed in which there is a noticeable absence of any reference to perversion, whereas psychasthenia is mentioned, and which ignores superbly the studies of psychiatrists (H. Ey), Foucault attempts to propose a coherence unifying this polymorphism. He pleads for an artificially created unity which blurs the frontiers with morality. He ends up by challenging, with the backing of phenomenology, the very notion of mental illness, even though phenomenologically oriented psychiatrists have never rejected it – quite to the contrary. As a whole, they were, and remain, in favour of preserving the organic aetiology at the basis of the clinical entities on which they have commented, and have repainted clinical material in the colours of philosophy, to which they rally, while extending its domain to mental pathology (Minkowski, Von Gebsattel, E. Strauss, Binswanger).[17] One can already note the accent placed on the role of the milieu, linked to a sociogenesis that is more ideological than respectful of the facts. In the account he gives of psychoanalysis, Foucault never fails to underline the responsibility of parents in castration anxiety ('the castration fantasies of parental threats'[18]). The exposition of psychoanalytic ideas is approximate. Psychoanalysis is subjected to a critique based on a phenomenological approach initially; then Foucault turns away from it.[19] The philosopher makes abundant references to the archaic,[20] without going into details. He appears to let himself be seduced by the idea of defence mechanisms borrowed from Anna Freud, but he soon pulls himself together and rejects the notion. He constantly opposes *evolution* (natural) and *history* (social), careful above all (he was not the only one at this time) to 'denaturalize' the psyche so as to anchor it rather on the side of anthropology, that is to say, of history. In so doing, he allows himself to be fascinated by the sirens of Jaspers. Foucault ignores the debates that animated psychiatry in his time, i.e. concerning the relations between neurology and psychiatry, and the psychogenesis of the psychoses and the neuroses – debates in which the best minds of post-Second World War psychiatry, under the direction of H. Ey, took part. And for good reason! He is totally oriented towards the aim of imposing a militant historical standpoint with the aim of making psychiatry and psychoanalysis pass for repressive social practices. His description of mental illness is thereby slanted, 'normalizing' the mad so as to highlight the pathology of society around him all the better. For Foucault needs a culprit to blame. Even if one adopts the phenomenological point of view, one has great difficulty in linking up his descriptions with the historical perspective that he proposes. In fact, Foucault uses phenomenology and historical study, first and foremost against psychoanalysis. One understands that, behind the critique of natural sciences (*Naturwissenschaft*), what hounds his discourse is Freud's theory of the drives which he wants nothing to do with. This refutation is not innocent.[21] For giving prominence to the history of madness is only justified on the condition that the right concepts are applied to it. However, Foucault dreams only of denouncing the 'moralizing sadism'[22] of some in order to turn attention away from the perverse structure and the sadism of certain pathologically defined structures. Everyone will remember, moreover, his commentary on '*Moi, Pierre Rivière* . . .', in which the psychiatrists of the time are accused of all the sins, even though, *in terms of the knowledge of the epoch*, the expertise with which they approached mental illness provided models worthy of the highest admiration.

For Foucault, Freud provided the perfect incarnation of a simplistic image of the father of the Oedipus complex, 'whose triumphant rivalry arouses both hate and amorous desire for identification'.[23] Hate, yes, and love? And yet, when the time came to settle accounts, he wrote, after having condemned just about everybody: 'Freud was the first to open up once again the possibility for reason and unreason to communicate in the danger of a common language, ever ready to break down and disintegrate into the inaccessible'.[24] After this acknowledgement, the work closes with a summary condemnation of the concept of the drive (at the time, one said instincts): 'A mythology built on so many dead myths'.[25]

How many times has one not read the expression 'the theory of the instincts is our mythology', cited with the aim of condemning Freud with his own arguments. There would be no reason to be surprised if it were not that these citations come from the pen of readers highly experienced in exegesis. One is surprised to see them making a misinterpretation so casually. To say that the theory of the instincts is our mythology is certainly not meant to come to the aid of those who reject it, but shows a will to explain that this status of myth is the only one which makes it possible to recognize the truth which it bears. Would one think of attributing to Freud the idea that, as it is only known to us via a myth (and then via a tragedy inspired by it), the story of Oedipus is pure nonsense? Foucault, rejecting the sham of the world of pathology, pleads in favour of 'the effective causality of a world which cannot, of itself, offer a solution to the contradictions to which it has given rise', a facile and demagogical confusion between the phenomenon of mental alienation and that of social alienation creating institutions which are supposed to cope with it, without succeeding. 'In alienating its freedom, the world cannot acknowledge its madness.'

One senses in these lines the prefiguration of the *Anti-Oedipus* of Deleuze and Guattari. A strange illustration of the 'concrete' a priori in which a whole generation would rush to turn its eyes away from a madness that it did not cease to attempt to ward off by all the intellectual means of the period. I do not think that the arguments had fundamentally changed when, at the end of his life, Foucault treated of *The History of Sexuality* which suddenly and surprisingly sings the praises of chastity. His genealogical historiography, by denouncing this dependence of power vis-à-vis truth, is reversed into a dependence of truth vis-à-vis power (Habermas). It draws on an irremediable subjectivism. As Habermas says, Foucault's critical analysis leads to an adhesion to a historiography 'narcissistically oriented toward the standpoint of the historian'.[26] Foucault's struggle against interiority is a vigorous incitement to turn oneself away from it,[27] without convincing us of the exactitude of the point of view that is supposed to replace it advantageously.

I am going to open a large parenthesis on philosophers who put language at the centre of their arguments. I will single out two: first, Wittgenstein, who in the end managed to cross the French frontier after reigning as master in the Anglo-Saxon world without his thinking crossing the channel; second, Derrida, whose relations with psychoanalysis are not very clear. These two authors, very different from each other, pose the problem of the relationship between their ideas and Lacan's, whose influence has extended beyond psychoanalysis to philosophy.

Wittgenstein[28]

Making an appraisal of the dispute between Wittgenstein and Freud is an enterprise which goes beyond my possibilities, so I will just be making a few remarks here so as not to sin by omission. The points of departure of the two theories cannot be more different. For Wittgenstein (§133, *Philosophical Remarks*[29]), it is simply a question of applying some extremely simple principles: 'which every child knows' to get out of the confusion that our language creates. As we are bewitched by it, it is up to us to clarify the symptoms of the true mental illness from which we suffer. At certain moments Wittgenstein even refers to the psychoanalytic method, even though he only had a very partial knowledge of psychoanalysis. For Freud, mental illnesses do not originate on the side of language. Wittgenstein reproaches him, as we know, for taking reasons for causes. In point of fact, the role of philosophy for Wittgenstein is not to produce new theories but to demonstrate more clearly *what we already know*. Which amounts to saying that there is no unconscious. The consequence thereof is that one can only speak of that which can be expressed in words. The rest must be silenced. It can be seen that this position repudiates definitively any theorization which tries to treat the question of affect and, more generally, all the phenomena implying a relation to the body. We are familiar with his remarkable developments on pain, in which he denounces the idea of a private language. As soon as I speak, however subjective the state to which I am referring may be, I yield to grammar. The complaint arising from pain is thus not a private matter. Verbal expression is linked to expressions of natural sensations which have a signification to the extent that what I say presupposes the reference to *public* criteria of linguistic usage. But when I read: 'Be Good, my Sorrow, quiet your despair',[30] does grammar exhaust the message? For Wittgenstein, the bewitching nature of our language (would this be the definition of poetry?) leads to an incessant struggle *against* language. With Wittgenstein, logical positivism reached its most extreme form. Philosophy suffers from the misappreciation (*méconnaissance*) of philosophy, from an incomprehension of the logic of language, a source of illusions. If, today, there is a renewed interest in France for Wittgenstein thanks to J. Bouveresse,[31] it is because his philosophy principally influenced the Anglo-Saxon world, including the philosophy of science. A psychoanalyst will have difficulty in accepting the idea of a total superposition between language apparatus and psychical apparatus. Getting to know psychical life outside language, even if a moment comes when one is obliged to formulate it through language and via language, is the challenge of psychoanalysis. Bewitchment by language? No doubt, but what about bewitchment by dreams, desire and jouissance? 'Language disguises thought' (*Tractatus* 4.002). What analyst would not agree? But rationalization, if it is recognized as such, does not say why I rationalize, why I disguise *myself*. For disguise is also very much transvestism. Is Swann bewitched by language or by Odette? Can desire be subjected to a rigorous examination by linguistic analysis? This is not very convincing.

Nevertheless, Wittgenstein finally undertook his own self-critique by denouncing the quest for an ideal language which is in contradiction with the search for a real language. He then created the theory of language games which would be taken up in the concepts of postmodernity (see further on). Wittgenstein finally decides to take into account the extra-lingusitic context. *Language always refers to its other, which is not language, if even it only reaches us by means of a linguistic formulation.* Against the idea of a representation of the state of things, which the *Tractatus* defends, the philosophical *Investigations* sets the idea of a game with an indefinite quantity of functions. Playing? That suits the psychoanalyst better, especially if he takes his inspiration from Winnicott. The consistency of the concept of language is finally called into question. It is interesting to note the place that Wittgenstein's work occupies in a country where psychoanalysis has experienced the impact of the ideas of another theoretician of language, J. Lacan. Now it is remarkable that Lacan constructed his theory from linguistics, that it is to say, from Saussure, Jakobson and Chomsky, without according the slightest interest to Wittgenstein. For a long time, Lacan's thought was unable to cross the Anglo-Saxon linguistic barrier. Could that be because Wittgenstein's thought stood in the way? At any rate, one can recognize Heidegger's influence in Lacan's work. Yet Heidegger and Wittgenstein, at opposite extremes from each other, shared between them the philosophical domain of their time.

Riceour

The portrait gallery of French philosophy does not allow us to identify any unity, and there will hardly be a sense of doing them justice since there will be many whom I will not be able to mention here. Thus, before going any further, tribute must be paid to Paul Riceour. He was the first to carry out a detailed and rigorous examination of Freud's work, subjecting it to a philosophical analysis.[32] In France, his work was coolly received in psychoanalytic circles, especially by Lacan and his disciples (Valabrega), for his conclusions did not seem to meet their expectations. And yet, no one before him – I mean no psychoanalyst – had taken the risk of embarking on such a project, namely, that of studying Freud, as one would study Descartes, Leibniz or Kant. It may have been that, after frequenting Lacan's *Seminar* for a time, he had not sufficiently recognized the genius of the Master of Sainte-Anne, something the latter did not fail to point out to him bluntly. In any case, he was often subjected to unjust critiques on account of the prejudice which holds that a philosopher can understand nothing of psychoanalysis. These critiques, which did not go unnoticed by Riceour and surprised him all the more in that he had gone about the task with a seriousness rarely encountered, were offset by the warm welcome that his work received in the United States, where he taught for part of the year. American psychoanalysts acclaimed this work of philosophy which showed them, with serenity, the limitations of their own interpretation of the inventor of psychoanalysis. For the first time, Freudian concepts were presented by articulating the symbolic and the economic. Ego psychology's often reductive conception of the Freudian corpus, cast in a medicalizing mould, was weakened by it.

Derrida

There is no more problematic case, in the study of the relations between philosophy and psychoanalysis, than that of Jacques Derrida. I shall grant him a more important place than the others, given his close relations with the psychoanalytic milieu. Even before his founding work *Of Grammatology* (1967), Derrida had quite close relations with Nicolas Abraham (psychoanalyst and philosopher claiming allegiance to Husserl) and Marika Torok.[33] The reading of *Of Grammatology* had an effect on certain psychoanalysts of the time, especially those who had taken an interest in structuralism. The *voice* and the *phoneme* had been the subject of the author's reservations vis-à-vis the *ousia* of speech. Two questions arise in relation to the ideas and concepts to which Derrida gives prominence. The first concerns their philosophical validity. I will say nothing about this since I am not competent to do so. The second is that of their impact on psychoanalysis. The positions taken by the author in *Of Grammatology* were bound to hold the attention of psychoanalysts. In proposing the idea of *archi-writing* as a leading concept, was he not approaching the concept of the *memory trace*, so essential to the thought of Freud who was constantly seeking to link it up with the memory system and to relate verbal memory traces with the other types of traces (thing memory traces)? At the outset, Derrida set about making a very detailed examination of Freud's theory.[34] He recognized that Freud was an exception, who did not fit into western metaphysics.

251

I will confine myself here to the work that Derrida published in 1996, *Resistances of Psychoanalysis*.[35] The *of* marks the distinction between the resistance *to* psychoanalysis (which Derrida flays in passing, even though he says he will not deal with this position, and the resistance *of* psychoanalysis to itself, which is what the author will focus on. The first essay, which is a rich text, proceeds in two phases. The first is an exhaustive investigation of certain texts of Freud on resistance concerning which Derrida proposes a personal interpretation; the second is an analysis of the relations between psychoanalytic thought and deconstruction, and is of a much more philosophical character, so I will not speak about it. Resistance as a psychical force does not just resist the recognition of meaning; it itself also has meaning, and Freud comes up against a limit to this meaning, owing to the very fact of resistance. Derrida turns, then, to the analysis of Irma's dream. Starting with Freud's style, which is nonetheless frank and self-critical, Derrida first condemns it insidiously, then more clearly. The deconstructor does not seem to understand that Freud is trying to give as sincere an account as possible of his state of mind when he returns to the day's residues. Of course, this is not the first time that Freud has been caught out for blatant authoritarianism, and even misogyny. But Derrida seems to miss Freud's strategy of sincerity presented without false candour in an attempt to account, as faithfully as possible, for the manner in which this humour can influence the structure of the dream. There are two different problems here. The first concerns Freud's attitudes in reality, which can justifiably be criticized; the second is that of undertaking as lucid, complete and objective an analysis as possible, in order to understand how the dream was formed after the dream-work has occurred. Derrida does not conceal the pleasure he derives from denouncing Freud's position, showing that the use of the concept of resistance applies to the patient's refusal to comply with the explanatory hypotheses, which Freud says, are 'my solution'. He considers, then, that this power struggle corresponds to a *polemos* and an *eros*; hence the condensed form *poleros* in seduction. Let us note well what Derrida's text will show, namely, *an unconscious identification of the deconstructor with Irma*. In other words, writing will reveal that the femininity of the victim Irma-Derrida serves as a support for the authoritarian and castrating virility of Freud (the aggressor). Another remark concerns the well-known question of the dream navel (*omphalos*). Derrida engages here in highly interesting reflections on the function and the nature of the omphalos. When Derrida, making use of the image of the meshwork, designates the spot where the dream wish grows up 'like a mushroom out of its mycelium' (Freud), it seems to me that Freud has put his finger on something here that could, in effect, be compared with a chiasmus, as Derrida contends: the psychic forces are transformed by passing from one side where psychical elaboration works on the dream *thoughts* to another where they have become dream *images*. One is astonished that the theoretician of *archi-writing* does not even raise this question. Starting with this omphalos, Derrida comes to the analysis of the deepest resistance, viewed as the place where the analysis should stop. He cites Freud while wondering if, when the latter writes, 'In the most well-analysed dreams, one must . . .', it is a question of a Factum or a Fatum, of an impassable limit or an injunction, of a dutiful, 'One must'. In the name of what? In fact, there is no indication in Freud of a prohibition against going further; what he seems to say is: 'One is forced to', 'One has no choice but to'. In fact, Derrida wants to present an image of Freud establishing a limit beyond which any progress would be a transgression, a limit in the face of which he has to withdraw, so as to show all the better that he, Derrida, is stopped by nothing. Which explains why he speaks of being proud of his resistance to psychoanalysis. 'In other words, I am not going to tell you a story, especially not the story of how I have heroically resisted analysis and, more radically, the Freudian analysis of analysis.'[36] Are we to understand by that that Derrida is laughing and that his modesty prevents him from passing himself off as a hero who does not deserve this title? Analysing Freud's attitude at the dawn of psychoanalysis, as it is presented in the *Studies on Hysteria*, Derrida cites: 'When the resistance is prolonged, when one has not succeeded in transforming the patient, the resister, into a "collaborator"', and Derrida adds, 'that is Freud's word'.[37] Let us deconstruct the deconstructor: everyone knows, surely, that the word collaborator did not have the same sense before the German occupation as it did after it. Right from the beginning of his article, he admits that, for him, resistance evokes 'the most beautiful word in the politics and history of this country'.[38] The allusion is transparent: whoever resists analysis is likened to those who resisted the Nazi occupation of his country. A blow below the belt. I do not know very well what the navel refers to inasmuch as it is 'impenetrable, unfathomable, unexplorable, unanalysable', but what I do know on the other hand is that these, at the very least, tendentious allusions could well be the navel of Derrida's thought with regard to psychoanalysis. One wonders about the double game, announced in the preface (p. vii), in which he apparently takes the defence of psychoanalysis against a 'sometimes subtle and refined' cultural resistance, 'an inventive or arrogant disavowal, often direct and massive on the scale of the whole of European culture which . . . seems still today to be rejecting, fearing and misunderstanding it now that its fashionable period (in fact, rather brief, is over', before going on to sing the praises, first, of the resistant patient, and then, under the guise of a denial, of the deconstructor of psychoanalysis. What Derrida does not want to understand is that the patient who resists analysis resists *so that the forces of guilt or destruction within him remain intact* – the forces *occupying the patient* opposing the efforts of his liberator. For it is these forces, through the compulsion to repeat, which are at the source of the production of the symptoms which poison his life and keep him in a state of alienation impeding any sort of lucidity. Derrida has at his disposal very direct sources of information concerning *psychoanalytic therapeutics*. The philosophical justification for the positions he adopts towards psychoanalytic thought do not concern us.

With Lacan, it is quite a different story. A verbal sparring match was organized between Lacan and Derrida in Baltimore, under the auspices of René Girard. In the essay entitled, 'For the Love of Lacan',[39] Derrida engages in a mixture of interminable confession, philosophical *disputatio* and psychoanalytic mimetism, which makes archive material of this text, as the author's preoccupations indicate. After Baltimore, Derrida was to continue a dialogue, in written form, with Lacan and sometimes, more generally, with psychoanalysis. Various traces of these exchanges testify to this, for instance, certain passages of *The Post Card* (1980) or, more specifically, 'Le facteur de la vérité' (reply to 'The Purloined Letter' by Edgar Alan Poe, a fundamental text for understanding Lacan's ideas).[40] With his usual sharp intelligence, Derrida deconstructs the role of the lack in Lacan's work, *a lack which is itself never missing*. The phallus is missing from its place, but the lack is never missing. But with 'For the Love of Lacan' Derrida crossed the Rubicon. Cutting the ground from under the feet of the eventual interpretation by a searching analyst of these debates or frolics, Derrida exclaims, counting on scandalized reactions: 'You see, I think that we loved each other very much, Lacan and I.'[41] The unconscious never loses its rights; they show through in writing even when one claims to be able to circumvent it by anticipating it. Are we to understand that it was Derrida who loved Lacan a lot or that he would have liked Lacan to have loved him a lot? I do not know if Lacan loved Derrida. But there can be no doubt that in his book Derrida admits to his passion for Lacan.

He tells us how pleased he was to be invited to take part in this tribute, and speaks, in 20 lines or so, of his liking for Lacan, an admission no doubt made easier by the fact that it was then a dozen years or so after Lacan's death and so the latter was no longer there to hear him. It is remarkable to note the extent of Derrida's fascination with Lacan, perhaps as much with his person as with his thought. Citing the title of one of his Seminars, 'L'Insu-que-c'est', which, of course deals with the sense of failure (the *insuccès*) that Lacan felt concerning his teaching, Derrida cannot resist the temptation to imitate him by using a formulation very much in his style. Returning to the subject of Baltimore, he writes: 'Baltimore (dance or trance and terror)',[42] a mimesis of the Lacanian procedure of dividing up the moneme. The fascination exerted by the psychoanalyst over the philosopher is acknowledged. 'Lacan is so much more aware as a philosopher than Freud, so much more a philosopher than Freud! Lacan's refinement and competence, his philosophical originality, have no "precedent" in the world of psychoanalysis.'[43]

This recognition did not earn Lacan his enthronement. No sooner had Derrida acknowledged his admiration for him than he set about refuting him. A few pages further on, in fact, he reproaches Lacan for being too much of a philosopher. He qualifies his work as a 'powerful, philosophical, philosophizing reconstitution of psychoanalysis'.[44] Derrida finds Lacan's discourse too philosophical, too much at home with the 'philosophers'.[45] Consequently, he considers that his work lends itself particularly to deconstruction. Let us admire the strategy. Freud is not enough of a philosopher; Lacan is, fortunately, but that is precisely why he should be deconstructed. The polemic opposing the two titans around the interpretation of Poe's 'The Purloined Letter' is a very strange one indeed. On one side we have a psychoanalyst who places at the beginning of his *Ecrits* a Seminar on a short story by Poe; and on the other, a philosopher who contests the psychoanalyst's thought which is based on this text. Psychoanalysis was supposed to have been born and to have developed around a practice using the method for the treatment of certain neuroses. Yet here, all reference whatsoever to the analysand has disappeared and they are fighting about a text! What is the point in encumbering ourselves with the soul states of analysands? Everything is much simpler if one forgets them – for the time of a polemic!

And yet, if an analysand is pushed out through the door, he will come back through the window. Derrida relates something René Girard had said concerning a commentary of Lacan about him. Concerning the philosophers' contributions, Lacan supposedly replied: 'Yes, yes, it's good, but the difference between him and me is that he does not deal with people who are suffering' (p. 67). Suffering serves as an ultimate argument when the philosophers appear to have the edge in the *poleros*! But it cannot really be said that people's suffering ever stopped Lacan from sleeping. Derrida thus shows that he is just as cunning as his interlocutor: 'I too deal with people who suffer – all of you, for example, and, as a philosopher, I am constantly involved with them. What difference is there, then, between a philosopher and a psychoanalyst?' Derrida reproaches Lacan, first and foremost, for his *phallo-logo-centrism*. Let us refrain from interpreting the saying by separating each of the monemes of which it is comprised. I shall not dwell on the eight reasons where he develops his objections, for the debate is too far removed from the heart of psychoanalytic experience which Derrida does not care about – and which he mistrusts. It does not lead to any opening which is likely to help us in our work.

When all is said and done, Derrida only sees in the psychoanalytic treatment an enterprise of normalization which disgusts him. It has to be admitted that psychoanalysis is the last of his concerns. He aims well beyond it, his work bearing witness to the wide scope of the field of application of his thought. Nonetheless, among the disciplines comprising contemporary knowledge, psychoanalysis seems to disturb him. For him it is complex, but not enough so; analytical, but not enough so; questioning, but not enough so, revolutionary, but not enough so. Therapeutic? That, he says, is not his problem.

Derrida only knows what he can deconstruct, namely, texts. Texts, however in–depth and painstaking they may be, will never be more than a misleading reflection of experience. One only has to think of an analytic session to realize just how flat the theory of it is.

Habermas

In *The Philosophical Discourse of Modernity* (1985), Jürgen Habermas sets out his own philosophy of communicative reason: 'Narrative tools can, if necessary, be stylized into a dialogically conducted self-critique, for which the analytic conversation between doctor and patient offers a suitable model.'[46] The reference to the psychoanalytic model, made on numerous occasions, is evident. Does this psychoanalysis, revised and corrected by communication theory, still have any relation to truth? Such a discursive function manages very well without the unconscious; it has only retained the envelope of psychoanalysis so as to rid itself more easily of its content. Certainly, Habermas wants to get out of logo-centrism, but he does not escape a naive ideological view of rationality (p. 314).

Freud is cited at least a dozen times in this work which starts with Hegel and culminates with himself. The Freudian discourse constitutes the axis of his thought. His theory of communicative reason has certainly been constructed on the model of psychoanalytic dialogue. Yet, what does one notice? In one sentence in this work, Habermas cites side by side Bataille, Lacan and Foucault. Foucault is accorded two chapters, Bataille one, and Lacan is forgotten, even if he is mentioned five times! Just like Freud, who, though widely cited, is not accorded a chapter. It is not reticence towards Freud or even towards Lacan. What this means, quite simply, is that Jürgen Habermas is incapable of writing a chapter on Freud or Lacan in this context, even though he recognizes their importance. It is this observation that has led me to my present idea – one that is perhaps pretentious. It is easy for anyone to expatiate *on* psychoanalysis, but when it is a matter of knowing what it is really about, it is quite a different matter. Unless, of course, one belongs to the world of the 'psy' (i.e. psychiatrists, psychologists, psychotherapists, psycho-sociologists, all professions which are connected with the 'psy' world). Even though not all these professions are necessarily in agreement with psychoanalysis, at least they are ploughing a common field. Naturally, there are many discussions, polemics, debates and divergent views at the heart of this milieu, but this is not the problem. What I mean is that experience of the field of 'psy' leads to a certain way of seeing things for which psychoanalysis provides only one interpretation – which one can approve or disapprove of – but which, nonetheless, does not give the impression of talking endlessly and unprofitably. Otherwise, they are simply discourses added to other discourses, without any real debate occurring on the fundamental questions[47] which arise from experience.

Having become obsolete, psychoanalysis now has to face up to a new protagonist in the cultural discourse, namely, *the neurosciences and the cognitive sciences*. The 'psy' has been hounded out by the 'neuro', just as the unconscious of the drives has been hounded out by the cognitive. Almost everything that constitutes so-called 'scientific' discourse knows nothing, in fact, of psychoanalysis.

Legendre[48]

Pierre Legendre is a jurist and law historian, which has not stopped him from discovering the interest of the experience of psychoanalysis. As a penetrating analyst of social phenomena, he recognizes the sovereignty of fantasy, which leads to nihilism and contributes to the development of obscurantism. He has no difficulty in concurring with Freud either on the question of religion or on man's obsessive fear of murder. All this calls for coherent interpretations that are frequently occulted by ideological positions and pious wishes, which are subjected here to pertinent critiques. One cannot help admiring the way in which the jurist has availed himself of the different forms of expertise he lacked in order to understand his object better – psychoanalysis being one of them. And it was the marginality of psychoanalysis, more than the officially recognized discipline, that attracted him. It is really comforting to hear him say that he does not inhabit the present but the past and the *distant* future. Psychoanalysts will be sensitive to the way in which Legendre takes the body into consideration. He deplores the way in which the state has abandoned its function as a guarantor of reason, yielding to the pressure of small groups. It is easy to accuse him of having reactionary opinions. In fact, Legendre refuses to lay down the law simply because certain sectors of opinion are restless because they feel their beliefs have been trivialized. He denounces the hedonistic logic which leads to a triumph of fantasy. He does not hesitate to see in it a distant consequence of Nazism. Without forcing the facts, one could liken Freud and Legendre in their common passion for the triumph of reason, since for Freud the analysis of the unconscious coincides with the analysis of insanity, which would like to impose its law. To say the contrary would be to run the risk of committing a nonsense.

Castoriadis

I cannot end this chapter without mentioning Cornelius Castoriadis,[49] a revolutionary militant, philosopher and psychoanalyst, who had the courage to undergo the experience of psychoanalysis, to discover its truth and its limits, and to practise analysis himself, that is to say, to speak of it other than by hearsay, by listening in the cure to the language of the imaginary realm (that is, of representations produced by the drives). But Castoriadis goes further: he postulates a *radical* imaginary realm thanks to which he surpasses Freud's drive hypothesis. For him, it is less a question of treating the effects of the imagination than of designating the source of meaning and signification. The author's preoccupations, which focus on socio-historical concerns, are not without their repercussions for the conception of the psychic. Thanks to the other, the narcissistic monad is 'opened up' through a process of socialization. Castoriadis is exemplary in that, having been much inspired by Marxist thought, he was able to free his thinking from it. Moreover, he has linked up his theorizations on the unconscious with those on consciousness by showing the place of the other. He has indicated how cogitative division can be understood as being analogous to the division of the I and of the other or as a division of the subject (conscious–unconscious) – presupposed by consciousness. Furthermore, he adopts a position against formalization without limits and brings imagination and human passion into play. Finally, he has made an encounter possible between psychoanalytic value and social value through the concept of autonomy which he proposed as a criterion of social analysis. One cannot avoid making the comparison with the same concept, at the individual level, proposed by Winnicott, which Castoriadis opposes to dependence in psychopathology. Lastly, the ego is no longer conceived of as the possessor of truth, but as a constantly renewed source and power of creation in which thought coincides with Eros.

Notes

1 *The Letters of Sigmund Freud to Eduard Silberstein (1871–1881)*, ed. Walter Boehlich, trans. A. J. Pomerans. Cambridge, MA: Belknap Press, 1990.

2 Anzieu, D. (1988). *L'auto-analyse de Freud et la découverte de la psychanalyse*, vol. 2. Paris: Presses Universitaires de France.

3 Aristotle *On the Soul (De Anima)*, trans. Hugh Lawson-Tancred. London: Penguin Classics, 1986.

4 Freud, S. (1941 [1938]). 'Findings, Ideas, Problems', *S.E.* XIII, 299.

5 Freud, S. (1895). *Project for a Scientific Psychology*. *S.E.* 1. 281–397.

6 The reader will find above, at the end of chapter six, 'Language, speech, discourse', a commentary by H. Meschonnic which draws on Spinoza.

7 Kant, E. *Anthropology from a Pragmatic Point of View*, trans. Victor Lyle Dowdell, Southern Illinois University, 1978.

8 Ibid. p. 20.

9 Ibid. p. 45.

10 Ibid. p. 131–132.

11 Ibid. p. 136.

12 Ibid. p. 250.

13 Ibid. p. 263–264.

14 Schopenhauer, A. The Metaphysics of Sexual Love. In: *The World as Will and Representation*, trans. E.F.J. Payne. New York: Dover Publications, 1958.

15 As far as Hegel is concerned, I refer the reader to my book *The Work of the Negative* (Free Association Books, 1999) where a chapter is devoted to him. I have left to one side the problem of the relations with Nietzsche, which requires a lengthy treatment. Further, the reference to Spinoza, often cited, has not been touched on here. I have preferred to emphasise the role of authors less frequently referred to in the literature.

16 Foucault, M. (1954). *Maladie mentale and psychologie*. Paris: Presses Universitaires de France. [English edition: *Mental Illness and Psychology*, trans. Alan Sheridan, foreword by Herbert Dreyfus. London: Harper and Row, Publishers, Inc., 1976.]

17 See A. Green, critique of the work *Existence* by R. May, E. Engel and H.F. Ellenberger. In *Evolution Psychiatrique*, 24 (3), pp. 471–506, 1959.

18 Foucault, M. *Mental Illness and Psychology*, ibid. p. 25.

19 Ibid. p. 101.

20 Ibid. p. 39.

21 This allusion to the author's private life is only justified in the measure that the philosopher's conceptions constitute a patent contradiction of what inhabited him. Moreover, at the moment of his death, those around him were far from ready to assume the sexual choices of the teacher of the Collège de France. My position criticizes a theoretical attitude which would like to pass itself off as being lucid and philosophically grounded, free of any subjective influence.

22 Ibid. p. 87.

23 Ibid. p. 26.

24 Ibid. p. 83.

25 Ibid. p. 99.

26 Habermas, J. (1985). *The Philosophical Discourse of Modernity*, p. 278. tr. Frederick Lawrence. Cambridge: Polity Press, 1987.

27 M. Foucault reiterated the same arguments in *Madness and Civilization* (1961), where he demonstrates a remarkable ambivalence towards psychoanalysis, his pendulum swinging between a grateful admiration and, almost immediately outright condemnation. Derrida, on the occasion of the thirtieth anniversary of the publication of Foucault's *Folie et déraison: Histoire de la folie à lâge classique:* Paris: Plon, 1961. [English edition: *History of Madness*], gave a lecture on 23 November, 1991 entitled 'To Do Justice to Freud: The History of Madness in the Age of Psychoanalysis'. See *Resistances of Psychoanalysis* (1966) trans. Kamuf, Brault and Naas, Standford University Press, 1998. This role as a dispenser of justice that Derrida assumed on this occasion would not prevent him, later, from showing a comparable ambivalence. In short, it was nothing but a quarrel between philosophers to see who knew best how to deal with psychoanalysis before turning away from it. I will come to the case of Derrida further on.

28 Wittgenstein, L. (1921). *Tractatus Logico-Philosophicus*, followed by *Philosophical Investigations*, 1953.

29 Wittgenstein, L. *Philosophical Remarks*, Ed. R. Rhees, trans. R. Hargreaves and R. White. Oxford: Blackwell, 1964; 2nd ed., 1975.

30 Translator's note: 'Sois sage, ô ma douleur, et tiens-toi plus tranquille', from Beaudelaire's sonnet 'Receuillement' in *Les Fleurs de Mal* (1868). [English edition: 'Meditation', *The Flowers of Evil*, trans, James McGowan. Oxford: Oxford World's Classics, p. 347.]

31 Bouveresse, J. (1976). *Le mythe de l'intérorité. Expérience, signification et langage privé chez Wittgenstein*. Paris: Editions de Minuit.

32 Riceour, P. (1965). *De l'interpretation. Essai sur Freud*. Paris: Le Seuil.

33 Maria Torok has left us the memory of a very talented, original and creative psychoanalyst. Her intuition was out of the ordinary.

34 Derrida's text, Freud et la scène de l'écriture was initially presented at my seminar

at the *Institut de psychanalyse* and published in *L'écriture et la différence*. Paris: Le Seuil, 1967. [English version: Freud and the scene of writing. In *Writing and Difference*, translated by Alan Bass. University of Chicago Press, 1978.]

35 Derrida, J. (1996). *Resistances of Psychoanalysis*, trans, P. Kamuf, P-A. Brault, and M. Naas, Stanford University Press, 1998.

36 Ibid. p. 25.

37 Ibid. p. 17.

38 Ibid. p. 2.

39 In *Resistances of Psychoanalysis*, transcription of a speech made during the meeting 'Lacan with the philosophers'.

40 Moreover, Lacan placed the 'Seminar on "The Purloined Letter"' at the beginning of his *Ecrits* (1966).

41 Ibid. p. 42.

42 Ibid. p. 47.

43 Ibid. p. 50.

44 Ibid. p. 55.

45 Ibid. p. 56. The title of the gathering, let us recall, was, 'Lacan avec les philosophes' (a meeting organized at UNESCO by the International College of Philosophy in May 1992), *Lacan avec des philosophes*, Deeds of the Colloquium published by Albin Michel in 1992.

46 Habermas, J. (1985). *The Philosophical Discourse of Modernity*, p. 299; trans. Frederick Lawrence. Cambridge: Polity Press, 1987.

47 The preceding paragraphs are mainly inspired by an article published in *Passages*, no. 102, relating a conference I gave on 24 November, 1999.

48 Legendre, P. (1981). *Jouir du pouvoir*. Paris: Editions de Minuit.

49 Castoriadis, C. (1999). *Figures du pensable. Les carrefours du labyrinthe*. Paris: Le Seuil.

16

SCIENTIFIC KNOWLEDGE

One of the most remarkable characteristics of contemporary psychoanalysis is the in-depth reflection on the knowledge of science, its nature, functions and criteria. This approach differs from that of philosophy, which has its own language and concepts.[1] Such reflection aims to provide food for thought for those for whom the problems of contemporary epistemology are important. The two types of thinking which share the same field as psychoanalysis are the biological and anthropological models.

Biological thinking: the neurobiological models

Neurobiology is striving to supplant psychoanalysis and to discredit it by declaring it to be unscientific, thus not very credible. In fact, its pretensions are already outmoded, epistemological reflection having pointed up their limits. Research into man is currently dominated by the neurobiological interpretation of consciousness. The unconscious of psychoanalysts is as a rule beyond the reach of neurobiologists. Within this general context, specific studies have been carried out into various subjects: dreams, memory, the emotions, and affect, among others. These are included in the surrounding theoretical constructions: Edelman's theory of the selection of neuronal groups; Henry Atlan's self-organization; the concept of the fluctuating central state (Panksepp); epigenesis and diverse versions of the body/mind problem.

In none of these groups does the progress of neurobiology call for a dramatic revision on the part of psychoanalysis. A few details may need straightening out. If we look into the matter more closely, it is rather the neurobiologists who find that they are obliged to take into consideration the criticisms that are addressed to them (by others than psychoanalysts) or that they address to each other. The recent creation of the review *Neuro-Psychoanalysis* now constitutes a forum for debating these questions.[2] But one swallow does not make a summer,

261

and as long as scientists refuse to emerge from their objectivist fortresses, remaining content to camp on their lines of defence, nothing will change. There would be nothing to find quarrel with if, behind their apparent modesty, there did not lie an exaggerated ambition in relation to the means at their disposal. They claim, in fact, to be able to resolve all – or almost all – the enigmas of the mind. Even if they are obliged to leave certain enigmas to one side, at least they have the feeling that they can pride themselves in front of others on the fact that their knowledge is guaranteed, proven, verified, even if they risk seeing it refuted a little later. This refutability has been turned into a criterion that obliges us to confine ourselves to the short-term present. They do not seem to realize that these results are obtained at the price of oversimplifications that are often improper. Consequently, their exchanges with psychoanalysts cannot avoid referring to the ideology underlying the scientific works and their desire to make a clean sweep of all areas of knowledge, which, in their eyes, can shed scarcely any light whatsoever on a field whose cumbersome trappings can only be cleared up by the scientific method. In fact, these positions are already rearguard; the really avant-garde scientific thinkers are developing more open points of view. This can be shown in a certain number of domains which, as a whole, form the pedestal of scientific thought:

1 *Genetics*, considered as the science which affirms that 'everything is hereditary'. On this point, ideas are changing. Under the influence of Henri Atlan, the idea of a genetic programme is contested.[3] The question now is more one of genetic strategies than of realizing the programme. We know, above all, that the nucleus, on which geneticists focus all their attention, is not the exclusive locus of the transmission of information.

2 *The 1 per cent which separates the genetic code of the anthropoids* from that of man forces us to reflect on the nature of these differences, by underlining the importance of the connections and regulations. This issue raises the question of the relationship between *animals and humans*. Minds are divided between those who have the tendency to place value on the separation between these two reigns and those who postulate the continuity between them (the neuroscientists). It is a remarkable fact that this division is also present among psychoanalysts. Freud was for continuity; Lacan for separation.

3 *The neurosciences and the philosophy of mind*. Essentially, this field takes up again the data on the knowledge of the brain. There is a clash here between the conceptions of the 'philosophers of mind' and those of the anti-reductionists. Some theorists plead in favour of taking a more rigorous approach which involves taking account of requirements for studying the psyche which cannot be ignored (Edelman).

4 *Consciousness and the unconscious*. It is striking to note the small degree of interest aroused by the knowledge of the unconscious. The neurobiologists say that the unconscious is what they are concerned with most of the time

since they are dealing with biological structures where any idea of consciousness is foreign. To put it in another way, the psychic unconscious is
drowned in the absence of consciousness which is the rule in biological
phenomena. Generally, no doubt, owing to the fact that ordinary scientific
procedures prove to be incapable of shedding any light in this domain, the
preference, with a few exceptions (Perry) is for ignoring it. Consciousness
remains the domain of incessant investigations. The theories put forward
on this subject can be of interest to the psychoanalyst but studies on dreams
(M. Jouvet[4]) show that hostility to psychoanalysis is still lively (A. Hobson[5]).
The studies of the psychoanalyst and researcher, L. Garma,[6] are worthy of
acclaim here.

5 *The paradigm of reason.* Consciousness and reason go together in the investigations of neurobiologists. Some of them do not hesitate to speak of 'neurones
of reason' (Changeux[7]). Paradoxically, this betrays an idealistic and intel-
lectualized view of the mind. This conception, the ideological bases of which
are not difficult to demonstrate, also presents the inconvenience of having
to separate the intellectual (rational) and the affective. The latter, driven out
from knowledge through the door, returns to claim its rights by the window.
It presents itself as a rival dimension of the former and contests its right
to pass itself off as a paradigm, namely of a body of knowledge purified of
its scoria. Not the least of the drawbacks is that one is faced here again with
an agonizing struggle between the intellect, incarnated by reason (neuronal)
and an emotional life that stands in a more direct relationship with affect
(hormonal). However justified this division may seem, albeit debatable in
many domains, it is perhaps necessary to try to go back to the source (unless
it is considered that this division is in its essence to be respected as such). The
question arises, then, of situating the place of the act and of its determinants
within this dichotomy. One thereby avoids discussing the status of the drive
(internal act). *Epigenesis*, the role of which used to be underestimated, is now
taken into consideration in all its importance (Prochiantz[8]). The relations
between what is innate and acquired are given greater clarification but are
less simplified.

6 *Emotions and affects.* This is the most recent of the domains of the mind,
envisaged from a neurobiological standpoint. But here, too, the diversity
of approaches scarcely admits of a unified theory. Pleasure and desire have
entered the field of neurobiological questionings (J.-D. Vincent[9]). Let us say,
briefly, that for some, the affective dimension accompanies all psychic
phenomena (A. Damasio[10]). Without emotion, there is no reason, no
motivation, no life; while for others, it is only a question of clarifying the
neurobiology of a class of psychic phenomena by demonstrating different
and specific circuits (Panksepp[11], Le Doux, etc.).

7 *The problem of representations.* What does representation refer to in biology,
psychology, sociology and psychoanalysis? And in this last discipline, what

does it mean for the different schools? There are two opposing theories, one of which is reductionism (Turing), and the other psychical complexity (Edelman). In the first case, an inscription on a magnetic strip can serve in its stead. In the second, phylogenesis has to be taken into account in the answer.

8 These diverse problems overlap in more general approaches concerning the evolutionist perspective and induce us to define the *specificity of man* more clearly. In this last domain *pre-history* is also involved. Among the functions which determine the gap between man and animals, language deserves to be given particular attention. We are faced again here, in a general way, with the eternal *mind–body problem*, with the incessant renewal of the data which constitute it and make it appear periodically in a new light.

Psychoanalysis has not remained insensible to the recent advances of science. Some authors have felt the need for new metaphors (G. and S. Pragier[12]), which we will find in thinkers who favour an open naturalism (Morin, Atlan, Prochiantz, Varela, Vincent, Danchin, Thom, etc.). Much remains to be done in order to convince the reductionists (most of whom refuse, moreover, to be described as such) of the distortions they impose on the facts and of the pseudo-knowledge which results therefrom.

The enumeration of the different areas of research shows that those areas in which a debate could be engaged do indeed touch upon the theory of psychoanalysis. But it seems that it is not sufficient to adopt a more or less tolerant attitude towards its approach. Researchers in neurobiology are far from genuinely recognizing the problematics of psychoanalysis.

K. Kaplan and M. Solms have had the merit of establishing the bases of *neuropsychoanalysis*. Their project of establishing a neuro-anatomy of the psychical apparatus is not lacking in ambition. There is nothing here that resembles a mechanism comparable to one that aims to describe 'the neurones of reason'. The agencies described by Freud, that is, the ego, id and superego, are frequently reproached for having scarcely any correspondence with anatomical localizations. This is nonetheless what the Solms try to do. By attaching these agencies to certain brain formations, they make them refer to anatomical structures, but ones that do not come within the realm of macroscopy and are united by common functions within the system.[13]

They situate the genesis and topography of the ego at the periphery of the body, at the extremity of the sense organs. The information received at this level is coded, analysed and synthesized according to myriad functional criteria in the grey matter of the marrow, the nuclei of the cranial pairs and the thalamus. This corresponds, roughly, to Freud's perceptual system. The peripheral perceptual apparatus provides the ego with its first protective barriers (probably of genetic origin), devoid of capacities of memory; the unimodal cortical zones are ideal anatomical points which, through fusion with the heteromodal cortical zones, form the first mnemic systems. The unimodal cortex registers the diverse qualities of perceptual consciousness. The mnemic systems of convexity retranscribe the information on the basis of inventories and in the light of functional criteria. The global principle comprises associative links of characteristics selected from the incoming information constituted into spatial and quasi-spatial models. For the Solms, what is involved is a structuring process of the ego according to phylogenetic selections. When an associative model is formed, it functions like a protective barrier. Even though these models are partly dependent on phylogenetic selections, they also concur with ontogenetic experience. This structuring occurs above all in the heteromodal cortico-thalamic zones. The system of thing-presentations is thus constituted, which, once introjected, exerts influence on the peripheral perceptual events. The stage of the earlier mnemic inscriptions takes place at the level of the left hemisphere. Concrete, total objects of a visuo-spatial primary type are associated here with quasi-spatial presentations of an audio-verbal type. The transcription, establishing thing-word connections as a process of symbolization, then takes place (Freud–Luria). These symbolic transcriptions provide a new protective barrier because they organize the infinite diversity of things into a lexicon of categories. Words protect us from things. If we turn towards the motor extremity of the apparatus (in the prefrontal region), the transition of the associations posterior to the anterior zones associates the lexical system with a system of logico-grammatical rules. The simultaneous models are transcribed into sequential programmes. They play an essential role in the structure of propositional language. At a deep level, the logico-grammatical and propositional codes serve to link and organize the drives arising from the inside. The prefrontal medio-basal zone, which merges with the limbic system, is the anatomical locus of this deep economic transformation. At this point, the structures corresponding to the ego and the superego enter into contact, resulting in a process of self-regulation. The bound energy engendered by this transformation furnishes the essential basis for all the ego's executive functions. Between this inhibiting nucleus of the ego and the primary motor cortex lies an intermediary region, which is the longest to mature. It codes the deep propositional sequences, by means of retranscriptions, into current models of motor activity. The 'ego' then exerts its influence on the neutromuscular system. Not only is the motor discharge controlled, but the perceptual discharge too, binding projection (preventing hallucination). This is the secondary process.

In short, the ego (as a totality) coincides anatomically with the separation between the internal and external worlds. The ego starts with unimodal perception (perceptual and motor) and ends in the ring of the limbic cortex. Its essential function is to serve as a mediator by establishing barriers between the internal and external worlds. These barriers (protective barriers) interpose memory between impulsion and action and are in the service of attention, judgement and thinking. Nevertheless, the anatomical frontiers of the ego must not be confused with its functional sphere of influence; just as in metapsychology, the topographical point of view must not be confused with the dynamic point of view. It should not be forgotten that the ego is at once the master and the servant of the forces it regulates. The 'id' has its epicentre in the grey matter surrounding the fourth ventricle, but its influence extends beyond that, to the hypothalamus in particular. The hypothalamus reacts to the vital needs of the subject via the intermediary of the autonomous and endocrine nervous systems. The ascendant activating system is influenced by the information from the posterior cortical regions, the values of which are modulated by desires and dangers and by programmes established with the aid of language in the anterior cortical regions. The id is thus indirectly influenced by reality, through the mediation of the ego. The incitements of the id seem to restrict access to the posterior cortical regions (perhaps because they direct their inhibiting activities towards the external world).

Motility and sensory experience are thus under the control of the ego, whereas the vital organs within the body fall under the domination of the id. Let us recall that the viscera emerge in the skin through the mucous orifices of the mouth, anus and genitals (erotogenic zones).

Let us move on now to the drives. The libido is rooted in the physical processes of certain tissues of the body. The drives of self-preservation might be related to the fundamental emotional systems of command described by Panksepp in 1998. The destructive drives will stand in relation to certain more primitive properties of the nervous tissue (which are formed in pathological states of equalization and inertia).

The Solms are aware of the gulf between their theories and reality, as well as of the contradictions contained in their description. There is no triumphalism here. It is but an introduction. As one reads them, one is struck by the ingenuity with which they succeed in harmonizing the two fields: psychoanalysis and neurobiology. This is a work that could only be undertaken by psycho-analysts. Finally, let us acknowledge fully our admiration for the Freudian invention which, coming solely from the head of its inventor, succeeded in constructing a body of ideas which is not in complete contradiction with science, 50 or 100 years after.

Certainly, some small modifications need to be noted. They all bear witness to a greater level of interactivity between the agencies. And we learn, for instance, that the ego can exert a certain influence on the id (repression?) But what is most remarkable, it seems to me, is the prominence given to separate structures for the data of the external world and of the internal world.

A few clarifications are necessary on the difference between soma and psyche. Let me begin by pointing out that the so-called 'somatic' manifestations do not form a univocal field. They cover functional phenomena, conversion, the symptomatology of the actual neuroses (including hypochondria), alexi-thymia, the delusion of the negation of organs (Cotard's syndrome) and, finally, psychosomatic pathology properly speaking. It is easy to highlight the role of affect in this polymorphism. Psychoanalysis proposes to draw a contrast between the soma and the corporal, reserving the latter term for manifestations presenting an entanglement with the psychic, and which only enter into relation with the somatic indirectly.

The question raised here is one of dualism and monism. I propose the idea of a *de facto monism* culminating in a *structural dualism* inferred from different modes of organization (the brain is organized differently from the liver or lungs).[14] A further point needs adding. When we speak of somatic factors, it is clear that they are also dependent on the brain, like the others. However, even the study of the brain distinguishes between periphery and centrality. One is therefore led to say that somatic and cerebral are not opposed and apply to periphery and centrality. There is no need to stipulate that the brain itself is divided into deep structures (fourth and third ventricles) and superficial structures, i.e. cortical and neocortical. P. MacLean has defended, on phylogenetic grounds, the idea of a *tri-unique brain*. What is important is to understand the necessity of co-ordinating structures that are phylogenetically different. Human specificity must be taken into consideration (prolonged dependence, loss of the oestrus, role of the similar other, order of signs).

Ameisen: Cellular suicide and death drive

One of the most controversial questions in Freudian theory is the mythical, fabulous and improbable 'death drive'. Among the accepted arguments, and I will not mention them all, would figure, as a supreme argument, the idea that biology shows nothing of the sort which could, from close up or far off, be linked up with the Freudian concept. Jean-Claude Ameisen sustains a thesis which comes singularly close to it: 'Today, we know that all our cells possess the power, at any moment, to self-destruct in a few hours.'[15] Cells constantly produce deadly substances in order to accomplish this task. It is the inhibition of these which guarantees life. 'Life proceeds from the negation of a negative event, self-destruction.' Here we are closer to Hegel than C. Bernard. This decon-struction, which results neither from an accident, nor from ageing, allows for the permanent reconstruction of our organism. Our life depends on the language of the signals which intervene in the process of making decisions. The adaptive aim is not absent. Cellular suicide prevents our defensive immune system from attacking our bodies, or prevents the cellular orientation towards the risk of organs becoming cancerous. This possibility has existed since our animal ancestors of a billion years ago. This cellular suicide is nonetheless linked to cellular interdependence, complexity and plasticity. Life is not such a wise and discerning phenomenon that it is enough to let it go uncontrolled. Death is useful. Depending on the circumstances, the mechanisms of self-destruction are sometimes used because they are necessary, and sometimes repressed. It is doubtless not impossible to imagine that, as a result of evolution, the mechanisms of death have been integrated with those of life. Freud said that our death was the result of internal conflicts. This observation proves, does it not, that he was right? Life and death share between them the activity of living beings. This is not the way things are expressed in laboratories where they prefer to speak of *protective* phenomena and *executory* phenomena.

These observations have diverse consequences. The first concerns the process of ageing, which I will not go into. The second concerns a phenomenon we are familiar with, namely, the death of neurones. Every cell is born, grows, ages, and dies. Reproduction is thus a generalized phenomenon. The old opposition between soma (mortal) and germen (immortal) is inexact. As for neurones, they were supposed to die without any possibility of regeneration. But, the contrary has been maintained since 1998. 'It is probable that, throughout our lives, original cells are presented in each of the regions of our brain, sleeping like spores which can only be drawn out of their sleep by death.' But there is more. It could be supposed that, since newborn neurones are without experience and the dead neurones take their experience with them, the latter would also be lost, and that an entirely new work of learning would become necessary. Yet, this is not the case. The neurones without a past 'are integrated within a network of educated neurones'. The functioning of the network as a whole imprints the 'past experience' rapidly into the neurones which have just been born, conferring on the organism 'the memory' of a history that it has never experienced. The plasticity of living substance, anthropoids and man is astonishing.

According to J.-M. Vidal,[16] animals possess systems of communication, but not a hierarchic language structure. The capacities acquired by experimental means are neither secondarized nor used between like creatures; they remain confined to the relation with the experimenter. I will pass over the other traits, for language is undoubtedly the most important issue. The rest has been the object of controversies (creation of tools and transmission of techniques; rites versus ceremonies; limitation of inbreeding vs. prohibition; limitation of aggressive forms of expression vs. culpability; attachment vs. love; self-perception vs self-consciousness). However, the question of language has to be nuanced. What animals are lacking, above all, is less the use of speech than the capacity *to tell stories*, that is, narrative. In other words, man invents stories. Thus, if his speech is silver, his lie is golden.

Let us turn now to the ideas of certain neurobiologists.

Panksepp: Primary and secondary emotions

Concerning recent studies on affect, an exchange has reunited Mark Solms and Edward Nersessian[17] (psychoanalysts) and J. Panksepp[18] (neurobiologist) who claims he is being conciliatory. This is undoubtedly the deepest reflection on the subject to date. The scientific point of view is affirmed here (rigorous empirical evaluation of propositions). The aim is to investigate: (a) the cerebral processes which synchronize the visceral and motor expressions of the emotions; (b) the key components in the mnemic and cognitive aspects; (c) to combine these experimental discoveries with the subjective relations of human beings. It is valuable to have dealings with a conciliatory rather than hostile investigator, and one who shows that he is open to certain Freudian propositions. But it is at the price of a good many confusions. Conciliation has its limits and it does not take much for the author to show his divergence with the psychoanalysts. He rejects the concept of drive (but speaks of the energies of the id). He continues to ask psychoanalysts (like Grunbaum!) to pass through the Caudine Forks of scientific verification. And if he brings together scientific techniques and the subjective experience of human beings, it is only to the extent that his 'robust' [*sic*] science can be found in human beings. It would not occur to him to start out from subjective human experience and to gravitate towards the scientific method. For a scientist, as for so many others, the wheat has to be separated from the chaff. The wheat, is the scientist; the chaff is what comes from clinical work or subjectivity. For the clinician, this division is not convincing. One cannot hold clinical work to be secondary, for it has its own specific richness. Panksepp no doubt means that the picture, so to speak, is polluted. He is not sure that the pathological constitutes a major path towards an understanding of the normal. The author's vision, far from being devoid of speculation, is evolutionist, no doubt attaching affect to the vertebrates in their struggle for life; later, other mechanisms will be added which require the reference to 'solidly constructed' cognitive processes (jealousy, shame) which are superimposed on basic emotions (without a cognitive connotation). This evolutionism seems somewhat simplified. The primary nature of the emotions requires us to understand the subcortical processes, particularly in eruptive manifestations. Here, Panksepp shows he is in favour of taking into account the expression of human manifestations. Pharmacological research can make an important contribution. A psychoanalyst will certainly agree with the assertion that 'the hemisphere of language seems to be master of confabulation and deception in its accredited role of communicating with others in the world' (Le Doux 1985). And thus we now have the right brain – the affective side! – once upon a time a poor relation and negligible quantity, decked out in all the virtues: more profound, more sincere. We speak, live and act with both sides of the brain together. How are we are to find our way in all this? Let us pay tribute to the researchers who work against the current as their themes of research are looked upon with suspicion!

Edelman: The selection of neuronal groups (Darwin and Freud)

In his major work, *Bright Air, Brilliant Fire*,[19] G. Edelman, an immunologist converted to neurobiology, offers, in my opinion, what is the most powerful and original synthesis of the relations between matter and mind. Edelman, who is interested in the sciences of recognition (recalling his past as an immunologist), proposes a definition of the latter. 'By "recognition", I mean the continual adaptive matching or fitting of elements in one physical domain to novelty occurring in elements of another, more or less independent physical domain, *a matching that occurs without prior instruction*'[20] (my italics). The immune system is capable of distinguishing between self and non-self. Neuronal recognition is selective. The position adopted by Edelman insists on the role of cerebral morphology to explain the functioning of the brain, in contrast with those (cognitivists, in particular) who claim that it can be disregarded. For morphology reflects evolution. By adapting the idea of a *selective construction*, structural variability can show how the brain carries out *categorizations*. These must take into account a certain number of factors, such as the existing links between physico-chemical, physiological and psychological processes. This is what Edelmann calls the *theory of the selection of neuronal groups (TNGS)*, which comprises two main notions: *selection and reentry*.[21] The TNGS rests on three tenets:

1 *The primary repertoire*: comprising a population of different neuronal groups in a given brain region set up by processes of *somatic selection*: 'the genetic code does not provide a specific wiring diagram for this repertoir'.[22]
2 *The mechanism of supplementary selection*: during behaviour certain synaptic connections are strengthened or weakened. Certain circuits are carved out. This is known as *selection through experience*; the strengthened synapses constitute the secondary repertoire.[23] The connections are matched.
3 The selective phenomena described in (1) and (2) have the effect of linking physiology and psychology by virtue of a process of *reentry*. This results in the constitution of maps due to the coordination of the repertoires (1) and (2). Reentrant signals are exchanged: 'This means that as groups of neurons are selected in a map, other groups in reentrantly connected but different maps may also be selected at the same time.'[24] And Edelman adds: 'In evolution, the main unit of selection is the individual animal (the phenotype).'[25] Stimulating and inhibiting sets are created, forming circuits. *No neurone is selected in isolation, no neurone can connect itself with another isolated neurone; no single neurone can present alone the properties that it acquires in a group.*

To these three tenets must be added *emergence*.

Let us consider categorization. 'Within a certain time period, reentrant signalling strongly connects certain active combinations of neuronal groups in one map to different combinations in another map'.[26] *This structuring occurs even though each map is receiving independent signals from the outside world.*[27]

The topographical connection will make it possible to correlate happenings at one spatial location in the world (without complementary instruction). The topography accounts for the correspondence between the maps, so that neighbouring locations on the map are also neighbouring locations on the sensory receptor sheet. The property of reentry allows for recursive syntheses (new properties emerging in the course of time through successive and recursive reentries (Figure 16.1)).

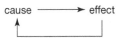

Figure 16.1

Categorization operates 'by coupling the outputs of multiple maps that are reentrantly connected to the sensorimotor behaviour of the animal.'[28] This is achieved through the intervention of a higher order structure called *global mapping*. It allows selectional events in its local maps. It also allows dynamic loops to be formed: 'sensorimotor activity over the whole mapping selects neuronal groups that give the appropriate output or behavior, resulting in categorization'.[29]

At this point the reference to value is introduced: 'The bases for value systems in the animals of a given species are already set by evolutionary selection.'[30] Regulating bodily functions is the first concern. Survival first. The great revolution proposed by Edelman resides in one phrase: the *simulator* (automaton # animal) 'categorizes only on the basis of experience'.[31] *Neither instruction, nor an order of relations.* Such is the effect of the *somatic* selection of neuron groups. 'Categorization is not the same as value, but rather occurs on value.'[32] It is the result of epigenesis. Selection makes possible the categorization arising from experience.

What is it that makes this theory so attractive for the psychoanalyst? I think it is because we can see neurological findings being linked up in a convincing manner with those arising from the individual experience of the animal, which does not simply obey instructions or a programme. By drawing on the theory of evolution, we have on the one hand facts relating to heredity and, on the other, neuron group selection. Natural selection has produced two different systems of somatic selection capable of recognition and leading to diverse phenotypic forms of behaviour.

Are these reflections to be regarded as alien to psychoanalysis? How are we to understand the place Freud gave to *perceptual identity*, a source of psychic recognition? And, above all, how can we avoid letting ourselves by confined by it?

Let us pass on now to the study of the higher functions of the brain. Consideration must be given to the relations between the terms of a fundamental triad formed by perceptual mental categorization, memory and learning. They are connected with value systems via the intermediary of parts of the brain other than those that carry out categorizations, such as the hedonic centres and the limbic system, which satisfy *sexual and nutritional homeostatic needs* and are dependent on hypothalamic, mesencephalic nuclei, and others. Learning occurs through the connection of global mappings and value centres. I will skip over memory for the moment. The ganglions of the stem are connected with hedonic centres (through the intermediary of one of their appendices, which plays a role in establishing long-term memory: the hippocampus).

Finally, we come to concepts. 'Concepts are *not* conventional or arbitrary, do *not* require linkage to a special community to develop, and do *not* depend on sequential presentation. Conceptual capabilities develop in evolution well before speech.'[33] They are enormously heterogeneous and general. They involve mixtures of relations concerning the real world, memories and past behaviour. The brain thus constructs maps of its own activity. 'The structures in the brain categorize parts of past global mappings according to modality, the presence or absence of movement and the presence or absence of relationships between perceptual categorizations.'[34] This results in a *mapping of different types of maps* (Babel's library!). This occurs independently of the sensory entries of the moment.[35] The role of the frontal cortex is important; however, at a higher level, we can observe that mapping is transcended. Memory 'frees' the brain of certain constraints limiting its functioning, opening the way to intentionality.

The object of Edelman's work is consciousness. What interests me in his elaboration, is the schema of the relations between the structures of the brain and psychical activity. His description of psychic states is acceptable for a psychoanalyst. Edelman is one of the rare authors who takes the trouble to set out the underlying assumptions of the theories put forward. He exposes in succession:

* the physics assumption
* the evolutionary assumption
* the *qualia* assumption (relative to the sensible quality of things).

The last of these calls for commentary: 'We cannot construct a phenomenal psychology that can be shared in the same way as a physics can be shared.'[36] The physico-psychical gap remains, for the physical world can be shared, unlike the psychological world. To put it in another way, in order to do physics, I appeal to *qualia* but, in intersubjective communication, I can exclude them, confident in the idea that my scientific interlocutors will be able to carry out the prescribed manipulations enabling them to arrive at comparable results. But in the study of consciousness, sensations (*qualia*) cannot be disregarded: 'No *scientific* theory of whatever kind can be presented without already assuming that observers have sensation as well as perception.'[37] As we are the only self-conscious animals (*sapiens sapiens*), 'we can take human beings to be the best canonical referent for the study of consciousness.'[38] One has to acknowledge the merit of a theory which accepts that it is impossible to bypass the *qualia* assumption which, in fact, is one of subjectivity. On the other hand, one can point out that, for all kinds of reasons, including those that reside in the existence of the unconscious, the reliability of the account given of *qualia* is debatable. Nonetheless, one relies on the individual to debate this, in the light of the fact that different phenomena, of which they are the centre, are *correlated*.

One then comes to a theorization which sets out to distinguish between primary consciousness and higher consciousness. Primary consciousness is restricted to phenomenal experiences limited to the measurable present. Higher consciousness presupposes the use of concepts. It is striking to find once again the dichotomy between primary and secondary processes, even though they are grounded differently here. Two systems in primary consciousness can be described:

1   The brain stem, together with the limbic (hedonic) system, concerned with appetite, sexual and ingestive behaviour, and defensive patterns. These are internal systems.
2   The thalamocortical system, regulating sensory experience, and helping to satisfy the aims of the first system. It is established by means of learning which favours categorization. Here, Edelman introduces into the correlations the concept of scene to speak of the categorization of happenings *without necessary physical or causal connections to others in the same scene.*

The first systems are connected to the body; the second system adjusts to the signals from the outside world – a change of value.

Primary consciousness depends on the evolution of three functions:

* a cortical system linked to the limbic functions
* a memory able to classify categories (value–categories)
* circuit allowing for continual reentrant signalling between the value-category memory and global mappings.

'With the appearance of the new reentrant circuits in each modality, *a conceptual categorization of concurrent perceptions* can occur *before* these perceptual signals contribute lastingly to that memory.'[39] A process (bootstrapping) is set up whereby a system constructs more useful and more powerful structures than those that were initially present. This is primary consciousness.

To summarize, the brain carries out a process of conceptual self-categorization matching past perceptual categories with signals from value systems, a process carried out by cortical systems capable of conceptual functions. This value-category system then interacts via reentrant connections with brain areas carrying out ongoing perceptual categorizations of external events. This is what is called the 'remembered present'.

Now for the conclusion: *a great division distinguishes between self and non-self systems*. It results from the relations between the limbic and thalamo-cortical systems. It is striking to notice the self-enclosed unitary self-sufficiency of this system capable of meeting the satisfaction of its needs. 'The self, or internal systems, arise from interactions between the limbic and the cortical systems. This differentiates them from outside-world systems that are strictly cortical.'[40] *It does not seem to me to be excessive to endeavour to find in the system of the self the concept of the drive as defined by Freud and the concept of the object inasmuch as it is connected with the external world*. It should nonetheless be added that the object also has a self, which enters into resonance with the self of the subject, not only in an empathic mode but also via its limbic system.

This architectural schema provides me with sufficient grounds to assert that it is the first time that I have encountered a neurobiological theory which appears to be compatible with psychoanalytic theory. Are value categories and reentrant imagination the most pertinent factors for such an encounter?

This said, a few further remarks may be added to reaffirm my agreement with his position. Let me recall, then, briefly that for Edelman the brain already possesses the necessary bases for semantic capacities; it is thus capable of forming concepts. The author's epigenetic conception of language leaves to one side any genetically programmed language-acquisition device. Syntax is the result of epigenesis, contrary to widespread opinion. It forms the link between pre-existent conceptual learning and lexical learning. As can be seen, *the concept precedes language*; according to Edelman, meaning arises from the interaction of value-category memory with *the combined activity of conceptual areas and speech areas*. I will not go into the details of the examination of higher order consciousness. Great attention is paid to 'the relating of speech symbols to the gratification of affective needs by conspecifics in parental, grooming or sexual interactions'.[41] The process of bootstrapping occurs at two levels: perceptual and semantic. Adaptation is relativized: 'The history of humanity since the evolution of hunter-gatherers speaks to both the adaptive and maladaptive properties of the only species with fully developed higher-order consciousness.'[42] Is not the counterpart of this the ego's opacity to itself? Edelman is uncommonly courageous in that he devotes a chapter to the unconscious and to Freud. We have finally arrived safe and sound, especially when we read: 'Against silly reductionism'.[43] Here Edelman reminds us that the system of meaning 'is almost never free of affect'.[44] Likewise, every attempt to reduce psychology to neuroscience necessarily ends in failure at a certain practical point.[45]

Reading Edelman is reassuring to the extent that he does not share with the cognitivists what he considers to be illusions; he even speaks of intellectual fraud (see the critical postface). He underlines the absurdity of the analogy between thought and logic.[46] I totally share his positions of principle on the necessity of taking into account a morphology shaped by evolution and the obligation to find a basis for speculations in the study of the brain. However, as he says himself, 'a theory of everything will certainly have to include both a theory of the mind and a fuller theory of the observer.'[47] With Edelman's work, biology is back on its feet again:

- no knowledge without morphology
- no morphology without evolution
- no description without categorization
- no categorization without values
- no values without interconnected maps and reentrant phenomena
- no unitary system without a self/non-self distinction
- no knowledge without conceptual semantics before language
- no meaning without memory
- no meaning without linkage between language and non-language
- no psychology without *qualia* and especially without affect
- no consciousness without the unconscious
- no brain without structural variability
- no entirely computational psychology
- no syntax without semantics
- no realism resting on determinism
- no objectivism without subjectivism
- no functionalism without materialism
- no intentionality without symbolic sensibility.

Metaphor triumphs, with a correspondence being established between a structure in one domain and a corresponding structure in another domain.[48]

The paradoxical conclusion is that cognitivism, which claims to be objectivist and materialistic, is the result of an *idealized* modelling. A long process of examination is needed to realize this and a lot of resistance has to be overcome to have it recognized.

For the moment psychoanalysts confine themselves to being witnesses to the enquiries of neurobiologists who often prefer, when they venture out of their field, to consult with phenomenologists (Varela).[49] One can, however, without undue optimism, hope that psychoanalysts will succeed better, in the long term, in making themselves heard, clinical practice remaining the touchstone for judging the relevance of a general theory. Notwithstanding these disappointments, I remain in favour – contrary to many others – of being open towards the biologists; for, although, for the moment, the bridges allowing psycho-analysis to dialogue with them only exist very exceptionally, this possibility has to be reserved for the day when the exchange can take place. If I am proposing that this space, which has been left provisionally almost empty, be conserved, it is because *I can see no advantage to be gained from constructing a psychoanalytic theory totally freed from knowledge on the soma.* Moreover, certain branches of psycho-analytic practice remain in touch with the reality of it: the psychotherapy of the psychoses, often practised jointly with chemiotherapies, and psychosomatics which forces us to reflect on the relation of psychoanalysis with medical disciplines; psychic treatment coexisting with medical treatment.

Admittedly, the day is still a long way off when we will have at our disposal a mode of thinking which is capable of uniting the knowledge of the mind (practical or theoretical) according to psychoanalysis and that which is derived from the study of the brain and the soma.[50] Certain portents leave room for hope, however.

The models of anthropology

Though psychoanalysis has, for the most part, deliberately ignored biology, there has been a long history of controversies between psychoanalysis and anthropology – the debate reflecting an altogether different state of mind. When they discuss psychoanalytic theses, anthropologists do not consider them as pseudo-knowledge, but rather as knowledge applied, ill-advisedly, to social groups, or even as a body of knowledge which they have the duty to refute or to argue with. Which is already a manner of recognizing it, since they fight against it. It also has to be said that a not inconsiderable part of Freud's work gives them matter for argument, whereas his positions with regard to biology are more a case of begging the question than of a genuine reflection; for, in the domain of biology, knowledge was very sparse in his time. And when this reflection occurred, it quickly turned towards metaphysics ('Beyond the Pleasure Principle').

Today, the situation has changed. After a period during which the ideas of Lévi-Strauss[51] dominated the field of anthropology (especially in France), other theorizations have emerged that are more receptive to the idea of a dialogue with psychoanalysis. I will include in this discussion the findings that have arisen from reflections on the present – the inevitable point of departure for all reflection. I will not, however, be reconsidering the problem of civilization, which has already been dealt with elsewhere. I will simply point to an insistent fact, which seems to me almost unquestionable – namely, the increasingly strong impact of violence, a fact that can justifiably be connected with instinctual life. But it as if these phenomena were being interpreted as the result of a certain cultural disorder which engendered them 'naturally'. As if it were normal that we are witnessing these understandable disturbances, without there being any need to ask ourselves questions either about their place in the psyche or about their relation to this cultural disorder. There is a refusal to analyse in any depth their origin, their psychical organization, or their connection with civilized activity. In other words, here as elsewhere, there is a refusal to accredit Freud's hypothesis of drive activity, even though no alternative explanation is put forward. When one thinks of how social prejudices form the basis of explanations for the most irrational, the most violent, and the most uncontrollable forms of behaviour, and how the latter re-emerge after a phase during which they seemed to have been understood or eliminated, whereas in fact they had simply been reduced to silence, one cannot fail to be persuaded of the resistance of the instinctual bedrock to the most 'civilized' social evolutions.

I will not return to the critique of structuralism, but will focus rather on the poststructuralist positions which interest me much more (Godelier, Juillerat, Héritier), while not overlooking the importance of other anthropological conceptions outside structuralism (Bateson, Geertz, Sahlins). These have been developed, in most cases, independently of any debate with psychoanalysis. A distinction must be made between what belongs to the central western tradition, historically and geographically, and that which belongs to other traditions (T. Laqueur, W. Doniger, G. Obeyesekere).[52] The debate can also be extended to phenomena which go beyond the facts of anthropology (see the studies of Cavalli-Sforza on the diffusion of languages following the the migrations of peoples). By going back to prehistory, psychoanalysis encounters unexpected sympathisers.[53] I will confine myself here to the discussion of recent theorizations encountered during the dialogue between anthropologists and psychoanalysts. This is centred on the question of the universality of incest and parricide, components of the Oedipus complex. The prohibition of incest appears indeed to be the rule of rules and is only contradicted in cases where the exception is clearly asserted as a privilege (Pharaohs) bringing those to whom it is granted nearer to the gods. The same is not true of parricide, which has scarcely been the object of such clear recognition and which arouses the scepticism of anthropologists. I have stated the reasons for this elsewhere. The prohibition of incest has to be constantly reasserted because the child's period of immaturity puts him in direct, carnal contact with the mother or whoever provides basic maternal care. From this has been inferred the idea of a necessarily and inevitably incestuous relationship which has to be constantly prohibited by a prescription at each new birth. This promulgation remains present in everyone's mind not only because it is necessary to keep the relationship of alliance in mind, but because the temptation of transgression is reactualized permanently by the excitations of the flesh. Infantile sexuality, which is unaware of social taboos, is inclined to transgression all the more easily in that the first objects, other than those on the subject's own body, are those connected with maternal care. As Freud says, the mother is the child's first seductress. But today, we know that it is not just the libido that is in question, especially when we distance ourselves from the ordinary conditions regulated by repression. I have defended the idea of a *maternal madness*, and described the passionate state of the mother (in resonance with that of the child), which is in no way pathological (it is when it does not take place that one notices the existence of an anomaly by default). *This madness (of love) is totally at variance with psychosis.*[54]

The existence of incest of the second type (between mother and daughter) has been described by F. Héritier.[55] F. Héritier starts out from the masculine/feminine difference between the sexes, as a fundamental dualistic category, an avatar of the more general pair identity/difference. But this pair is transcended by one fact: women have the capacity to give birth to children, that is to say, to children either of the same sex or of a different sex. Here an opposition can be inferred between the flesh (the fluids) and the act of begetting (which can be consanguineous). By means of sperm and milk, flesh and blood create a new pair. The taboo sometimes concerns the sharing of identical humours – this is incest of the second type. Even though F. Héretier conducted her inquiries independently of psychoanalysis, they refer to it.

Maurice Godelier is in agreement with Freud in attributing sexuality with a major role. Like Freud, he recognizes that the mutation which makes sexual desire a constantly present force – and not a periodic one, as in animals – carries with it a danger of disorder and social disorganization, whence the imperious necessity of regulating it (by prohibiting incest) and of repressing it. This prohibition is thus not limited simply to protecting society; it *produces* society, too. I will conclude these observations on incest by pointing out that, in the Oedipus complex, the mother is the only pole of the triangle to have a carnal relationship with the two others. The existence of a *Muttercomplex* is thus in no way secondary to the *Vatercomplex*.

On the question of parricide, there is a difficulty. By way of a response to anthropologists who say they do not observe it – though Frazer gives examples of it – one can say that parricide does not need to be mentioned; it is included in the prohibition pertaining to homicide of which it is simply a particular case. Furthermore, unlike incest, the danger of which is reactivated with each new birth by the bodily excitations involved in rearing, parricide not only has to be repressed but annulled. *Speaking about it, even for the purpose of prohibiting it, is to admit that the mere idea of this act can inhabit the mind of someone who is not a monster.* Which is why, for instance, it is not mentioned in Solon's code of laws. Repression, then, is deeper here, and the return of the repressed can scarcely be envisaged. However, I think that however complete the repression purports to be, traces of it subsist. Scarcely any society exists with beliefs that do not include feelings of fear, respect, devotion, and submission to *spirits*. If parricide exists, it should not be looked for in the explicit reference to the act and to desires towards the real father, but rather in the fear of retaliation on the part of the dead. In other words, parricide can only be envisaged through its consequences, *once accomplished*. The dead father is to be feared much more than the living father; for, associated with his image are feelings of guilt, which make one fear his manifestation in the beyond. The projections concerning him are marked by the terror of his vengeance. Instead of being carried out on the father himself, it is directed towards the symbolic father, who observes us and judges us from on high, even though he is not explicitly designated as the one who possesses the mother and has the right to enjoy her.

Among anthropologists, no one has undertaken a more detailed and precise study of the relations between anthropology and psychoanalysis than Bernard Juillerat;[56] nor, for that matter, one that has been more productive of original solutions. The light had to come from an anthropologist who had escaped the influence of C. Lévi-Strauss sufficiently, and who has been able to stand back enough to be able to reopen questions in an impasse. In his last works, C. Lévi-Strauss – after a long period of silence which could have passed for neutrality, and which allowed Lacan to make use of the backing of anthropological structuralism to justify his own conception of the unconscious, even though nothing permitted the legitimization of this patronage – the master of structural anthropology, finally brought himself, after Lacan's death, to say what he thought of psychoanalysis.[57] It soon became obvious, that he remained, even more so than at the outset, profoundly hostile to its ideas. Nonetheless, those who claimed allegiance to him (to some degree or other) did not always follow him in his conclusions. But before Juillerat, no one had undertaken a complete examination of the different aspects of the conflict. One of the advantages of Juillerat's inquiry is that it is not confined to examining Freud's ideas, but embraces the principal authors of the psychoanalytic literature. His conclusions have the merit of adopting a freer position towards the prejudices invoked for postponing or refusing dialogue. Juillerat writes: 'The mythological materials of societies without writing, which are available today and are often close to the myths of Antiquity, confirm that the cultural realm of imagination spontaneously thinks of the evolution of the relations between men and women in the form of successive stages, based alternatively on co-operation and conflict, and inspired by timeless fantasies aroused by sexual differentiation.'[58] The implicit postulate (which makes it possible to avoid pronouncing in favour of either of the prescriptions) is the argument whereby the theorization of psychoanalysis, elaborated on the basis of analysing *individual* patients, is set in opposition to the theorization of the imaginary formations of *societies* without writing which are still accessible today, not in the form of past history as if it were the product of a cold history, but of an imaginary formation that is still alive. As Juillerat, who rejects this old objection, points out, there are no universals without variants and there is no diversity without a common basis.[59] His merit is that he shows how anthropological and psychoanalytic criteria differ. The reference to the social, which is of prime importance for anthropologists, reveals the same facts as are advanced by psychoanalysis but in a different way.

Let us take the example of the maternal uncle, which, for Lévi-Strauss, is the starting-point of any theory of attitudes because he is assumed to be the representative of the group. Anthropologists are so concerned with *denaturalizing* the relations of kinship that they need a referent which excludes any interpretation referring to a 'natural' relation. But denaturalizing does not necessarily mean sociologizing. Psychoanalysts consider the maternal uncle differently. They are not only concerned with his role as a representative of the group, but also with his role as the counterpoint to the marriage relationship. In the latter, conflict is inevitable between the child and the one who enjoys certain rights with respect to the mother. Hence the necessity for he who comes from the same womb as the mother – and who, accordingly, is also subject to the prohibition of incest – to play a moderating role, without however having a carnal relation with the mother. His role is to regulate the exchanges with the child. Which means that the difference of generations (between parents and children) is tempered by the intervention of a man from an earlier generation, but who does not benefit from the privileges of the marriage, namely, the sexual relationship. The maternal uncle is, then, an *intercessor* between the different consanguineous generations and a marriage relationship, of which he is the guarantor without being the sexual beneficiary. It can be seen, then, that the reference is social *and* psychic, for the system of attitudes, in its complete form, has to take account of its psychic repercussions, even if their coding only uses social references. Those which pertain to the psychic dimension play their role nonetheless *by making them all refer back to sexuality.*[60] There is a difference here between what anthropologists consider to be socially acceptable (hostility included) and socially prohibited. The collateral relation is a consanguineous relationship but it cannot in itself sum up consanguinity as a whole, which manifests itself even more in the non-collateral relations of the marriage relationship. The social position concerning sexuality shows that it is sexuality that determines attitudes and which is at the root of every system. No preoccupation that is centred on maintaining the reference to exchange can overlook the link between attitudes and affects (accepted or inhibited) and, beyond them, with the drives. Juillerat clearly shows that the inspiration for Lévi-Strauss's atom of kinship is to be found in Troubetzkoy and the phonemic system. The occultation of affects is an attempt to resolve the insoluble problem. All the anthropological reflections on the Oedipus complex 'forget' that Freud speaks of a *double* Oedipus complex, positive and negative, of which only vestiges remain.

The preoccupation with denaturalization sacrifices aspects of a problem of great interest, and it was left to F. Héritier to show that it is so-called 'natural' ties that offer a rich material for symbolization. In fact, one has to understand the constituents of the Oedipal corpus which is at once a *complex, a structure and a model.*[61] It is history and structure. Ultimately, Juillerat opposes a *closed* atom of kinship (according to psychoanalysis) and an *open* structural atom (according to anthropology).

The analysis of Lévi-Strauss's work is very revealing. By taking the structural phonology of someone like Troubetzkoy as a model and applying it to his own domain, Lévi-Strauss illustrates admirably two a priori. The first is the anti-naturalist obsession, which is at the basis of the identity of anthropology.

Lévi-Strauss draws on the elementary forms of language, whose social nature is accepted, and the place of meaningfulness recognized. He attempts, then, to ground the bases of anthropology on a social model: a system of designations (language), a system of attitudes (reduced to a system comparable to that of phonology, thus language at an elementary level). But language is neither entirely independent of nature nor entirely diverted by the social. The second a priori is the obsession with constructing a system (unconscious) independent of any signification, in the sense of content. And it was this double obsession that gave birth to anthropological structuralism which had a twofold aim: (1) to do without any reference to the signified in its conception of the unconscious, and (2) to avoid any possibility of anthropology being reduced to a natural discipline. Here, then, the atom of kinship is considered as a minimal anthropological reality without any link with nature and, when it refers to attitudes, it is considered to have no link with a psychically determined mental content. It remains to be demonstrated that other solutions exist which, while affirming the gap with nature, do not deny their links with it (loss of the oestrus) and defend the idea of an unconscious whose contents serve as symbolic formations relating to human facts connected with *metaphorized* natural functions.

Reflections on both models

These reflections on the biological and anthropological models, both of which would like to annex the psychoanalytic model, considering it as a secondary derivation which proceeds from each of them, have made it possible to show how, in fact, it is irreducible for them. Three questions have to be raised before I conclude:

1 What is the humanity of man?
2 What is the state of our knowledge about man?
3 How does psychoanalysis fit into this knowledge?

A recent work comes to our assistance as far as the first question is concerned.[62] Local answers are all the more tempting in that they avoid the need to form an opinion on those that have a global character and are currently discredited. I will concentrate on those which interest me the most, namely, the acquisition of the capacity for symbolization (Morin), or establishing relations with others (A. Jacquard). Some authors underline the relation with the drives and insist on 'the genius of the instincts' (Marcel Moreau). Other references suggest a touch of belief; they mark the place of speech in the constitution of the human being and his relation with the verb, demonstrating his liberation from nature (an obsession! 'we are not beasts'). Others will see this frontier of the human dimension in the invention of the arts. Finally, there are some who confess that they are no longer able even to utter the word 'human' (Bonnefoy). This admission of the enigma, at a time when knowledge appears to be developing so considerably, is revealing.

I will now turn to the important work of E. Morin, which makes an appraisal of the spirit of contemporary knowledge. Edgar Morin has made himself the defender of hypercomplex thought, which changes the modalities for comprehending the corpus submitted to knowledge. In an attempt to embrace the different aspects at play, Morin tries to evaluate the different levels involved: living entities – individual human beings – the social dimension – the species. He identifies the instruments of hypercomplex thought:

- *hologrammatic*: the part is in the whole, which is in the part
- *recursive*: which comprises a loop in which the causes produce effects which have repercussions on the causes
- *dialogical*: uniting the terms of a relation that is both complementary and antagonistic.

Why this complication? Because, contrary to the idea of a *Homo sapiens*, then a *Homo sapiens sapiens*, Morin recognizes the existence of a *Homo sapiens demens*.[63] His theorization, which resists any sort of simplifying modification, claims to organize a plural mode of thinking governed by the laws of organization–disorganization. This vision concurs with Freud's last theory of the drives. Morin opposes the model of *low complexity* to that of *high complexity*.[64] In the latter, we notice that the accent is placed on pluralism, autonomy, the multiplicity of communications, the hierarchy of levels of organization (with a strong polyarchic and anarchic component), weak constraints, the prevalence of the strategy over the programme with value being placed on creative capacities, etc. The complex organization accepts uncertainties, liberties, disorder, antagonisms, rivalries. This leads, ultimately, to considering the individual as 'the centre of consciousness in and for society. The individual mind-brain is more complex than society, more complex than the Earth, more complex than the galaxy'.[65] Morin's thought is probably nearer to psychoanalysis than he suspects.

The unconscious and science

During a symposium on 'The Unconscious and Science',[66] I tried to analyse the dispute between science and psychoanalysis. The subject of science and the subject of psychoanalysis are not identical. The former is a 'purified' subject, which is not the case of the latter. Objectification and subjectivity have always been opposed. Psychoanalysis objectifies the subjective during the production of the analytic discourse. Moreover, objective knowledge is a source of controversies among scientists (Popper, Kuhn, Lakatos, Feyerabend). *Scientific knowledge is not knowledge about objective reality but only knowledge of that which lends itself to treatment by the scientific method, in contradistinction to knowledge of the psyche which has to account both for that which is treatable by the scientific method and that which is not.* In any case, the attempt to do without subjectivity in scientific knowledge has been denounced by G. Edelman. This point has been the object of a systematic attack, explicit in someone like Lévi-Strauss who would like to 'be finished with the subject'. Such an attitude fails to explain the coexistence, in the same man, of the scientist and the non-scientist (beliefs, religion, diverse expressions of spiritualism). On the other hand, an openly mechanistic approach (Changeux) claims to avoid reductionism. Reductionism reduces the psychic to the biological, then the biological to the physico-chemical and, finally, to mathematics, the purest science if ever there was one – and the only one that is rigorous. One cannot pass over in silence the seduction exerted on a good many psychoanalysts (Lacan and his school) by the idea of mathematizing psychoanalysis with the fantasy of a signifier 'without remainder'. From his starting-point with mirrors, Lacan arrived at the signifier (getting rid of the sign and signified) and finally discovered the matheme. Affect? Excluded. The result of this orientation was that the pastor lost some of his most promising lambs (Granoff, Perrier, Valabréga, Laplanche, Pontalis, Aulagnier, Rosolato, and even Leclaire). As for mathematical theory, R. Thom gave a more than curious picture of psychoanalysis and one that was open to some of its ideas.

It is remarkable that this orientation occurred at a time when epistemology was abandoning its extremism and was proposing open models (Von Foerster, Atlan, Varela, Vincent, Edelman). In psychoanalysis, other authors (Bion, Winnicott) offered us ways out of the Freudian or Kleinian confinement.

Faced with the complexity of reality, Edgar Morin proposes a *method*. He points out that no one can do without general ideas and that great ideas are not born from within a discipline with limited frontiers. They result from a vision. What justifies the thinking on complexity is that all knowledge is incomplete owing to multidimensionality. To look for a total knowledge would be the worst of illusions. What matters, on the contrary, is to organize knowledge, to articulate its different facets. Likewise, to search for a single foundation would be another illusion. Determinism is an error, for it rejects the unforeseeable. The selection of theories is carried out in the name of the pleasure principle more than in that of the reality principle, in the ideology of the human sciences.

Let us look a little closer at Morin's *method*. 'We human beings know the world via the messages transmitted by our senses to our brain. The world is present inside our mind, which is inside the world.'[67] One is struck here by the similarity of Morin's words with certain sentences at the end of *The Future of an Illusion* in which Freud takes the defence of science.[68] Morin proposes an incompressible tetragram, order/disorder/interaction/organization. He points out that 'knowledge not only presupposes an undoubted separation from the external world, but also presupposes a certain degree of separation from oneself.'[69] He goes on to propose a definition of the paradigm: 'A paradigm is a type of logical relation (inclusion–conjunction–disjunction–exclusion) between a certain number of major categories.'[70] The *scienza nova* strives to base itself on an ontology which puts the relation before the substance, puts the emphasis on emergences, establishes interferences as composite, constructed phenomena, endowed with a certain autonomy. The metasystem is open. Complexity is not incompatible with a paradigm of simplicity. Psychic organization tends towards degradation, whereas living organization tends towards development. The universe commences as a disintegration, and it is by disintegrating that it organizes itself (disorder and order). Let us recall the three principles: (1) the dialogical principle; (2) the principle of recursivity; (3) the hologrammatic principle. The resulting causality can be seen from three angles: linear, circular, retroactive and recursive. What is striking in Morin's thought is not just that it is capable of including different dimensions of knowledge; for a psychoanalyst, it is first and foremost that he finds in it a mode of thinking that is evocative of the psychic mechanisms relative to the two domains conscious–unconscious. Basically, without knowing it, Freud was a precursor of the theories of complexity. This has gone almost unnoticed because his successors elaborated theories in which this seems not to have been recognized. A return to linear thinking is occurring surreptitiously. The future will depend on the way in which psychoanalysts will seek to engage with this thinking on complexity.

H. Atlan follows a convergent approach. With biology as its starting-point, self-organization attempts to define the mental object. Henri Atlan's ideas have often been the object of debates within psychoanalytic circles. Pierre Marty has discussed certain aspects of it; G and S. Pragier refer to it explicitly in their work on new metaphors. I myself have examined the repercussions of these conceptions for psychoanalysis.[71] I have also made use of a model borrowed from Heinz von Foerster,[72] whose thought is close to that of Atlan, though the ends to which I have put it are different from those it had initially. The definition of mental objects, from the angle of neurobiology, has also been one of the aims pursued by Jean-Pierre Changeux. But the latter, at the opposite extreme of complexity, claims allegiance to La Mettrie, a militant in favour of mechanism. Among the efforts towards a synthesis, one can mention those of André Bourguignon.[73] The central theorem of von Foerster and Atlan is the establishment of the principle of order from noise.

Here one finds again one of the ideas most frequently advanced by the theoreticians of biology (chaos theory, where chaos appears as the regressive stage prior to the establishment of a change of organisation which constitutes a progression by creating a new state of order). Changeux has followed the same approach, while remaining faithful to his mechanistic options.

Postmodernity

J. F. Lyotard has studied the condition of knowledge in postmodern societies.[74] Postmodernity is characterized by incredulity towards 'metanarratives'; that is to say, grand theoretical syntheses. This mutation is based on the adhesion to the progress of technologies applied to language-related disciplines. These are marked by prejudices that confuse explanation with 'clear' communication and the concern to cleanse it of all ambiguity. The analysis of knowledge, in this modernity, widens the gap with the knowledge of psychoanalysis. The method is based here on *language games* (Wittgenstein). However, though the Saussurian or Chomskian models underlay the reflections of certain theoreticians of psychoanalysis, here it is more with Wittgenstein that one should seek its inspiration. The linguistic reference is based on the pragmatic model (J. Austin, J. R. Searl). I had sensed the fortune in store for this model,[75] having come, as it did, to the rescue of a general polemic in which not the slightest mention is made of the theories of conflict at the centre of Freud's work. The struggles of language games became the regulators of the system. All of this led to a *pragmatics of narrative knowledge (savoir)*. Science is considered as a subset of learning (*connaissance*), but my investigations show that this feigned modesty dissimulates poorly hegemonic ambitions with respect to knowledge. There is a consensus that recognizes the pre-eminence of narrative knowledge in the form of traditional knowledge. In psychoanalysis a similar point of view has been defended. But knowledge of this type can only come about once a psychoanalysis is finished, and never before.[76] Or it can only be a question of fragments of narratives, eroded from within by free association. Nevertheless, certain psychoanalysts, like Donald Spence, have been attracted by the reference to narrativity. They have had little following. Free association breaks the narrative. It seems to me that, when the issue is one of understanding the analytic relationship, the theory of games is but one form of intellectualist abstraction amongst others, still haunted by the cognitivist postulate but, in my view, unsuited to accounting for the processes involved in the conflict, which are accessible thanks to the transference. It is not the studies of the school of Palo Alto (P. Watzlawick) which will make me think the contrary. Once the effect of curiosity has passed, these works, albeit frequently cited, occupy a very limited place today in psychiatry and psychopathology. Of course, it will be recognized that the process of interactional exchange does not depend on the denotative; nor does it depend on prescriptive statements, since the principle of prescription of the fundamental rule is in fact a principle of non-prescription through the rule of 'saying everything without omitting or selecting anything' in what comes to the mind. For such is the paradox of free association. The analyst knows perfectly well that such a prescription cannot be observed, though it remains fundamental.

Having attempted to forge links between psychoanalysis and the biological and anthropological models, it is surprising to observe once again its deterritorialization. Yet, I believe the issue is less one of an essential inevitability than of an obstinate refusal to enter deeply into this mode of thinking (with notable exceptions: Edelman, Vincent, Juillerat, Morin, etc.). It is true that psychoanalysis remains, in itself, alien to the postmodern preoccupation with increasing power. Roger-Pol Droit[77] even sees human beings as sharing a 'higher' weakness which seems to me to be in line with the aims of psychoanalytic treatment.

We are clearly straying a long way from the question that has become prevalent, i.e. 'What's the use?' Do not count on me to reply, 'There isn't any.' On the contrary, my idea would be to turn the question round, in good analytic tradition, on the questioner, and to ask: 'What is your purpose in asking the question?' This is the best way to set about answering it. But to do this, one would have to begin by admitting that the instruments of traditional thought are useless in this case. As for those that might eventually have their use, once analysed rigorously, they lead to this mode of thinking about the hypercomplex, a domain in which psychoanalysis has no difficulty in recognizing itself. We should call as witnesses those whom we regard as being capable of helping us to formulate the meaning of our research. They have not been obsessed by the idea of neutralizing psychoanalysis or of attempting to skirt around it; they have not continued to hope for its decline so as to be rid of it. They have accepted the need for dialogue. Apart from those already mentioned, let us not forget René Thom, and particularly the concepts that he has defended concerning *saillance* and *prégnance*. P. Medawar thinks, for his part, that success in a particular field of knowledge is 'having ideas'. One still needs to be open to those ideas which seem far removed from the body of knowledge which one started out with and which sometimes result in it being called into question. For surely a powerful idea is one that destabilizes you and confronts you with what has not been thought about? Having ideas does not always lead to an increase in power. On the contrary, experience often shows that the conditions of success for an increase in power lie in the scorn or negligence of ideas.[78] Nazism was extremely powerful, to the point of dominating Europe; it cannot be said that it did much to further scientific discussion. True enough, some will reply: but what is going to happen ultimately? Ultimately, we do not know if there will still be anyone left to give an account of it.

Notes

1 They do sometimes coincide. See J.-F. Lyotard (1979). *The Postmodern Condition: A Report on Knowledge*, p. 40 (trans. G. Bennington and B. Massumi, Manchester University Press) which I will discuss further on.

2 See, for instance, the article by Lawrence Krunstadt, a neurobiologist from New York University Psychoanalytic Institute, on the theories of Allan Hibon, who is resolutely hostile to psychoanalysis, in *Neuro-Psychoanalysis*, 2001, 3, pp. 85–101.

3 Atlan, H. (1998). *La fin du tout génétique*. Paris: INRA Editions, 1999.
4 Jouvet, M. (1992). *Le sommeil et le rêve*. Paris: Odile Jacob.
5 Hobson, A. (1992). *Le cerveau rêvant*. Paris: Gallimard.
6 Garma, L. Aperçus sur les rêves et les activités mentales du dormeur dans la clinique du sommeil. *Revue française de psychosomatique*, 1998, no. 14, pp. 15–32.
7 Changeux, J.-P. Les neurones de la raison. *La Recherche*, June 1992. See, also, A. Green, L'homme machinal: à propos de *L'homme neuronal* de J.-P. Changeux, *Le temps de la réflexion*, 4, pp. 345–369; and: Un psychanalyste face aux neurosciences, *La Recherche*, no. 247, October 1992, pp. 1166–1174.
8 Prociantz, A. (1995). *La biologie dans le boudoir*. Paris: Odile Jacob.
9 Vincent, J.-D. (1986). *Biologie des passions*. Paris: Odile Jacob; and, *La chair et le diable*. Paris: Odile Jacob, 1996.
10 Damasio, A.R. (1995). *L'erreur de Descartes. La raison des émotions*. Paris: Odile Jacob.
11 Panksepp, J. Emotions as viewed by psycho-analysis and neuroscience: An exercise in consilience. *Neuro-Psychoanalysis*, 1999, 1, pp. 5–15. The entire number is devoted to emotions with an introduction and very open discussion, in which I took part.
12 Pragier, G. and Faure-Pragier, S. Un siècle après *L'Esquisse:* Nouvelles métaphores? Métaphores du nouveau: Report to the 50th Congress of French-speaking psychoanalysts, Madrid, 1990, *Revue française de psychanalyse*, 6–1990: Psychanalyse et sciences: nouvelles métaphores; and A. Green, Penser l'épistemologie de la pratique, reprinted in *Propédeutique*. Paris: Champ Vallon, 1995.
13 Kaplan, K. and Solms, M. (2000). *Clinical Studies in Neuro-Psychoanalysis*. London: Karnac Books.
14 See, Green, A., Psychique, somatique, psychosomatique. In: *Somatisation, psychanalyse et sciences du vivant*. Paris: Esterel, 1994, pp. 167–186.
15 Ameisen, J.-C. (1999). *La sculpture du vivant. Le suicide cellulaire et la mort créatrice*. Paris: Le Seuil. See, too, by the same author: Au coeur du vivant, l'autodestruction, *Le Monde*, 1999.
16 Vidal, J.-M. (1992). Evolution du psychisme et évolution des organismes. In *Darwinisme et société*, ed. P. Tort. Paris: Presses Universitaires de France.
17 Freud's theory of affect. Questions for neuroscience. *Neuropsychoanalysis*, 1999, 1.
18 Panksepp, J. Emotions as viewed by psycho-analysis and neuroscience. An exercise in conciliation. *Neuro-Psychoanalysis*, 1999, 1, pp. 15–35. Cf. the discussion which followed (A. Damasio, A. Green, J. Le Doux, A. Schore, H. Shevrin, C. Yorke).
19 Edelman, G. (1992). *Bright Air, Brilliant Fire. On the Matter of the Mind*. New York: Basic Books. The title is a citation from Empidocles; and the book is dedicated to Darwin and Freud.
20 Ibid. p. 74.
21 Ibid. p. 75.
22 Ibid. p. 83.
23 Ibid. p. 83.
24 Ibid. p. 85.
25 Ibid. p. 85.
26 Ibid. p. 87.
27 Ibid. p. 87.

28 Ibid. p. 89.
29 Ibid. p. 90.
30 Ibid. p. 90.
31 Ibid. p. 93.
32 Ibid. p. 94.
33 Ibid. p. 108.
34 Ibid. p. 109.
35 Ibid. p. 110.
36 Ibid. p. 114.
37 Ibid. p. 115.
38 Ibid. p. 115.
39 Ibid. p. 119.
40 Ibid. p. 120.
41 Ibid. p. 132.
42 Ibid. p. 135.
43 Ibid. p. 165.
44 Ibid. p. 170.
45 Ibid. p. 175.
46 Ibid. p. 242.
47 Ibid. p. 208.
48 Ibid. p. 247.
49 Varela, F. Sciences cognitives et psychanalyse. *Journal de psychanalyse de l'enfant*, 1993, 14, pp. 313–327.
50 I refer the reader here to my book *La causalité psychique*. Paris: Odile Jacob, 1995, pp. 16–106.
51 For a discussion of his ideas, see *La causalité psychique*. Paris: Odile Jacob, 1995, p. 155.
52 See the references in *La causalité psychique*.
53 See the monograph on *Psychanalyse et Préhistoire. Monographies de la Société psychanalytique de Paris*. Paris: Presses Universitaires de France, August 1994.
54 Green, A. (1995). *La causalité psychique*. Paris: Odile Jacob.
55 Héritier, F. Inceste et substance. In *Incestes*. Paris: Presses Universitaires de France, 'Petite Bibliothèque de Psychanalyse', 2001.
56 Juillerat, B. (2001). *Penser l'imaginaire. Essai d'anthropologie psychanalytique*. Payot-Lausanne.
57 Lévi-Strauss, C. (1985). *La potière jalouse*. Paris: Plon. [*The Jealous Potter*. Translated by Benedict Chorier, University of Chicago Press, 1988.]
58 Ibid. p. 42.
59 Ibid. p. 52.
60 Ibid. p. 116.
61 See Green, A. (1992). Oedipe, Freud et nous. In *La déliaison*. Paris: Les Belles Lettres,
62 *L'humanité de l'homme*, under the direction of Jacques Sojcher, Editions du Cercle d'Art, 2001. Let us note the participation of Antoine Vergote, a psychoanalyst (attached to the Lacanian movement) and Catholic theologian.
63 Morin, E. (2001). *La méthode*, vol. 5: *L'humanité de l'humanité*, p. 107. Paris: Le Seuil.
64 Ibid. p. 177.
65 Ibid. p. 187.

66 *L'inconscient et la science*, under the direction of P. Dorey. This colloquium brought together C. Castoriadis, H. Atlan, R. Thom and A. Green. On this occasion, my contribution attempted to treat the subject of the 'Misrecognition of the Unconscious'. See *L'inconscient et la science*. Paris: Dunod, 1991, pp. 140–220.

67 Morin, E. (1950). *Introduction à la pensée complexe*. ESF Editeur, p. 117.

68 Freud, S. (1927). *The Future of an Illusion*. S.E. XXI, 55–56.

69 Morin, E. ibid. p. 146.

70 Ibid. p. 147.

71 Green, A. *Les théories de la complexité, autour de l'oeuvre de H. Atlan*, Colloque de Cerisy, under the direction of F. Fogelman Soulé. Paris: Le Seuil, 1991; and Autoorganisation et psychanalyse: la psychanalyse et la science, dialogue avec H. Atlan. In: *Médecine et hygiène*, 50, 1992, pp. 2370–2377.

72 Von Foerster, H., Note pour une épistémologie des objets vivants. In: *L'unité de l'homme*. Paris: Le Seuil, p. 401.

73 Bourguignon, A. (1989). *L'homme imprévu*. Paris: Presses Universitaires de France; and (1994) *L'homme fou*. Paris: Presses Universitaires de France.

74 Lyotard, J.-F. (1979). *The Postmodern Condition: A Report on Knowledge*, Manchester University Press, 1984.

75 'Why are psychic processes said to have a meaning?' A lecture given to the Paris Psychoanalytic Society (contribution to a symposium held in Lyon in 1998).

76 Green, A. Méconnaissance de l'inconscient. In: *L'Inconscient et le sens*, under the direction of R. Dorey. Paris: Dunod.

77 Droit, R.-P. Faiblesse et barbarie. L'histoire des fondements. In: *L'humanité de l'humain*, pp. 101–109. Paris: Editions Cercle d'Art, 2001.

78 J.-F. Lyotard looks upon the possibility of terror as being a consequence of the computerization of societies (ibid. p. 107).

PROVISIONAL CONCLUSIONS

What do these orientations mean? Where are they leading? Seen from a certain distance, it seems to me that what is happening is a reaction to the disillusionments produced by certain earlier ideological choices. The justification of 'scientificity', which is concerned with the search for 'objective' meaning, was intended to be a response to the limits reached by existential phenomenology which took over from the philosophies of consciousness. However, without realizing it, these were shaken by the discovery of the unconscious. With hindsight, it might be asked whether these phenomenologies were not suffering from the illusions of consciousness. There was a willingness to recognize the unconscious, but on the condition that it paid a price. The price Freud proposed was unacceptable, so one had to choose instead its Saussurean, or even biological version. The Saussurean unconscious came after the studies of the Vienna circle (Troubetzkoy), which saw salvation only in formalism. Wittgenstein, for his part, lent his support to the critique of the unconscious with his theory of logical positivism. One could not 'explain' what language referred to; one could only say what things looked like through its bewitching effects.

Another major disappointment was Marxist thought and the terrible revelation concerning the blindness of the intellectuals who had adhered to it. Their involvement meant that they had blotted out, more or less deliberately, the crimes of those who were supposed to have drawn inspiration from this system of thought in order to justify their actions (F. Furet[1]). The liberation from Marxist thought and its illusions based on the so-called scientific character of historical materialism led to a denunciation of history and its teleological versions. Once history had been relegated to the wings of the intellectual scene, structure occupied the terrain left vacant. Who does not recall the controversies of the time? Lévi-Strauss took Sartre to task, finding an ally in Merleau Ponty (who played an important role in the rediscovery of Saussure[2]). Lévi-Strauss then endeavoured to neutralize Riceour whose corpus of reference was not societies without writing, but rather the writing of western societies. Derrida jumped over this debate. In fact, the neo-Kantism advocated by Lévi-Strauss (return to analytic reason and repression of dialectical reason) paved the way for the cognitivism to come. The new ideology aligned itself with science (Monod). The human sciences were keen to show that they had emerged once and for all from childhood and laid claim to the respectability belonging to objective knowledge, in the image of the exact sciences. Hence the interest of recognizing linguistics as a pilot science; for, as phonology showed, it knew how to rise to a level devoid of subjectivity, while flourishing in the sphere of what is significant. It was even thought that syntax (Chomsky) could be advantageously substituted for semantics. It was subsequently realized that this ambition was called into question (Benveniste).

This sophistication scarcely covered up the abdication it revealed regarding a study of meaning. For if the signified is governed by the unconscious and, what is more, by an unconscious rooted in drive activity (anchored in the somatic), there can be no question of abandoning the conceptual signifieds by accepting to replace them by drive movements linked to the body. An ambivalent position emerged concerning the animal inheritance of man, organized by his infantile history, underlining the limitations and even the failure of our will (and thus of all voluntarism). The *secondary* character of the elaborations of our consciousness remains. Such then – in an overview whose lack of precision and eventual confusions I am conscious of – is the history which is not recounted, but which can be made out behind the sparring matches which have followed one after the other.

Psychoanalysis has traversed this period of intellectual history, following various paths depending on the country or on the influences of its most creative figures. Nor has it failed to tear itself apart into opposing groups for good or bad reasons. It has pursued its growth along sometimes diverging lines of orientation. It has resisted the attacks of its opponents who have changed in appearance, but not in attitude, depending on the epoch concerned. Its imminent death has constantly been predicted, but it is still there.

Today, it still continues to be subjected to arrogant offensives from horizons which are more or less closely influenced by the hypnotic fascination of technical feats. Fortunately, other paths exist which attract us, solicit us, and push us to remain faithful to our intellectual investments and our human responsibilities.

It may even be hoped that psychoanalysts will one day rediscover their taste for speaking together. Far from claiming to find the path leading to the truth, we will finally recognize, like Machado, that the truth is the path.

Notes

1 Furet, F. (1995). *Le passé d'une illusion. Essai sur l'idée communiste au XXe siècle.* Paris: Robert Laffont/Calmann-Lévy.
2 Green, A. La psychanalyse devant l'opposition de l'histoire et de la structure. *Critique*, no. 194, July 1963.

BIBLIOGRAPHY

Ameisen, J.-C. (1999) *La sculpture du vivant. Le suicide cellulaire et la mort créatrice*, Paris: Le Seuil.

—— (1999) Au cœur du vivant, l'autodestruction, *Le Monde*, 14 October.

Anzieu, D. (1988) *L'auto-analyse de Freud et la découverte de la psychanalyse*, Paris: Presses Universitaires de France, 2 vols.

—— (1994) *Le penser*, Paris: Dunod.

Aristotle *On the Soul (De Anima)*, trans. H. Lawson-Tancred, London: Penguin, 1986.

Atlan, H. (1991) *Les théories de la complexité*, autour de l'œuvre d'H. Atlan, Cerisy Colloquium, under the direction of F. Fogelman-Soulé, Paris: Le Seuil.

—— (1999) *La fin du tout génétique*, Paris: INRA Éditions.

Avtonomova, N. (1991) Lacan avec Kant: l'idée du symbolisme, in N. Avtonomova *Lacan avec les philosophes*, Paris: Albin Michel.

Balier, C. (1996) *Psychanalyse des comportements sexuels violents*, Paris: Presses Universitaires de France.

Baranes, J.-J., Sacco F. et al. (2002) *Inventer en psychanalyse. Construire et interpréter*, Paris: Dunod.

Baranger, W. (1999) *Position et objet dans l'œuvre de Melanie Klein*, Paris: Érès.

Bayle, G. (1989) Des espaces et des temps pour l'objet (clivage structurel et clivage fonctionnel), *Revue française de psychanalyse* 53, 4: 1055–67.

Bergmann, M. (2000) *The Hartmann Era*, New York: Other Press.

Bion, W. R. (1962) *Learning from Experience*, London: Heinemann.

—— (1963) *Elements of Psychoanalysis*, London: Heinemann.

—— (1967) *Second Thoughts*, London: Heinemann.

Botalle, C. and Botella (2001) (2001) *La figurabilité psychique*, Lonat: Delachaux and Niestlé; English edition: *Psychic Figurability: Mental States without any Representing*, trans. A. Weller, London: Routledge.

—— (2001) Figurabilité et régrédience, *Revue française de psychanalyse* 4: 1149–1240.

Bott, Spillius E. (2001) Développements actuels de la psychanalyse kleinienne, *Revue française de psychanalyse*, special edition 'Courants de la psychanalyse contemporaine', under the direction of André Green: 253–64.

Bouquet, S. (1997) *Introduction à la lecture de Saussure*, Paris: Payot.

Bourguignon, A. (1989) *L'homme imprévu*, Paris: Presses Universitaires de France.

—— (1994) *L'homme fou*, Paris: Presses Universitaires de France.

Bouveresse, J. (1976) *Le mythe de l'intériorité. Expérience, signification et langage privé chez Wittgenstein*, Paris: Editions de Minuit.

Bouvet, M. (1967) Dépersonnalisation et relations d'objet, in M. Bouvet *La relation d'objet. Œuvres psychanalytiques*, vol. 1, Paris: Payot.

Cahn, R. (1991) *L'adolescent dans la psychanalyse. L'aventure de la subjectivation*, Paris: Presses Universitaires de France.

Castoriadis, C. (1999) *Figures du pensable. Les carrefours du labyrinthe*, Paris: Le Seuil.

Castoriadis-Aulagnier, P. (1975) *La violence de l'interpretation*, Paris: PUF; English edition: *The Violence of Interpretation*, trans. A. Sheridan, London: Routledge and Institute of Psychoanalysis, 2001.

Changeux, J.-P. (1992) Les neurones de la raison, *La Recherche*, June.

Combe, C. (2002) *Soigner l'anorexie*, Paris: Dunod.

Cournut, J. (1983) Deuils ratés, morts méconnues, *Bulletin de la SPP* 2: 9–26.

Damasio, A.-R. (1995). *L'erreur de Descartes. La raison des émotions*, Paris: Odile Jacob.

Darmsteter, A. (1979) *La vie des mots*, Paris: Le Champ Libre (first published 1887).

Denis, A. (1995) Le présent, *International Journal of Psychoanalysis* 59: 1083–91.

—— (1995). Temporality and modes of languages, *International Journal of Psychoanalysis* 76: 1109–19.

Derrida, J. (1967) Freud et la scène de l'écriture, in J. Derrida *L'écriture et la différence*, Paris: Le Seuil; English edition: Freud and the scene of writing, in *Writing and Difference*, trans. A. Bass, London: Routledge, 1978.

—— (1967). *De la grammatologie*, Paris: Minuit. English edition: *Of Grammatology*, trans. G. C. Spivak, Baltimore: Johns Hopkins University Press.

—— (1975) 'Le facteur de la vérité', *Poétique* 21: 96–147.

—— (1980) *La carte postale: De Socrate à Freud et au-delà*, Paris: Aubier-Flammarion.

—— (1996) *Résistances de la psychanalyse*, Paris: Galilée; English edition: *Resistances of Psychoanalysis*, trans. P. Kamuf, P.-A. Brault and M. Naas, Palo Alto: Stanford University Press, 1998.

Diatkine, G. (2000) Surmoi culturel, *Revue française de psychanalyse* 64, 5: 1523–88.

Donnet, J.-L. (1995) Le concept freudien et la règle fondamentale, in *Le Surmoi*, vol. 1, Paris: Presses Universitaires de France, 'Monographies de la Revue française de psychanalyse'.

—— (2001) De la règle fondamentale à la situation analysante, *Revue française de psychanalyse* 1: 243–57.

Donnet, J.-L. and Green, A. (1973) *L'enfant de ça. Pour introduire la psychose Blanche*, Paris: Editions de Minuit.

Droit, R.-P. (2001) Faiblesse et barbarie. L'histoire des fondements, in R.-P. Droit *L'humanité de l'humain*, Paris: Éditions Cercle d'Art.

Edelman, G. (1992) *Bright Air, Brilliant Fire. On the Matter of Mind*, New York: Basic Books.

Engler, R. (2002) Bibliographie saussurienne, in *Cahiers F. de Saussure*, Paris: Gallimard.

Faimberg, H. (1996) Listening to listening, *International Journal of Psycho-Analysis* 77, 4: 667–77.

Fairbairn, W. R. (1976) *Psychoanalytic Studies of the Personality*, London: Tavistock Publications, Routledge & Kegan Paul.

Fenichel, O. (1976) A review of Freud's analysis terminable and interminable, *International Review of Psycho-Analysis*, 109–16.

Ferenczi, S. (1932) *The Clinical Diary of Sandor Ferenczi*, ed. J. Dupont, trans. M. Balint and N.Z. Jackson. Cambridge, MA: Harvard University Press 1988.

Fonagy, I. (1983) *La vive voix*, Paris: Payot.

—— (2001) *Attachment Theory and Psychoanalysis*, New York: Other Press.

Foucault, M. (1954) *Maladie mentale et psychologie*, Paris: Presses Universitaires de France; English edition: *Mental Illness and Psychology*, trans. A. Sheridan, foreword Herbert Dreyfus, London: Harper and Row, 1976.

Freud, A. (1936) *The Ego and Mechanisms of Defence*. Revised edition, *The Writings of Anna Freud*, Vol. II. New York: Intl. Universities Press Inc.

Freud, S. *The Letters of Sigmund Freud to Eduard Silberstein (1871–1881)*, ed. W. Boehlich, trans. A. J. Pomerans, Cambridge, MA: Belknap Press, 1990.

—— (1891) *On Aphasia*, London and New York: International University Press, 1953.

—— (1895) *Project for a Scientific Psychology, Standard Edition (S.E.) Complete Psychological Works of Sigmund Freud*, London: Hogarth Press (1950–1974), S.E., I: 281–397.

—— (1900a) *The Interpretation of Dreams*, S.E. IV and V: 1–621.

—— (1908) Character and anal eroticism, S.E. IX: 169.

—— (1909) 'Notes upon a case of obsessional neurosis', S.E. X: 155.

—— (1913) The disposition to obsessional neurosis, S.E. XII: 313.

—— (1914c) 'On narcissism: An introduction', S.E. XIV: 69.

—— (1917) On transformations of instinct as exemplified in anal eroticism, S.E. XVII: 127.

—— (1919h) The Uncanny. S.E. XVII: 217–52.

—— (1920g) 'Beyond the pleasure principle', S.E. XVIII: 7.

—— (1921) *Group Psychology and the Analysis of the Ego*, S.E. XVIII: 105.

—— (1921c) 'Group psychology and the analysis of the ego', S.E. XVIII: 69.

—— (1923b) *The Ego and the Id*, S.E., XIX: 3–66.

—— (1924c) The economic problem of masochism, S.E. XIX: 157.

—— (1924e) The loss of reality in neurosis and psychosis, S.E. XIX: 183.

—— (1925h) Negation, S.E. XIX: 233–9.

—— (1926f) 'Psychoanalysis: Freudian School', *Encyclopaedia Britannica*, 13th ed., S.E. XX: 261.

—— (1926d [1925]) *Inhibitions, Symptoms and Anxiety*, S.E. XX: 75–174.

—— (1927c). *The Future of an Illusion*, S.E. XXI: 1–56.

—— (1927e) 'Fetishism', S.E. 21: 149.

—— (1933a [1932]) *New Introductory Lectures on Psychoanalysis*, S.E. XXII: 1–182.

—— (1937c). Analysis terminable and interminable, S.E. XXIII: 209–53.

—— (1937d). Constructions in analysis, S.E. XXIII: 255–69.

—— (1938) *An Outline of Psycho-Analysis [Preface]*, S.E. XXIII: 144.

—— (1940a [1938]) *An Outline of Psychoanalysis*, S.E. XXIII: 139–207.

—— (1940e) 'Splitting of the ego in the process of defence', S.E. XXIII: 273.

—— (1940b [1938]). Some elementary lessons in psycho-analysis, S.E. XXIII: 281.

—— (1941[1938]) Findings, ideas, problems, S.E. XXIII: 299.

Furet, F. (1995) *Le passé d'une illusion. Essai sur l'idée communiste au XX siècle*, Paris: Robert Laffont/Calmann-Lévy.

Garma, L. (1982) Aperçus sur les rêves et les activités mentales du dormeur dans la clinique du sommeil, *Revue française de psychosomatique* 14: 15–32.

Gibeault, A. (1989) Destins de la symbolisation, *Revue française de psychanalyse* 53, 6: 1493–1617.

Godel, R. (1957) *Les sources manuscrites du* Cours de linguistique générale *de F de Saussure*, Genève: Droz.

Green, A. (1959) Critique de l'ouvrage *Existence* de R. May, E. Engel et H.F. Ellenberger, *Evolution psychiatrique* 24, 3: 471–506.

—— (1963) La psychanalyse devant l'opposition de l'histoire et de la structure, *Critique*, 194, juillet.

—— (1964) Névrose obsessionnelle et hystérie, leur relation chez Freud et depuis: étude clinique, critique et structurale, *Revue française de psychanalyse* 28, 5/6: 679–716.

—— (1966) L'objet *a* de J. Lacan, sa logique et la théorie freudienne, *Cahiers pour l'analyse*; repris dans *Propédeutique*, chap. 6, Paris: Champ Vallon.

—— (1970) 'L'affect', rapport présenté au XXX Congrès des psychanalystes de langues romanes, *Revue française de psychanalyse* 1970–34: 8851169; also in *Le discours vivant: la conception psychanalytique de l'affect*, Paris: Presses Universitaires de France, 1973.

—— (1973) *Le discours vivant*, Paris: PUF; English edition: *The Fabric of Affect in the Psychoanalytic Discourse*, trans. A. Sheridan, London: Routledge, 1999.

—— (1975) L'analyste, la symbolisation et l'absence dans le cadre analytique; also in *La folie privée*, Paris: Gallimard, 1990; English edition: *On Private Madness*, London: Hogarth Press, 1986.

—— (1975) The analyst, symbolization and absence in the analytic setting, *International Journal of Psycho-Analysis* 56; also in *On Private Madness*, London: Hogarth, 1986.

—— (1976) Le concept de limite, in A. Green *La folie privée*, Paris: Gallimard, 1990; English edition: The borderline concept, in *On Private Madness*, London: Hogarth Press, 1986.

—— (1979) Le silence du psychanalyste, *Topique*, 23.

—— (1980) La mère morte, in A. Green *Narcissisme de vie, narcissisme de mort*, Paris: Éditions de Minuit, 1983; English edition: The dead mother, trans. K. Aubertin, *Life Narcissism, Death Narcissism*, trans. A. Weller, London: Free Association Books, 2001.

—— (1980) Passions et destins des passions, *Nouvelle Revue de psychanalyse* 21; also in *On Private Madness*, London: Hogarth Press, 1986.

—— (1984) Le langage dans la psychanalyse, in A. Green, R. Diatkin, E. Jabès, M. Fain, and I. Fonagy *Langages. 2nd Rencontres psychanalytiques d'Aix-en-Provence*, Paris: Les Belles Lettres, pp. 19–250.

—— (1986) Réponses à des questions inconcevables, *Topique* 37: 11–30.

—— (1988) Démembrement du contre-transfert, in J.-J. Baranes, F. Sacco et al. *Inventer en psychanalyse. Construire et interpréter*, Paris: Dunod, 2002.

—— (1988) Du sens en psychosomatique, in A. Fine and J. Schaeffer (eds) *Interrogations psychosomatiques*, Paris: Presses Universitaires de France.

—— (1989) De la tiercéité, in *Les monographies de la Revue française de psychanalyse;* also in *La pensée clinique*, Paris: Odile Jacob, 2002.

—— (1990) Penser l'epistémologie de la pratique, *Revue française de psychanalyse* 54: 1533–41.

—— (1992) Auto-organisation et psychanalyse: la psychanalyse et la science, dialogue avec H. Atlan, *Médecine et hygiène* 50: 2370–77.

—— (1992) Un psychanalyste face aux neurosciences, *La recherche* 247: 1166–74; *Penser l'épistémologie de la pratique*, reprinted in *Propédeutique*, Paris: Champ Vallon, 1995, pp. 311–20.

Green, A. (1992) L'homme machinal: à propos de *L'homme neuronal* de J.-P. Changeux, *Le temps de la réflexion* 4: 345–69.

—— (1992) Œdipe, Freud et nous, in A. Green *La déliaison*, Paris: Les Belles Lettres.

—— (1992) Un psychanalyste face aux neurosciences, *La recherche* 23, 247: 1166–74.

—— (1993). L'analité primaire, in *Monographies de la Revue française de psychanalyse*: 'La névrose obsessionnelle'; also in *La pensée clinique*, Paris: Odile Jacob, 2002.

—— (1993). Masochism(s) and narcissism in analytic failures and the negative therapeutic reaction, in A. Green *The Work of the Negative*, London: Free Association Books, 1999.

—— (1993) Méconnaissance de l'inconscient, in R. Dorey (ed.) *L'inconscient et la science*, Paris: Dunod.

—— (1994) Psychique, somatique, psychosomatique, in A. Green *Somatisation, psychanalyse et sciences du vivant*, Paris: Esterel, pp. 167–86.

—— (1994) *Un psychanalyste engagé*, p. 148, Paris: Calmann-Lévy.

—— (1995) De l'objet non unifiable à la fonction objectalisante, *Propédeutique*, Paris: Champ Vallon.

—— (1995) L'objet et la fonction objectalisante, *Propédeutique*, Paris: Champ Vallon.

—— (1995) Note sur les processus tertiaires, *Propédeutique*. *La méta psychologie revisitée* (annexe D), Paris: Champ Vallon (first published 1972).

—— (1996) La sexualité a-t-elle un quelconque rapport avec la psychanalyse?, *Revue française de psychanalyse* 60: 840–48.

—— (1997) Le langage au sein de la théorie générale de la représentation, *Pulsions, représentations, langage*, Lonat: Delachaux and Niestlé.

—— (1997) Ouverture à une discussion sur la sexualité dans la psychanalyse contemporaine, *Revue française de psychanalyse* 61: 225–32; reprinted in *Les chaînes d'Éros, Actualités du sexuel*, Paris: Odile Jacob, 1997; English edition: *The Chains of Eros*, London: Rebus Press, 2000.

—— (1998) Démembrement du contre-transfert, in J.-J. Baranes, F. Sacco et al. (eds) *Inventer en psychanalyse. Construire et interpréter*, Paris: Dunod, 2002.

—— (1998) L'intersubjectif en psychanalyse. Pulsions et/ou relations d'objet, Lanctôt, 1998; reprinted in *La pensée clinique*, Paris: Odile Jacob, 2002; trans. A. Weller: The intrapsychic and the intersubjective in psychoanalysis, *Psychoanalytic Quarterly* LXIX, 2000.

—— (1999) Sur la discrimination et l'indiscrimination entre affect et représentation. Report presented to the 10th International Congress of Psychoanalysis, Santiago; reprinted in *La pensée clinique*, Paris: Odile Jacob, 2002.

—— (1999) The intuition of the negative in 'Playing and Reality', in A. Green *The Dead Mother. The Work of André Green*, London: Routledge.

—— (2000) La mort dans la vie, in J. Guillaumin (ed.) *L'invention de la pulsion de mort*, Paris: Dunod.

—— (2000) The central phobic position: a new formulation of the free association method, *International Journal of Psychoanaysis* 81: 429 (first published 1988, *Revue française de psychanalyse* 3/2000).

—— (2001) Mythes et réalités sur le processus psychanalytique. Le modèle de *L'interprétation des rêves*, *Revue française de psychosomatique* 20: 75–96.

—— (2002) A propos de certaines tentatives d'analyse entreprises suite aux échecs de la psychothérapie. Le syndrome de désertification psychique, in F. Richard et al. (éds), *Le travail du psychanalyste en psychothérapie*, Paris: Dunod.

—— (2002) Preface, in F. Richard et al. (eds) *Le travail du psychanalyste en psychothérapie*, Paris: Dunod.

—— (in press) Linguistique de la parole et psychisme non conscient, in *Cahiers de l'Herne. Ferdinand de Saussure*.

Green, A. and Wallerstein, R. (2000) *Clinical and Observational Psychoanalytic Research: Roots of a Controversy*, London: Karnac.

Greenson, R. (1977) *Technique et pratique de la psychanalyse*, Paris: Presses Universitaires de France.

Guignard, F. (1986) Le sourire du chat. Réflexions sur le féminin à partir de la pratique analytique quotidienne, *Bulletin de la SPP* 9: 3–18.

Guiraud, P. (1978) *Dictionnaire érotique*, Paris: Fayot.

—— (1978) *Sémiologie de la sexualité*, Paris: Fayot.

Habermas, J. (1985) *Der philosophische Diskurs der Moderne: Zwölf Vorlesungen*, Frankfurt: Suhrkamp Verlag; English edition: *The Philosophical Discourse of Modernity*, trans. F. Lawrence, Oxford: Polity Press, 1987.

Heimann, P. (1950) On countertransference, *International Journal of Psychoanalysis* 31.

Héritier, F. (2001) Inceste et substance, in F. Héritier *Incestes*, Paris: Presses Universitaires de France,

Hobson, A. (1992) *Le cerveau rêvant*, Paris: Gallimard.

Jackson, J.-E. (2001). Capacité négative, in J.-E. Jackson *Souvent dans l'être obscur*, Paris: J. Corti.

Jacobson, R. (1963) Linguistique et poétique, in R. Jacobson *Essais de linguistique générale*, Paris: Editions de Minuit.

Jouvet, M. (1992), *Le sommeil et le rêve*, Paris: Odile Jacob.

Juillerat, B. (2001) *Penser l'imaginaire. Essai d'anthropologie psychanalytique*, Lausanne: Payot.

Kant, E. (1978) *Anthropology from a Pragmatic Point of View*, trans. V. Lyle Dowdell, Illinois: Southern Illinois University.

Kaplan, K. and Solms, M. (2000) *Clinical Studies in Neuro-Psychoanalysis*, London: Karnac.

Kernberg, O. (2001) Psychanalyse, psychothérapie psychanalytique et psychothérapie de soutien: controverses contemporaines, *Revue française de psychanalyse*, special edition: 'Courants de la psychanalyse contemporaine', dir. André Green: 15–36.

Kristeva, J. (1993) *Les nouvelles maladies de l'âme*, p. 302, Paris: Fayard; English edition: *New Maladies of the Soul*, p. 204. trans. R. Guberman, New York: Columbia University Press, 1995.

Lacan, J. (1966) *Écrits*, Paris: Le Seuil; English edition: *Ecrits: A Selection*, trans. A. Sheridan, London: Tavistock, 1977.

Laplanche, J. (1990) *Nouveaux fondements de la psychanalyse* (avec *Index général des problématiques*), 2nd edn, Paris: Presses Universitaires de France.

Laplanche, J. and Pontalis, J.-B. (1967) *The Language of Psychoanalysis*, trans. D. Nicholson Smith, London: Hogarth Press, 1973.

Lavallée, G. (2001) Le potentiel hallucinatoire, son organisation de base, son accueil et satransformation dans un processus analytique, *Revue française de psychosomatique* 19: 123–44.

Lebovici, S. (1961) La relation objectale chez l'enfant, *La psychiatrie de l'enfant* III: pt 1.

Le Doux, J.E. (1996) *The Emotional Brain: The Mysterious Underpinnings of Emotional Life*, New York: Simon & Schuster.

Legendre, P. (1981) *Jouir du pouvoir. Traité de bureaucratie patriote*, Paris: Éditions de Minuit.

Lévi-Strauss, C. (1916) *Course in General Linguistics*, trans. W. Baskin, New York: McGraw-Hill, 1959.

—— (1985) *La potière jalouse*. Paris: Plon; English edition: *The Jealous Potter*, trans. B. Chorier, Chicago: University of Chicago Press, 1988.

Lyotard, J.-F. (1979) *La condition postmoderne*, Paris: Éditions de Minuit; English edition: *The Postmodern Condition: A Report on Knowledge*, trans. G. Bennington and B. Massumi, Manchester: Manchester University Press.

McDougall, J. (1978) *Plaidoyer pour une certaine anormalité*, Paris: Gallimard; English edition: *Plea for a Measure of Abnormality*, London: Free Association Books, reprinted 1990.

Marty, P. (1976) *Les mouvements individuels de vie et de mort*, Paris: Payot.

—— (1980) *L'ordre psychosomatique*, Paris: Payot.

Meltzer, D. (1967) *The Psycho-Analytic Process*, London: Karnac.

Meschonnic, H. (2002) *Spinoza. Poème de la pensée*, Paris: Maisonneuve and Larose.

Morin, E. (1950) *Introduction à la pensée complexe*, Paris: ESF Editions.

—— (2001) *La méthode, vol. 5 L'humanité de l'humanité*, Paris: Le Seuil.

Neyraut, M. (1974) *Le transfert*, Paris: Presses Universitaires de France.

Normand, C. (2000) *Saussure*, Paris: Les Belles Lettres.

Ogden, T. (1994) *Subject of Analysis*, New York: Jason Aronson.

Panksepp, J. (1999) Emotions as viewed by psychoanalysis and neuroscience: an exercise in conscience, *Neuropsychoanalysis*, 1, 1: 5–15.

Peirce, C.S. (1955) *Philosophical Writings of Peirce*, ed. J. Buchler, p. 99–100, New York: Dover.

—— (1992) *Reasoning and the Logic of Things*, Cambridge MA: Harvard University Press.

Perron-Borelli, M. (1997) *Dynamique du fantasme*, Paris: Presses Universitaires de France.

Pontalis, J.-B. (1999) *La force d'attraction*, Paris: Le Seuil.

Pragier, G. and Faure-Pragier, S. (1990) Un siècle après *l'Esquisse:* nouvelles métaphores? Métaphores du nouveau, report to the 50th Congress of French-speaking psychoanalysts, Madrid, *Revue française de psychanalyse* 6.

Prochiantz, A. (1995) *La biologie dans le boudoir*, Paris: Odile Jacob.

Rastier, F. (2001) *Arts et sciences du texte*, Paris: Presses Universitaires de France.

Reich, W. (1933) *Character Analysis*, New York: Organe Institute Press, 1945.

Renik, O. (1993) Analytic interaction. Conceptualizing technique in the light of the analyst's irreducible subjectivity, *Psychoanalytic Quarterly* 72: 4.

Richard, F. (2001) *Le processus de subjectivation à l'adolescence*, Paris: Dunod.

Ricœur, P. (1965) *De l'interprétation. Essai sur Freud*, Paris: Le Seuil.

Rosenfeld, H. (1971) A clinical approach to the psychoanalytic theory of the life and death instincts: an investigation to the aggressive aspects of narcissism, *International Journal of Psycho-Analysis* 52: 168–78.

Rosolato G. (1969) *Essais sur le symbolique*, Paris: Gallimard.

Roussillon, R. (1991) *Paradoxes et situations limites en psychanalyse*, Paris: Presses Universitaires de France.

Sauguet, H. (1969) Introduction à une discussion sur le processus psychanalytique, *Revue française de psychanalyse* 33: 699–718.

Saussure, F. de. (1916) De l'essence double du langage in F. de Saussure *Ecrits de linguistique générale*, eds. S. Bouquet and R. Engler, Paris: Gallimard, 2002.

Saussure, F. de (1916) *Écrits de linguistique générale*, Paris: Gallimard, 2002.

Schopenhauer, A. (1958) The metaphysics of sexual love, in A. Schopenhauer *The World as Will and Representation*, trans. E.F.J. Payne, New York: Dover.

Schulz-Keil, H. (1988) A trip to Lacania, *Hystoria* 6, 9: 226–45.

Sebeok, T. (1974) Comment un signal devient signe, in T. Sebeok *L'unité de l'homme*, Paris: Le Seuil, p. 64–78.

Shapiro, M. (1982) Léonard et Freud, M. Shapiro *Style, Artiste, Société*, Paris: Gallimard.

Smadja, C. (2001) L'évolution de la pratique psychanalytique avec les patients somatiques, in A. de Mijolla (ed.) *Évolution de la clinique psychanalytique*, Bordeaux: L'Esprit du temps.

Spitz, R. (1966) *The First Year of Life*, New York: International Universities Press.

Tuckett, D., King, P. and Steiner, R. (eds) (1991) *The Freud–Klein Controversies 1941–1945*, London: New Library of Psychoanalysis.

Varela, F. (1993) Sciences cognitives et psychanalyse, *Journal de psychanalyse de l'enfant* 14: 313–27.

Vidal, J.-M. (1992) Évolution du psychisme et évolution des organismes, in P. Tort (ed.) *Darwinisme et société*, Paris: Presses Universitaires de France.

Viderman, S. (1970) *La construction de l'espace analytique*, Paris: Denoël.

Vincent, J.-D. (1986) *Biologie des passions*, Paris: Odile Jacob.

—— (1996) *La chair et le diable*, Paris: Odile Jacob.

Von Foerster, H. (1974) Note pour une épistémologie des objets vivants, in E. Morin and M. Piatelli-Palmarini (eds) *L'unité de l'homme*, Paris: Le Seuil, pp. 401–17.

Wallerstein, R. and Green, A. (2000) *Clinical and Observational Psychoanalytic Research: Roots of a Controversy*, London: Karnac.

Widlöcher, D. (1996) *Les nouvelles cartes de la psychanalyse*, Paris: Odile Jacob.

Winnicott, D. W. (1954) Metapsychological and clinical aspects of regression within the psychoanalytical set-up, in D.W. Winnicott *Collected Papers: Through Paediatrics to Psycho-Analysis*, London: Hogarth Press, 1958.

—— (1971) The use of the object and relating through identifications, in D.W. Winnicott *Playing and Reality*, London: Routledge

—— (1971) Fear of breakdown, *International Review Psychoanalysis* 1: 103–7.

Wittgenstein, L. (1921) *Tractatus Logico-Philosophicus*, trans. D.F. Pears and B.F. McGuiness, London and New York: Routledge, 2001.

—— (1964; 2nd edn 1975) *Philosophical Remarks*, ed. R. Rhees, trans. R. Hargreaves and R. White, Oxford: Blackwell.

INDEX

Entries in **bold** refer to figures/diagrams.